AIDS AND THE LUNG

AIDS and the Lung

EDITED BY

STEPHEN J.G. SEMPLE MD, FRCP

Professor Emeritus of Medicine,
Visiting Professor of Medicine,
Department of Medicine,
Charing Cross and Westminster Medical School;
and Honorary Consultant,
Hammersmith Hospitals Trust

AND

ROBERT F. MILLER MB, BS, FRCP

Senior Lecturer,
Division of Pathology and Infectious Diseases,
University College London Medical School,
Mortimer Market Centre,
Mortimer Market, London

FOREWORD BY

MICHAEL W. ADLER

**Blackwell
Science**

1997

© 1997 by
Blackwell Science Ltd
Editorial Offices:
Osney Mead, Oxford OX2 0EL
25 John Street, London WC1N 2BL
23 Ainslie Place, Edinburgh EH3 6AJ
350 Main Street, Malden
  MA 02148 5018, USA
54 University Street, Carlton
  Victoria 3053, Australia

Other Editorial Offices:
Arnette Blackwell SA
  224, Boulevard Saint Germain
  75007 Paris, France

Blackwell Wissenschafts-Verlag GmbH
  Kurfürstendamm 57
  10707 Berlin, Germany

  Zehetnergasse 6
  A-1140 Wien
  Austria

First published 1997

Set by Excel Typesetters Co., Hong Kong
Printed and bound in Great Britain
by Hartnolls Ltd., Bodmin, Cornwall

The Blackwell Science logo is a
trade mark of Blackwell Science Ltd,
registered at the United Kingdom
Trade Marks Registry

DISTRIBUTORS

Marston Book Services Ltd
PO Box 269
Abingdon
Oxon OX14 4YN
(*Orders*: Tel: 01235 465500
         Fax: 01235 465555)

USA
Blackwell Science, Inc.
Commerce Place, 350 Main Street
Malden, MA 02148 5018
(*Orders*: Tel: 800 759 6102
         617 388 8250
         Fax: 617 388 8255)

Canada
Copp Clark Professional
200 Adelaide Street West, 3rd Floor
Toronto, Ontario M5H 1W7
(*Orders*: Tel: 416 597-1616
         800 815-9417
         Fax: 416 597-1617)

Australia
Blackwell Science Pty Ltd
54 University Street
Carlton, Victoria 3053
(*Orders*: Tel: 3 9347 0300
         Fax: 3 9347 5001)

A catalogue record for this title
is available from the British Library

ISBN 0-632-03623-0

Library of Congress
Cataloging-in-publication Data

AIDS and the lung / edited by
Stephen Semple and Robert Miller.
      p.   cm.
   Includes bibliographical references
     and index.
   ISBN 0-632-03623-0
   1. Respiratory infections. 2. AIDS
     (Disease)—Complications.
   I. Semple, Stephen J. (Stephen John)
   II. Miller, Robert, FRCP.
     [DNLM: 1. Acquired Immunodeficiency
       Syndrome—complications.
     2. HIV Infections—complications.
     3. Lung Diseases—complications.
   WC 503.5 A2879 1997]
   RC740.A35   1997
   616.2′407—dc21
   DNLM/DLC
   for Library of Congress   96-44118
                                          CIP

Contents

Contributors

R.P. BRETTLE, MD, FRCP (ED), *Consultant Physician and Reader in Medicine, Regional Infectious Disease Unit, Royal Infirmary NHS Trust, City Hospital, Greenbank Drive, Edinburgh, EH10 5SB*

R.J. COKER, MB, BS, MRCP, *Consultant Physician, St Mary's Hospital Trust, Praed Street, London, W2 1NY*

R. DINWIDDIE, MB, FRCP, DCH, *Consultant Respiratory Paediatrician, Great Ormond Street Hospital for Children, London, WC1N 3JH and Honorary Senior Lecturer, Institute of Child Health, University of London*

M.A. JOHNSON, MD, FRCP, *Consultant Physician in General Medicine, Thoracic Medicine, Clinical Director HIV/AIDS, Royal Free Hospital NHS Trust, Pond Street, London, NW3 2QG*

R.F. MILLER, MB, BS, FRCP, *Senior Lecturer, Division of Pathology and Infectious Diseases, University College London Medical School, Mortimer Market Centre, Mortimer Market, London, WCIE 6AU*

D.M. MITCHELL, MA, MD, FRCP, *Consultant Physician and Honorary Senior Lecturer in Medicine, St Mary's Hospital Trust and Imperial College School of Medicine, Praed Street, London, W2 1NY*

V. NOVELLI, MB, BS, FRCP, FRACP, *Consultant in Paediatric Infectious Diseases, Great Ormond Street Hospital for Children, London, WC1N 3JH and Honorary Senior Lecturer, Institute of Child Health, University of London*

A.L. POZNIAK, MD, FRCP, *Senior Lecturer, Department of Genitourinary Medicine, Kings College School of Medicine and Dentistry, London, SE5 9RS*

N.M. PRICE, BSC, MB, MRCP, DTM&H, *Registrar in Respiratory Medicine and Infectious Diseases, Hammersmith Hospital, DuCane Road, London W12*

S.J.G. SEMPLE, MD, FRCP, *Professor Emeritus of Medicine, Visiting Professor of Medicine, Department of Medicine, Charing Cross and Westminster Medical School, London, W1N 8AA and Honorary Consultant, Hammersmith Hospitals Trust*

Foreword

None of us looking after our first patients with AIDS in 1983 could have imagined what the future held. This new virus has impinged upon everyone, whether they are infected or not. It has led to fierce moral and political debate, new alliances and types of relationships between patients, doctors and healthcare workers, and models of care which have acted as examples in all other areas of medicine. Finally, the basic clinical, behavioural and epidemiological research effort has been colossal with, again, spin-offs for other diseases.

Looking after patients with HIV infection and AIDS is a complex issue and one which with new therapeutic advances, particularly antiviral agents, is constantly changing. The lung is a major focus for infection and tumours for those suffering from HIV/AIDS. In this light, the current text is extremely important for those who wish to have a detailed and up-to-date knowledge of AIDS and the lung.

M.W. Adler

Preface

This book is one of the outcomes of the profound impact of the AIDS epidemic in the mid-1980s on The Middlesex Hospital and Medical School in general and the Department of Medicine in particular. At that time the infecting agent was unknown, clinical management uncertain, short- and long-term prognosis undefined and the risk to medical and nursing staff of acquiring infection undetermined. The clinical problems initially were dominated by disorders of the lung. Subsequently, although the pattern of HIV disease has changed, respiratory disorders remain the most common complication encountered and they are still the most frequent mode of presentation.

This book is designed to cover a broad outline of the epidemiology, pathogenesis, clinical presentation and treatment of infection with HIV-1 with special reference to the lung. It is not intended primarily for the expert working in an AIDS referral centre although we hope that some of the reports, especially about the less common manifestations of HIV infection, might be of interest. Rather, we hope this book will be of practical value to the physician who sees a few patients sporadically and requires background knowledge needed for the identification and management of patients infected by HIV. This group of physicians includes those who hold a consultant post as well as those in training and should provide a basis for the MRCP(UK).

Chapters 3–11 deal with the majority of pulmonary disorders which occur as a consequence of HIV infection. The exception is Chapter 7 devoted to the pulmonary complications of drug abuse but its relevance to HIV disease is obvious.

Chapters 1 and 2 provide a general background to the epidemiology and pathogenesis of HIV infection although particular attention is paid to pulmonary disorders. The widespread review of many of the pathogenic and protective mechanisms associated with HIV infection described in Chapter 2 may not be of interest or required by all readers but a summary of its contents is provided.

Acknowledgements

Thanks to: Dr John Clarke, Research Virology, St Mary's Hospital Medical School; Professors Mike Adler and Anne Johnson, Department of Sexually Transmitted Diseases, University College London Medical School; Dr Ann Wakefield, Molecular Infectious Diseases, Department of Paediatrics, Institute of Molecular Medicine, Oxford.

S.J.G. Semple
R.F. Miller
London

1 Epidemiology of HIV infection and AIDS

S.J.G. SEMPLE

1.0 AIDS and HIV infection worldwide

The World Health Organization (WHO) estimates that 18–19 million adults and more than 1.5 million children have been infected with HIV-1 since the late 1970s [1]. The WHO estimates that 17 million adults were infected with HIV and alive in 1994 (estimated prevalence) and Fig. 1.1 shows their geographical distribution [2]. Figure 1.2 illustrates the contrast between the number and distribution of AIDS cases as reported to the WHO with that estimated to have occurred when allowance is made for underdiagnosis, incomplete reporting, delay in reporting and other available data on HIV infection around the world [1]. Of the cumulative reported cases, 39% occurred in the USA, 12% in Europe and 34% in Africa. In contrast, of the estimated cumulative cases, 7% occurred in the USA, 4% in Europe and 75% in Africa (Fig. 1.2).

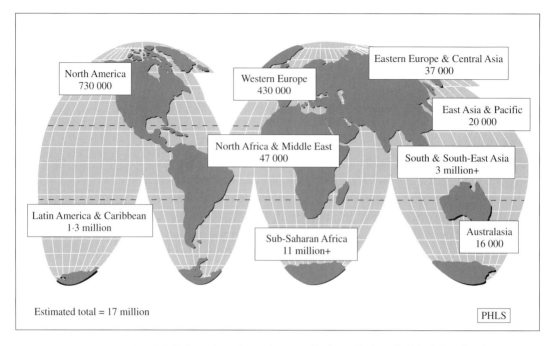

Fig. 1.1 Estimated number and geographical distribution of adults infected with HIV and alive late 1994 (estimated total 17 million). Figure from an original supplied by Dr A. Nicoll, Public Health Laboratory Service, London. Source of information [1].

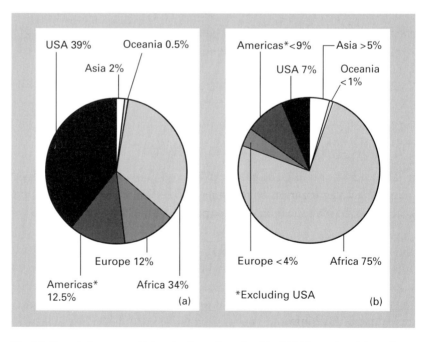

Fig. 1.2 Cumulative reported (a) and estimated number (b) of AIDS cases in adults and children by late 1995. Figure from an original supplied by Dr A. Nicoll, Public Health Laboratory Service, London. Source of information [1].

A cumulative total of 1 291 810 cases of AIDS in adults and children had been reported to the WHO by December 1995 but, because of deficiencies in reporting, this does not reflect the true cumulative total, which has been estimated to be 6 million [2]. There was an increase of 19% in the cumulative total of cases of AIDS between 1994 and 1995 but there was considerable variation in the increase between regions. The proportional increases were 11% in the Americas, 21% in Oceania, 22% in Europe, 26% in Africa and 167% in Asia. Of the increase in Asia, 80% of the reported cases occurred in Thailand [1].

AIDS is a disease of poverty, both globally and within individual societies [3]. Africa has suffered the heaviest burden of disease, with sub-Saharan Africa accounting for two-thirds of the estimated cases worldwide and over 90% of cases in women and children [3]. Of increasing concern is the recent growth of the epidemic in South and South-East Asia, which is predominantly heterosexual in nature. In India the prevalence of HIV infection is very high among female sex workers and men attending clinics for sexually transmitted diseases (STDs), especially in those who had recently had contact with sex workers. A more worrying finding in India has been the high prevalence of HIV in monogamous married women, pointing to a spread of infection into a section of the community not considered to be members of a 'high-risk group' [4].

The primary method of transmission (three-quarters) of HIV infection is through unprotected homo- and heterosexual intercourse but mother-to-child transmission is growing in importance. From a global perspective, 80% of infection in the world is spread by sexual intercourse, 70% heterosexual and 10% homosexual. At present, the only tried means of limiting the spread of HIV infection are the promotion and distribution of condoms, treatment of conventional STDs, transmission of information through the media and schools, maintenance of a safe blood supply and needle-exchange programmes for injecting drug users.

Any epidemiological study of HIV infection, whether it be within a single country or continent or worldwide, requires a reliable and widely acceptable categorization of the stages of HIV infection as well as the criteria for the identification of those people with AIDS.

1.1 Classification system for HIV infection and AIDS

A classification system for HIV infection and for AIDS is important for research and public health practice. Categorizing the clinical conditions and stages of HIV infection makes it possible to compare directly reports from different centres and countries on clinical trials and other research projects. Categorization also facilitates efforts to determine current and future healthcare needs.

The classification system described here is the 1993 revised classification system for HIV infection and the expanded surveillance case definition for AIDS among adolescents and adults [5]. It originates from the Centers for Disease Control (CDC) in the USA. The classification system is based on a combination of the clinical presentations of HIV infection together with the level of the CD4 cell count. Within this system of classification the criteria for identification of people with AIDS (referred to as the case definition of AIDS) have been expanded. Although the content of the revised classification is not changed in many respects from previous publications from the CDC [6,7], it does include important modifications and additions. Account of these changes introduced in 1993 must be taken when comparing the incidence and prevalence of AIDS before and after that year. In comparing the incidence of AIDS between countries, it is also necessary to determine the classification system in use at the time and in particular whether the 1993 expanded case definition of AIDS has been accepted in its entirety.

The case definition of AIDS for surveillance purposes is intended to provide consistent and comparable data for public health purposes. Clinicians should not necessarily rely on this definition alone to diagnose serious disease caused by HIV infection in individual patients. Such a diagnosis may be made on clinical grounds and laboratory findings characteristic of HIV infection.

Prior to 1993 the 1987 classification system for HIV infection and AIDS was used [6,7]. AIDS was defined on the basis of the development of a variety of clinical conditions, of which there were 23. These included *Pneumocystis carinii* pneumonia (PCP), Kaposi's sarcoma, cytomegalovirus (CMV) disease and toxoplasmosis of the brain, among others. The 1993 revised classification system for AIDS [5] takes into account the clinical importance of the CD4 T-lymphocyte count as a marker for HIV-related immunosuppression and the consequent implications for prophylaxis and clinical management. The choice of ranges of CD4 counts was determined on clinical grounds. People with counts between 200 and 500 cells/μl are in the range where antiretroviral therapy will be considered, while counts below 200 cells/μl is one of the indications for prophylaxis against *P. carinii*. Prior to the 1993 revised classification, these were a group of patients with counts below 200 cells/μl with severe HIV-related disease but without an AIDS-defining condition according to the 1987 criteria. Such patients required medical care and this must be taken into account in determining the resources needed in any healthcare system. It is estimated that, for every patient with an AIDS-defining condition according to the 1987 criteria, there will be one HIV-infected person without one of these conditions but with a CD4 count below 200 cells/μl.

Table 1.1 Tinted area shows the AIDS surveillance case definition. It includes the clinical conditions indicating AIDS (category C) as well as the CD4 count which defines AIDS, i.e. < 200 cells/μl. From [5].

CD4 T-cell categories	Clinical categories		
	A Asymptomatic, acute primary HIV or PGL	B Symptomatic (but not A or C)	C AIDS-indicating conditions
1 > 500 cells/μl	A1	B1	C1
2 200–400 cells/μl	A2	B2	C2
3 < 200 cells/μl— AIDS-indicating T-cell count	A3	B3	C3

The new system is based on three clinical categories and three ranges of CD4 T-lymphocyte counts. This produces a matrix of nine mutually exclusive categories, as shown in Table 1.1.

• *Category A*. This includes asymptomatic HIV infection, acute primary HIV infection with an accompanying illness and persistent generalized lymphadenopathy (PGL).

• *Category B*. The symptomatic conditions in this group include oropharyngeal candidiasis and constitutional symptoms, such as fever or diarrhoea lasting for more than 1 month. Also included are oral hairy leucoplakia, herpes zoster, idiopathic thrombocytopenic purpura and peripheral neuropathy.

• *Category C*. These are the clinical conditions indicative of AIDS which provide one of the criteria for the case definition of AIDS. Conditions included in this group are shown in Table 1.2. Three new clinical conditions were added in 1993, namely pulmonary tuberculosis, recurrent pneumonia and invasive cervical cancer. Pneumonia is considered to be recurrent when it occurs more than once a year. Diagnosis rests on radiological evidence of acute pneumonia and culture from a clinically reliable specimen of a pathogen that typically causes pneumonia (other than *P. carinii* or *Mycobacterium tuberculosis*). Laboratory confirmation of a causative organism for one of the episodes of pneumonia is not mandatory for a diagnosis of recurrent pneumonia.

The diagnosis of one or more of the clinical conditions in category C (Table 1.2) which is indicative of AIDS may be definitive or presumptive. Definitive diagnostic evidence will be derived from histology, cytology and culture of the appropriate fluid or tissue. While a definitive diagnosis is preferable, there will be circumstances where a presumptive diagnosis is acceptable, particularly where the presentation of the disease is typical, where it is difficult or hazardous to obtain a biopsy specimen or where the

Table 1.2 Conditions included in the 1993 AIDS surveillance case definition (category C).

Candidiasis of bronchi, trachea, lungs or oesophagus
Pneumonia, recurrent
Pneumocystis carinii pneumonia
Mycobacterium avium complex or *Mycobacterium kansasii*, disseminated or
   extrapulmonary
Mycobacterium tuberculosis, any site (pulmonary or extrapulmonary)
Mycobacterium, other species or unidentified species, disseminated or extrapulmonary
Herpes simplex: chronic ulcer(s) of greater than 1 month's duration, bronchitis,
   pneumonitis, oesophagitis
Cytomegalovirus disease (other than liver, spleen or nodes)
Cytomegalovirus retinitis (with loss of vision)
Cryptococcus, extrapulmonary
Coccidioidomycosis, disseminated or extrapulmonary
Cryptosporidiosis, chronic intestinal
Isosporiasis, chronic intestinal (>1 month's duration)
Histoplasmosis, disseminated or extrapulmonary
Kaposi's sarcoma
Lymphoma, Burkitt's (or equivalent term)
Lymphoma, immunoblastic (or equivalent term)
Lymphoma, primary of brain
Salmonella septicaemia, recurrent
Wasting syndrome due to HIV
Toxoplasmosis of brain
HIV-related encephalopathy
Progressive multifocal leucoencephalopathy
Cervical cancer, invasive

patient's condition does not permit the performance of definitive tests. Conditions where a presumptive diagnosis is likely to be made on occasion include PCP, toxoplasmosis of the brain, CMV retinitis with loss of vision, disseminated mycobacterial disease and candidiasis of the oesophagus [5]. The presumptive diagnosis will be based on characteristic clinical findings, laboratory abnormalities and response to treatment. For example, a presumptive diagnosis of PCP can be made with a history of dyspnoea or non-productive cough of recent onset together with the following: (i) a chest X-ray with diffuse bilateral interstitial 'shadowing'; (ii) arterial hypoxia (partial pressure of oxygen (Po_2) <70 mmHg, <9.3 kPa) or widened arterial–alveolar oxygen tension gradient or low transfer factor; and (iii) no evidence of bacterial pneumonia.

The majority of patients with a clinical condition indicative of AIDS will also have a positive HIV-antibody test. In a few patients, a laboratory test for HIV will not have been performed or will have given inconclusive results. However, if the disease indicative of AIDS (category C, Table 1.2) is definitive, the individual will meet the criteria for the case definition of AIDS. This will not apply where there is immunosuppression due to causes other than HIV infection, e.g. long-term systemic steroid therapy, various malignancies or a congenital immunodeficiency syndrome [5].

1.1.2 Summary of the case definition of AIDS for surveillance purposes

There are two criteria which meet the case definition for AIDS. The first is a CD4 cell count below 200 cells/μl. Individuals may not have a clinical condition indicative of AIDS (category C) and yet if the CD4 count is below 200 cells/μl they will still meet the case definition of AIDS (see A3 and B3 in Table 1.1). The second criterion depends upon the diagnosis of a clinical condition indicative of AIDS (category C, Tables 1.1 and 1.2). The CD4 cell count may be below 200 cells/μl (C3, Table 1.1) or may be greater than 200 cells/μl (C1, C2, Table 1.1) but the latter does not exclude the individual from the case definition of AIDS where there is a disease indicative of AIDS (Table 1.2).

In Europe, a CD4 count below 200 cells/μl is not accepted as a case definition of AIDS so that persons in the clinical categories A and B (Table 1.1) would not be included even if their CD4 cell count was below 200 cells/μl. The reason a CD4 count below 200 cells/μl is not accepted is that not all countries in Europe provide regular measurements of CD4 cell counts on HIV-infected people.

1.2 Cumulative total, prevalence, incidence and future projections of HIV infection and AIDS in England and Wales [8]

1.2.1 Epidemic of HIV infection followed by epidemic of AIDS

The peak of the annual incidence of HIV infection among homosexuals was in 1983, with a sharp fall-off thereafter to a constant, relatively low level; this is a classic example of an epidemic progressing to an endemic (Fig. 1.3). The epidemic of AIDS follows roughly 10 years later because that is the average time between infection and the development of full-blown AIDS.

1.2.2 State of the epidemic of HIV infection and AIDS at the end of 1994 [8]

A cumulative total of 11 520 cases of AIDS are estimated to have arisen in England and Wales by the end of 1994 since 1979. Of these, 8315 are estimated to have died (72%) and about 3210 were alive. The steep rise in deaths from AIDS between 1988 and 1993 appears to be stabilizing in male homosexuals from the data obtained in 1994. However, there is

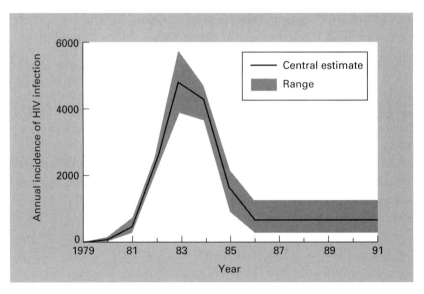

Fig. 1.3 Estimate of the annual incidence of HIV infection in England and Wales to 1991 with a peak incidence around 1983. Reproduced from *Communicable Disease Report* 1993; 3 (Supplement 1): S10.

evidence that the marked decline in HIV transmission that occurred between 1983 and 1987 has not been sustained, with transmission increasing from 1988 onwards [9]. If this resurgence continues, it will have a substantial effect on long-term AIDS projections in male homosexuals.

There have been a total of 3469 HIV infections reported by the end of 1994 which have arisen through sexual intercourse between men and women (heterosexual exposure). Of these, 403 have been acquired from partners with a high risk of HIV infection, such as injecting drug users and bisexual men. However, 2991 cases were probably not acquired from high-risk partners and 91% of these infections were acquired abroad, where sexual intercourse between men and women is the usual route of HIV transmission.

The incidence of HIV infection among injecting drug users in England and Wales peaked around 1985 and then declined sharply by the second half of the decade—a surprising change in a group normally resistant to health education. The annual incidence of AIDS in this category for 1993 and 1994 was about 100 each year.

1.2.3 Prevalence and recent incidence of HIV infection at the end of 1993 [8]

It is estimated that 21 900 adults were infected with HIV at the end of 1993; 12 350 infected through male homosexual exposure, 6800 men and women infected through heterosexual exposure and 2050 men and women infected through injecting drugs. About 3000 adults were alive with AIDS.

1.2.4 Projections for new AIDS cases to 1999 [8]

Future projections of the number of people who will be diagnosed as suffering from AIDS can be calculated by the method of 'back calculation'. This method is based on: (i) the number of people diagnosed per month as suffering from AIDS (obtained from surveillance data); and (ii) the incubation period between HIV infection and a diagnosis of AIDS (obtained from cohort studies). From these data an 'epidemic curve' of HIV infection is derived by estimating the number of people infected with HIV (prevalence) which is necessary to account for the number of people observed as suffering from AIDS. From knowledge of the epidemic curve of HIV infection and the incubation period, forward projection of the number of people diagnosed as suffering from AIDS over the ensuing years can be obtained. In addition to an estimate of the total number of people with a diagnosis of AIDS, the number within different exposure categories (e.g. injecting drug users, heterosexuals) can be estimated. The uncertainty of AIDS projections can be reduced by using data from different sources to derive HIV prevalence, together with the choice of the most appropriate mathematical methods and models for the final estimations. Added data include information obtained on HIV prevalence from unlinked anonymous serosurveillance programmes and the number of people infected with HIV but without AIDS receiving treatment and prophylaxis. Allowance is also made for the delayed and under-reporting of AIDS cases.

It is anticipated that there will be approximately 2025 new cases of AIDS in 1997 and 2010 in 1999. Breaking these numbers down into exposure categories for the same 2 years reveals estimates of 1305 and 1235 for homo/bisexual males, 410 and 525 for heterosexually exposed people and 140 and 155 for injecting drug users. It is anticipated that new AIDS cases in homo/bisexual males may fall by 7% between 1995 and 1999 but will rise by 25% where there is heterosexual transmission (Fig. 1.4). New AIDS cases among injecting drug users are projected to increase by 29% between 1995 and 1999. The incidence of AIDS in children will rise to 45 new cases in 1997 and 55 in 1999.

1.2.5 Deaths from AIDS and the prevalence of AIDS and other severe HIV disease [8]

The prevalence of AIDS is expected to increase by 15% from 3485 cases

9

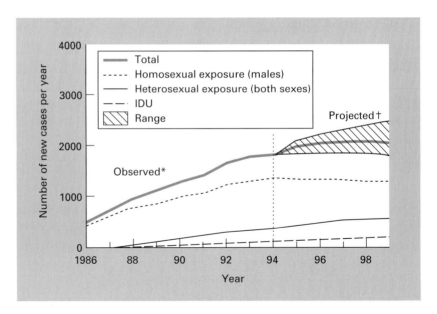

Fig. 1.4 Observed (1986–94) and projected (1995–99) annual incidence of AIDS (England and Wales, data to end 1994). * Adjusted for reporting delay and 13% underreporting; † adjusted for 13% underreporting. IDU, intravenous drug use. Reproduced from [8].

at the end of 1995 to 4010 at the end of 1999. The number of deaths from AIDS is expected to rise from 1600 in 1995 to over 1900 by 1998. However there is likely to be one person alive with severe HIV disease but without AIDS who requires medical care for each living AIDS case during 1995–99. Severe HIV disease is usually associated with CD4 cell counts below 200 cells/µl and in the USA such cell counts are accepted as one of the criteria for a diagnosis of AIDS, although this has not been adopted in Europe and the UK (see section 1.1).

The geographical distribution of the prevalence of AIDS cases in England and Wales is shown in Fig. 1.5, which illustrates the well-known concentration of AIDS cases in the Thames region.

1.2.6 Uncertainties in the predictions of prevalence and incidence of HIV infection and AIDS

In male homosexuals the uncertainty rests on the impact of any changes in sexual behaviour [9]. During the early to mid-1980s it is likely that HIV transmission fell due to the adoption of safe practices in sexual intercourse, presumably because of awareness of the appalling prognosis for patients with AIDS. However, as stated above, transmission of HIV has probably increased since 1989, which places considerable uncertainty on future predictions.

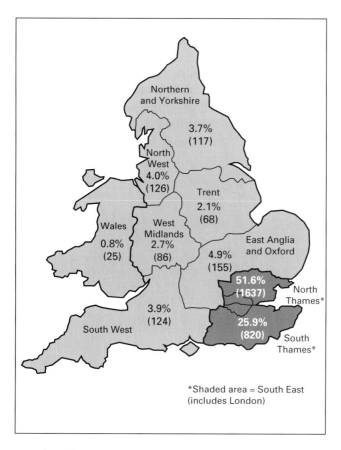

Fig. 1.5 Geographical distribution of percentage (regional total) of prevalent AIDS cases at September 1995. Reproduced from [8].

At present, no effects of treatment or prophylaxis on the various estimates have specifically been allowed for. With the advent of combination antiretroviral therapy it is likely that treatment effects will have to be taken into account, especially in determining the incubation period before the diagnosis of AIDS.

There are uncertainties in the future course of the epidemic among heterosexuals in England and Wales because it is dominated by infection acquired overseas. However, heterosexual transmission is growing internationally and the risk is that such infections may lead to indigenous transmission within the heterosexual community in the UK.

1.2.7 AIDS in Europe [10]

The incidence of AIDS may have reached a plateau in Germany and Switzerland but there is no evidence of a fall in Spain, Italy and France. In Germany and the UK the incidence of AIDS is comparatively lower than in the majority of other European countries. In Spain, Italy and France a greater proportion of HIV infection has been in injecting drug users compared with Germany and the UK, where HIV infection due to male homosexual exposure has been relatively large.

1.3 Prevalence and incidence of HIV infection and of AIDS in the USA

Approximately 58 000 people in the USA were diagnosed with AIDS in 1991 and projections made in 1992 were that 60 000–70 000 cases would be diagnosed annually to 1994 with an increase of a few per cent each year [11]. After allowing for the change in case definition in 1993 this projection has been shown to be broadly correct, albeit at the lower end of the range [12]. The number of people infected with HIV in the USA was estimated to have been between 500 000 and 900 000 in 1991 (quoted in [11]), while the number of people alive and diagnosed with AIDS was estimated to have been approximately 90 000 in January 1992, with a projected rise to 120 000 in January 1995.

It was anticipated that the expanded case definition for AIDS of 1993 [5] would profoundly affect the incidence of AIDS during that year. The purpose of the expansion was to identify people with severe disease/immunosuppression in the absence of a disease indicative of AIDS according to the 1987 criteria (see categories A3 and B3, Table 1.1). Such people represent a significant claim on healthcare resources, requiring prophylaxis, antiretroviral treatment and treatment of other HIV-related diseases. These diseases include those in category B, together with pulmonary tuberculosis, recurrent pneumonia and invasive cervical cancer, which were not included in the 1987 classification. Back-calculation models estimate the prevalence of severe immunosuppression (includes those diagnosed as AIDS in the 1987 definition) as approximately 115 000–170 000 in January 1992 to 130 000–205 000 in January 1995. The estimated incidence of AIDS under the 1987 surveillance definition for 1993 is 52 000–61 000 but under the expanded definition the estimate is 95 000–118 000, an increase of 80–100%. The large increase will not persist in 1994, falling to an increase of approximately 10% [11]. The reason for this is that reporting in 1993 will include a 'backlog' of prevalent cases with a CD4 count < 200 cells/µl who have not yet fulfilled the 1987 definition. When this group go on and develop AIDS according to the 1987 definition, they will not be reported again. In effect, the new reporting criteria bring forward in time the diagnosis of AIDS. A major cause for concern in the USA is that in January 1992 it was estimated that those receiving healthcare were under 50% of all severely immunosuppressed people [11].

1.3.1 Update: trends in AIDS diagnosis and reporting under the expanded surveillance definition for adolescents and adults—USA 1993 [12]

In the USA 105 990 cases of AIDS were reported in 1993; 56 400 were based on the new reporting criteria, of which 90% were based on the CD4 criteria alone [12]. To estimate the trend in the incidence of AIDS it is necessary to determine what would have occurred if the surveillance definition had not been expanded. This was done by determining the length of time between the occurrence of a specific CD4 cell count and the development of an AIDS-defining opportunistic infection (AIDS-OI) under the 1987 criteria. The estimated AIDS-OI is the sum of the observed AIDS-OI incidence and the incidence based on estimated dates of diagnosis for people reported with AIDS based only on the CD4 criteria. This allows a closer comparison between the AIDS pandemic in Europe and the USA.

In 1993 the estimated incidence of AIDS-OI was 62 000 cases, a rise of 3% on 1992. Figure 1.6 shows the rise in cases from 1986 to 1993 which, as predicted, is 'flattening off', rising by a few per cent per year. The estimated number of AIDS-OIs diagnosed in 1993 decreased by 1% among homo/bisexual men but increased by 8% among injecting drug users and by 23% among people infected through heterosexual contact. As the impact of the expanded case definition continues to decline, the total number of cases for 1994 will be less than in 1993 [12].

Over the 5-year period 1989–94 the rates of AIDS-OI for men who have sex with men increased by 31% (from 12.1 to 15.9 cases per 100 000 males) but the rates varied by race/ethnicity. The rate increase

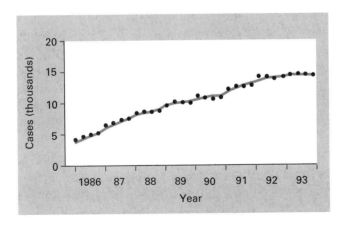

Fig. 1.6 Estimated AIDS opportunistic illness incidence, adjusted for delays in reporting by quarter-year of diagnosis—USA 1986–93. Reproduced from [12].

for black men was 79%, Hispanic men 61% and white men 14%. The most startling and dramatic changes occurred in an analysis of AIDS-OI cases in three cities — New York, Los Angeles and San Francisco — over the same 5-year period. In all three cities, the rate for white men decreased by 20, 16 and 3%, respectively, but the rate for black men increased by 49, 48 and 53%, respectively. Since 1981, these three cities have accounted for 27% of all AIDS cases occurring in men who have sex with men [13].

AIDS acquired heterosexually in 1993 and AIDS among women in the USA have been reported but the incidence has included cases based on the expanded AIDS surveillance case definition so the figures are not strictly comparable with the above analysis of AIDS-OI. However, some general trends in incidence in these two groups can be determined. In 1994, 18% (14081 cases) of AIDS cases occurred among women, which is nearly a threefold increase in the proportion of cases among women compared with 1985. The rates per 100000 population in 1994 for black and Hispanic women were 16 and 17 times higher than those for white women [14]. In 1993, cases of AIDS attributed to heterosexual contact increased 130% in 1993 over 1992 but this was predominantly due to the expanded case definition. However, this was still greater than in all other exposure categories (homosexuals, injecting drug users, etc.), which was 109% in 1993 over 1992. The increase in AIDS due to heterosexual contact was proportionately greater for men and women who were non-Hispanic blacks and for Hispanics than for non-Hispanic whites [15].

1.3.2 Death rates from HIV infection by age, sex and race—USA

The death rate caused by HIV infection in 1991 in the USA was 29850 (1% of all deaths) and the cumulative deaths from 1987 to 1991 inclusive was 2165000 [16]. Of the deaths in 1991, 3% were in those aged less than 25 years, 74% were in the age group 25–44 years and 23% were at 45 years or older. Among people aged 25–44 years HIV infection was the third leading cause of death in 1991, accounting for 15% of all deaths. Figure 1.7 shows the death rates from 1982 to 1991 among men aged 25–44 years from different causes, with deaths due to HIV approaching those due to accidents. During this time death rates remained stable apart from that due to HIV infection. Although the death rate for men was seven times that of women in 1991, the rate in women increased from 1985 onwards; the proportionate increase in death rate was greater for women than for men. In the age group 25–44 years the death rates were higher in black and Hispanic people than in white people for both men and women [16].

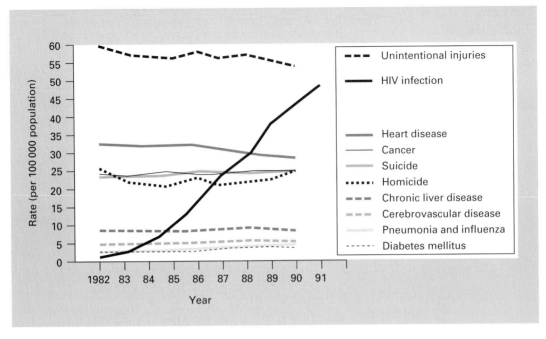

Fig. 1.7 Death rates in the USA 1982–91 for men aged 25–44 years from different causes. Reproduced from [16].

1.4 Cellular, serological and clinical markers for progression to AIDS and for risk of *Pneumocystis carinii* pneumonia

The CD4 cell count remains the best single predictor of progression to AIDS, although the ratio of CD4 to CD8 cells is also good. Other markers that have been assessed are the serum neopterin and β_2-microglobulin levels and levels of immunoglobulin A (IgA), interleukin 2 (IL-2) receptors and p24 antigen. The last three markers had little predictive power but the combination of the CD4 cell count and the serum neopterin had a greater predictive power than any single markers [17].

The risk of PCP in the absence of prophylaxis has been assessed in a multicentre AIDS cohort study [18] in people who were seropositive for HIV-1 but did not have AIDS as defined by the CDC surveillance case definition of 1987 [7]. During a 2-year follow-up of 1665 participants, 10% had their first episode of PCP. The risk of PCP was greatly increased in people with a CD4 count of 200 cells/mm^3 or below and this was significantly and independently increased in patients who developed thrush or fever. The majority of patients who were symptomatic developed PCP within 6 months even if their CD4 counts were over 200 cells/mm^3. Thus prophylaxis against PCP was recommended for patients with CD4 counts at or below 200 cells/mm^3 and for patients who were symptomatic [18].

1.4.1 The major histocompatibility complex and HIV infection

Associations have been reported between the major histocompatibility complex (MHC) and the acquisition of and response to HIV infection. In a critical review of these associations it has been pointed out that the results of studies in this field were often inconclusive and conflicting [19]. Often too few subjects with an accurately estimated duration of infection and long enough follow-up were available to provide a sufficiently wide range of disease-free intervals. Examination of each MHC gene individually may not be adequate because genetic markers governing other components of the immune system may reduce or enhance the effect of an individual gene. However, in the future, conflicting results may be reconciled by using molecular methods (oligonucleotide typing) rather than relying on serological typing alone [19].

In spite of these reservations there is evidence that the MHC of the host is related to the clinical and immunological response to HIV infection, although the precise relationship is yet to be determined. In a cohort of 106 homosexual men, with a known date of seroconversion, it was found that subjects with fever and skin rash during primary HIV infection showed an increased frequency of human leucocyte antigen (HLA)-B62. Subjects with a rapid decline in CD4 cell count were associated with an increased frequency of HLA-B35. The strongest association was between HLA-DR1 and Kaposi's sarcoma [20].

From a large hospital cohort of HIV-positive patients, mainly injecting drug users, a subgroup was identified with a good estimate of the time when they seroconverted [21]. This subgroup was followed over the time period 1985 to 1994. Clinical end-points chosen to indicate disease progression were death, the diagnosis of AIDS and the development of one of the complications of HIV disease listed in stage IV of the CDC classification system which was in operation at the time this study started [6]. In this subgroup, the haplotype A1–B8–DR3 was associated with an increased relative risk of dying (3.7, confidence interval (CI) 1.9–7.2), developing AIDS (3.1, CI 1.6–6.0) and progression to stage IV (1.9, CI 1.1–3.2). The relative risks were obtained by a comparison with subjects in this subgroup who were not A1–B8–DR3. In those subjects typed as B27, a reduced rate of progression to stage IV was found but no conclusion on the other clinical end-points could be made as the number of subjects was small and none died or developed AIDS. Immunological progression in the subgroup was assessed on an analysis of CD4 cell loss with time. A1–B8–DR3 was associated with a faster rate of CD4 loss and B27 with a slower rate when compared with subjects without these HLA antigens.

The authors speculate on the mechanism whereby patients with B27 have a slow progression of their disease [21]. The analysis makes the assumption that autoimmunity is part of the pathogenesis of AIDS (see Chapter 2, section 2.5.3). Autoimmunity may arise because part of the viral protein (glycoprotein gp120) mimics the HLA-DR β chain for class I presentation. Where this mimicry is close, as in the DR β_1 chain, the protein is recognized as 'self' when presented by HLA-B27 and no immune response is subsequently directed against the MHC of the host, i.e. there is no autoimmunity. In the case of the DR3 chain associated with A1–B8, the mimicry is poor, tolerance is lost and an immune response results, which is ultimately directed against the MHC-derived peptides of the host.

1.5 HIV-1 infection and AIDS in the era of prophylaxis

Improvement in the management of patients infected with HIV by earlier diagnosis, better treatment and the use of prophylaxis is likely to alter the clinical presentation and course of the disease. Such changing patterns of disease in patients with AIDS have important implications for healthcare provision and future medical research. In a study of 347 predominantly homosexual men with AIDS between 1982 and 1989, the proportion of patients who developed PCP dropped from 56 to 24% although it still remained the index diagnosis of AIDS in half of new patients. Kaposi's sarcoma decreased as the index diagnosis from 30 to 20% over this period but as a cause of death it rose from 14 to 32%. Lymphoma accounted for an increased proportion of deaths while PCP as a cause of death decreased from 46 to 3%. The median survival increased from 10 months in 1984–86 to 20 months in 1987 [22]. In another study, a comparison was made of HIV-1 antibody-positive patients presenting with a respiratory illness to a major UK centre in 1986–87 and 1990–91. No patient received zidovudine or prophylaxis for PCP in the earlier year. PCP remained the commonest respiratory disease, 68% of all diagnoses in the 1986–87 period and 48% in 1990–91. However, bacterial infections and Kaposi's sarcoma were seen more commonly in 1990–91 [23].

A more direct analysis of the effect of prophylaxis was studied in a cohort of 844 patients with AIDS of which 138 men received prophylaxis with zidovudine as well as prophylaxis for PCP. In spite of prophylaxis, 39 (28%) had PCP at some time. Four illnesses occurred more frequently in men who received prophylaxis than in those who did not (706 men). These illnesses were the wasting syndrome (involuntary weight loss with chronic diarrhoea or weakness with fever), CMV disease and oesophageal candidiasis. Collectively these four diseases accounted for the initial AIDS diagnosis in 42.7% of those on prophylaxis compared with 10.7% in those that were not. It is not certain from this study which prophylactic regimen was responsible for the result or whether it was a combination of both. However, the change in the pattern of illnesses was more closely related to the use of PCP prophylaxis than zidovudine. A final conclusion of the study was that prophylaxis may have delayed the onset of AIDS by 6–12 months [24].

In another study from North America, an analysis was made of the effect on the pattern of hospital admissions of prophylaxis against PCP with inhaled pentamide. There was a statistically significant decrease in the number of admissions due to PCP (from 48 to 29%) with a rise due to other infectious causes (from 52 to 71%); the total admissions were the same in the year before prophylaxis (1988–89) as in the year after (1989–90). The increase in infectious causes was primarily non-respiratory although there was a modest increase in respiratory-tract infection which was not due to PCP. In spite of a significant drop in admissions due to respiratory disease (from 50 to 41%), it remained the most frequent single cause. Dealing with the respiratory causes of admission alone, it was found that the drop in PCP as a cause was almost exactly offset by a rise in bacterial pneumonia [25].

1.5.1 Long-term survival in HIV-1 infection

Studies on long-term asymptomatic survivors are important in that they may reveal characteristics associated with a good prognosis as well as defining the immunological responses which appear to be most beneficial in combating HIV. The association of a particular immunological response to infection with a good long-term prognosis suggests that the onset of advanced disease may not be random and that there is more to long-term survival than statistical probability [26].

In a cohort study of homosexual men infected with HIV, a group were identified who remained asymptomatic after diagnosis for 7 years and this group was compared with those who developed symptoms during the same period [27]. As might be expected, it was found that the slope of the decline in CD4 cell count with time was higher in the long-term asymptomatic men than in those who progressed. In addition, those who remained asymptomatic were characterized by greater T-cell reactivity to stimulation with monoclonal CD3 antibodies, by seropositivity for antibodies to HIV core proteins and by the absence of hepatitis B markers [27].

In a cohort study of HIV-infected subjects with haemophilia an estimate has been made of the probability of a number of subjects remaining free of AIDS for up to 25 years [28]. The cohort consisted of 111 men followed for a median length of follow-up of 10.1 years with a median number of CD4 counts of 17. Prediction of the development of AIDS was made by using a linear extrapolation of the regression slopes of the CD4 counts. AIDS was defined in the model as when the CD4 count fell to 50×10^6 cells/l on extrapolation. The choice of this cell count was based on previous findings that AIDS occurs on average at about 50×10^6 cells/l. Prophylaxis from 1989 was provided against *Candida* and PCP and anti-retroviral drugs when the CD4 count fell below 200×10^6 cells/l.

Against this background, the model predicted that 25% (CI 16–34%) would survive for 20 years after seroconversion and 18% (CI 11–25%) for 25 years without developing AIDS. Such people may require antiretroviral drugs for as long as 20 years. If this prediction is substantiated and is applicable to the other categories of HIV-infected people, it is perhaps the first encouraging epidemiological study in a disease with otherwise such a devastating prognosis.

References

1 WHO. AIDS data as at 30 June 1995 and current global situation of the HIV/AIDS pandemic. *Weekly Epidemiological Record* 1995; **70**: 193–200.

2 WHO. AIDS data as at 15 December 1995 and current global situation of HIV/AIDS pandemic. *Weekly Epidemiological Record* 1995; **70**: 353–360.

3 Johnson A.M., De Cock K.M. What's happening to AIDS? *British Medical Journal* 1994; **309**: 1523–1524.

4 Rodrigues J.J., Mehendale S.M., Shepherd M.E. *et al.* Risk factors for HIV infection in people attending clinics for sexually transmitted diseases in India. *British Medical Journal* 1995; **311**: 283–286.

5 Centers for Disease Control. 1993 Revised classification system for HIV infection and expanded surveillance case definition for AIDS among adolescents and adults. *Morbidity and Mortality Weekly Report* 1992; **41** (No. RR-17): 1–19.

6 Classification system for human T-lymphotropic virus type III/lymphadenopathy-associated virus infections. *Morbidity and Mortality Weekly Report* 1986; **35**: 334–339.

7 Centers for Disease Control. Revision of the CDC surveillance case definition for acquired immunodeficiency syndrome. *Morbidity and Mortality Weekly Report* 1987; **36** (Suppl. 1S): 1S–15S.

8 The incidence and prevalence of AIDS and prevalence of other severe HIV disease in England and Wales for 1995 to 1999: projections using data to the end of 1994. *Communicable Disease Report* 1996; **6**: R1–R24.

9 Hunt A.J., Davies P.M., Weatherburn P., Coxon A.P.M., McManus T.J. Changes in sexual behaviour in a large cohort of homosexual men in England and Wales. *British Medical Journal* 1991; **302**: 505–506.

10 AIDS and HIV-1 infection worldwide. *Communicable Disease Report* 1995; **5**: 97–98.

11 Projections of the number of persons diagnosed with AIDS and the number of immuno-suppressed HIV-infected persons, United States, 1992–1994. *Morbidity and Mortality Weekly Report* 1992; **41** (No. RR-18): 2–24.

12 Update: trends in AIDS diagnosis and reporting under the expanded surveillance definition for adolescents and adults. United States, 1993. *Morbidity and Mortality Weekly Report* 1994; **43**: 826–831.

13 Update: trends in AIDS among men who have sex with men. United States 1989–1994. *Morbidity and Mortality Weekly Report* 1995; **44**: 401–404.

14 Update: AIDS among women. United States 1994. *Morbidity and Mortality Weekly Report* 1995; **44**: 81–84.

15 Heterosexually acquired AIDS. United States 1993. *Morbidity and Mortality Weekly Report* 1994; **43**: 155–160.

16 Update: mortality attributable to HIV infection/AIDS among persons aged 25–44 years — United States, 1990 and 1991. *Morbidity and Mortality Weekly Report* 1993; **42**: 481–486.

17 Fahey J.L., Taylor J.M.G., Detels R. *et al*. The prognostic value of cellular and serologic markers in infection with human immunodeficiency virus type 1. *New England Journal of Medicine* 1990; **322**: 166–172.

18 Phair J., Muñoz A., Detels R. *et al*. The risk of *Pneumocystis carinii* pneumonia among men infected with human immunodeficiency virus type 1. *New England Journal of Medicine* 1990; **322**: 161–165.

19 Kaslow R.A, Mann D.L. The role of the major histocompatibility complex in human immunodeficiency virus infection — ever more complex. *Journal of Infectious Diseases* 1994; **169**: 1332–1333.

20 Klein M.R., Keet I.P.M., D'Amaro J. *et al*. Associations between HLA frequencies and pathogenic features of human immunodeficiency virus type 1 infection in seroconverters from the Amsterdam cohort of homosexual men. *Journal of Infectious Diseases* 1994; **169**: 1244–1249.

21 McNeil A.J., Yap P.L., Gore S.M. *et al*. Association of HLA A1–B8–DR3 and B27 with rapid and slow progression of HIV disease. *Quarterly Journal of Medicine* 1996; **89**: 177–185.

22 Peters B.S., Beck E.J., Coleman D.G. *et al*. Changing disease patterns in patients with AIDS in a referral centre in the United Kingdom: the changing face of AIDS. *British Medical Journal* 1991; **302**: 203–206.

23 Pitkin A.D., Grant A.D., Foley N.M., Miller R.F. Changing patterns of respiratory disease in HIV positive patients in a referral centre in the United Kingdom between 1986–7 and 1990–1. *Thorax* 1993; **48**: 204–207.

24 Hoover D.R., Saah A.J., Bacellar H. *et al*. for the Multicentre AIDS Cohort Study. Clinical manifestations of AIDS in the era of *Pneumocystis* prophylaxis. *New England Journal of Medicine* 1993; **329**: 1922–1926.

25 Chien S.-M., Rawji M., Mintz S., Rachlis A., Chan, C.K. Changes in hospital admission pattern with human immunodeficiency virus infection in the era of *Pneumocystis carinii* prophylaxis. *Chest* 1992; **102**: 1035–1039.

26 Rutherford G.W. Long term survival in HIV-1 infection. *British Medical Journal* 1994; **309**: 283–284.

27 Keet I.P.M., Krol A., Klein M.R. *et al*. Characteristics of long-term asymptomatic infection with human immunodeficiency virus type 1 in men with normal and low CD4+ cell counts. *Journal of Infectious Diseases* 1994; **169**: 1236–1243.

28 Phillips A.N., Sabin C.A., Elford J., Bofill M., Janossy G., Lee C.A. Use of CD4 lymphocyte count to predict long term survival free of AIDS after HIV infection. *British Medical Journal* 1994; **309**: 301–312.

2 Pathogenesis of infection with HIV

S.J.G. SEMPLE

2.0 HIV-1

HIV-1 is a member of the retrovirus family, being classified with the lentiviruses (LV), which cause chronic degenerative diseases and an immunodeficiency syndrome but are non-oncogenic (non-transforming). The LV are quite distinct from the oncoviruses, which are not cytopathic, are transforming and include the leukaemia and sarcoma groups of viruses. Finally, there are the spumaviruses, which cause syncytial formation and cell lysis in cell culture but apparently cause no disease in humans who are infected with this subfamily of the retroviruses.

Another group of human T-cell lymphotropic retroviruses has also been isolated, initially from West Africans. This virus is referred to as HIV-2 and is associated with a syndrome similar to AIDS.

HIV has three principal genes (Fig. 2.1) [1]: *gag* encodes the core proteins p24, p17, p7 and p6, *pol* encodes the polymerases (reverse

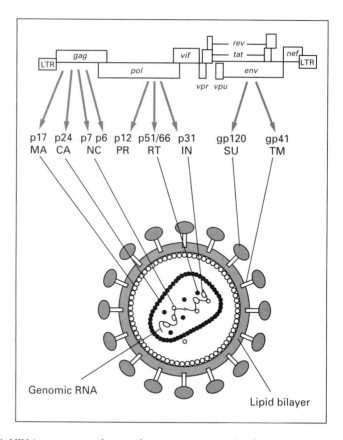

Fig. 2.1 HIV-1 genes: *gag, pol, env, vif, vpr, vpu, tat, rev* and *nef*. MA, matrix proteins; CA, capsid proteins; NC, nucleocapsid proteins; RT, reverse transcriptase; PR, protease; IN, integrase; SU, envelope surface protein; TM, envelope transmembrane protein; RNA, ribonucleic acid. Redrawn from [1].

transcriptase, protease and integrase) and *env* encodes the envelope protein of the virus, glycoprotein gp160, which is made up of two proteins, gp120 and gp41. The regulatory genes are *tat*, *rev* and *nef*. Transactivator (*tat*) enhances viral replication by encoding a protein acting on the promoter sequence of the long terminal repeat (LTR) of HIV, while the *rev* gene encodes a protein that promotes translation of viral messenger ribonucleic acid (mRNA). The product of the *nef* gene appears to have an inhibitory effect on viral replication. The product of the accessory gene *vif* (virion infectivity factor) is required for cell-free viral transmission, and virions generated in its absence are less efficient in establishing an infection. The product of the *vpr* gene (virion protein R) enhances rapid growth in the virus. The *vpu* gene produces the virion protein U, which is involved in virion transport, assembly and release.

There is considerable genetic variability of the HIV-1 virus. Nine clades (subtypes) have been identified (A–H and O), based on deoxyribonucleic acid (DNA) sequencing of the envelope protein of the virus, gp160. The envelope glycoproteins were chosen to determine the genotype of the virus because neutralizing antibodies are thought to be directed against epitopes of these glycoproteins. The geographical distribution of some clades is limited; for example, clade E is highly prevalent in South-East Asia, whereas B is dominant in North America and Europe. However, because of the movement of people between continents, it is not surprising that there is now evidence of the introduction of diverse genetic subtypes into the western hemisphere [2,3].

By cross-neutralization techniques it is possible to correlate genetic diversity (genotypes) with antigenic diversity (serotypes). This is done by measuring the inhibition of infection of monocytes *in vitro* by a virus of known genotype by serum or plasma from an HIV-infected person of the same or different serotype. As expected, strong neutralization activity has been observed when genotype and serotype are the same but weak activity when they diverge [4].

These findings are critical for vaccine development. A vaccine against clade B may be effective in Europe and the USA for the majority of people but is unlikely to be effective in South-East Asia. Indeed, with the introduction of diverse strains into the western hemisphere, it is likely in the future that vaccine development will have to take account of genotype diversity. This will certainly be true if the vaccine is to be used worldwide rather than targeted at one particular genographical region. There is, however, already encouraging evidence that neutralizing antibodies against a segment of gp41, one of the membrane glycoproteins, might provide the basis for a vaccine against both the B clade and strains outside this clade [5].

2.1 Entry of HIV in humans

The most obvious way for free virus or HIV-infected cells to enter the body is through an epithelium or mucosa damaged during sexual intercourse or childbirth or punctured by a hypodermic needle, voluntarily or inadvertently. However, it has been proposed, on the basis of experiments *in vitro*, that transmission can take place across an intact epithelium by cell-to-cell transfer of HIV from infected lymphocytes or macrophages to mucosal cells [6]. The means whereby the virus or infected cells gain access to the blood and the lymphoreticular system is critical for the strategy of vaccine development. Cell-to-cell transfer of virus was demonstrated using infected lymphocytes and uninfected epithelial cells from the small intestine. The experiments revealed that, when infected lymphocytes were added to a cell culture of epithelium, the lymphocytes became attached to the epithelial surface and virions were seen to be sequestered between interdigitating microvilli extending from lymphocyte and epithelial cells. Viral budding from the lymphocytes was polar, that is, directed towards the epithelium, and infection of the epithelium by HIV was subsequently demonstrated. Cell-to-cell transfer was independent of the CD4 receptor, which is the usual and best-known route of entry of HIV into cells. In the *in vitro* preparation used in these experiments, the viral particles were isolated in the confined space between infected lymphocytes and mucosal cell so that they could not be reached by antiviral serum added to the *in vitro* preparation [6]. If this isolation operates *in vivo*, this will enable HIV to evade immune detection by neutralizing antibodies.

2.2 Virus infection of cells

The receptor for HIV is the CD4 molecule, which is expressed on many cells but particularly the subset of T lymphocytes referred to as helper cells (Th) [7–12]. However, other receptors have been identified: galactosyl ceramide on brain and gut cells and the Fc and complement receptors.

The T-cell receptor is a heterodimeric molecule comprising an α and a β chain linked by a disulphide bond. The variability of the amino acid sequences of the α and β polypeptides determines the specificity of antigen binding and this domain is encoded by rearrangement of the variable (V), diversity (D) and joining (J) genes (Fig. 2.2). In addition, there are regions of the variable domain of the T-cell receptors with even greater variability (and hence greater specificity for antigen), referred to as the complementary determining regions (CDRs). The initial steps to virus infection of cells consist of attachment, fusion and nucleocapsid entry. These steps

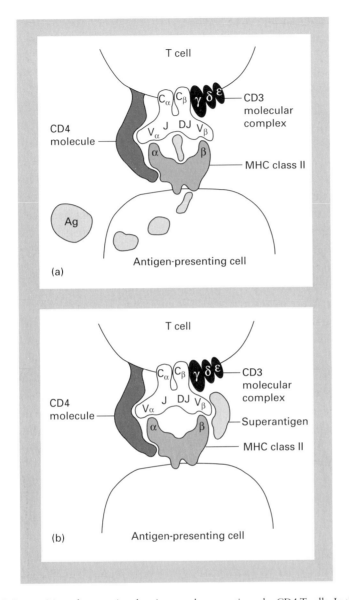

Fig. 2.2 Recognition of conventional antigens and superantigens by CD4 T cells. In the
upper panel, all the variable elements of the α and β chains of the antigen receptor are
involved in the recognition of the conventional antigenic peptides. In the lower panel, the
recognition of superantigen involves the variable region of the β chain of the T-cell antigen
receptor and virtually any MHC class II molecule. V, variable; J, joining; D, diversity;
Ag, antigen. Reproduced by permission of the authors and the *New England Journal of
Medicine* [42].

depend on the interaction and binding of components of the glycoproteins
of the HIV envelope (gp120/gp41) with the CD4 receptor.

There are areas of homology between amino acid chains of gp120
and critical areas of the amino acid sequences for binding on the CD4

receptor. The binding sites on the CD4 receptor are for the major histo-compatibility complex (MHC) class II molecules of the antigen-presenting cell (APC) (Fig. 2.2). Because of the homology of amino acid sequences of gp120 and gp41 and MHC class II molecules, these components of the HIV envelope may be immunologically silent, i.e. non-immunogenic [13].

The mechanism of viral entry has not been completely elucidated but may be dependent on phagocytosis, which is CD4-independent, as well as upon cells with the appropriate receptors for HIV infection, which are monocytes, macrophages (including alveolar macrophages (AMs)), follicular dendritic cells (FDCs), dendritic cells in blood, fibroblasts, Langerhans cells in skin and B lymphocytes. One model for viral entry into cells describes the interaction in stages between two envelope glycoproteins of the virus, gp41 and gp120, with the V_1 domain of the CD4 receptor [14]. The model is derived from experiments *in vitro* reported in the literature observing the effects on the binding of HIV glycoproteins with the CD4 receptor, using anti-CD4 monoclonal antibodies, soluble CD4 and recombinant CD4 proteins with mutations. Figure 2.3(a) depicts the molecular

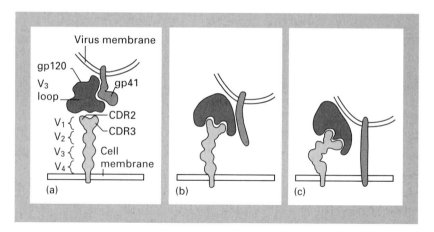

Fig. 2.3 Stages in the entry of HIV virions into CD4 cells. (a) The envelope glycoprotein of the HIV is gp120 (dark shading), which contains the CD4-binding sites. The glycoprotein gp41 (medium shading) is embedded in the envelope membrane of the virion and is non-covalently linked to gp120. The V_3 loop of gp120 is shown. The CD4 is shown (light shading) with the CDR2 and CDR3 (complementary determining regions), which react with gp120. The CD4 has four immunoglobulin-like domains, a transmembrane segment and an intracytoplasmic tail.
(b) Molecular conformational changes in gp120 and its V_3 loop ensure binding of this glycoprotein to the CD42 and three domains of the CD4 receptor. A bend in CD4 is shown because antibodies to this region inhibit infection after the initial binding process [14].
(c) The final step involves a further conformational change ('collapse') of the CD4 molecule, with dissociation of gp120 from gp41, freeing the hydrophobic amino-terminal domain of gp41, which fuses with the cell membrane, allowing viral entry. This cartoon is reproduced from reference [14].

structures involved in viral entry. The CD4 receptor consists of four extracellular immunoglobulin (Ig)-like domains, together with CDR2 and 3, a transmembrane segment and an intracytoplasmic tail. The HIV envelope glycoproteins are gp120 and gp41, which are non-covalently linked. The glycoprotein gp41 is embedded in the envelope membrane of the virion. Full engagement of CD4 with gp120 depends on molecular conformational changes in gp120 and its V_3 loop, together with CDR2 and three regions of the CD4 receptor; this is illustrated as shape changes in the molecules in the cartoon of Fig. 2.3(b). The final step is a further conformational change in the V_3/V_4 region of the CD4 receptor, which breaks the link between gp120 and gp41, freeing the hydrophobic amino-terminal of gp41 to fuse with the target cell membrane, allowing viral entry (Fig. 2.3c).

After entry of the virus, genomic RNA is then transcribed into DNA by reverse transcriptase and is subsequently circularized and integrated into the host genome by a virus-encoded enzyme (viral integrase). At this stage of the HIV life cycle, the HIV genome is designated DNA provirus. Considerable quantities of unintegrated viral DNA remain in the cell cytoplasm. There is little HIV replication unless the cell is activated, when viral proteins and genomic RNA are assembled at the cell surface and virions are formed by budding (Fig. 2.4) [15]. This process results in cell lysis.

2.3 Immunological defence against HIV-1

Primary infection with HIV-1 is followed by detectable humoral and cellular immune responses to the virus and a prolonged period of clinical latency. These responses include neutralizing antibodies, antibody-dependent cell cytotoxicity (ADCC), activation of the complement system, cytotoxic T lymphocytes (CTLs) and natural killer (NK) cells. The difficulty is in defining the importance of each system of defence against the virus and whether any of them may be redundant or even pathogenic. However, it seems reasonable to assume *a priori* that the initial clearing of the virus and some of the infected cells from the peripheral blood (but not necessarily from the tissues) may be due to the normal immunological mechanisms for the defence against viral infections.

2.3.1 Neutralizing antibodies

The ability of antibodies to neutralize isolates of HIV-1 has been tested by sera from patients and from animals immunized with a recombinant envelope protein of the virus, gp120–gp41 [16]. Human sera were obtained from patients in Britain and Uganda. The human sera effectively

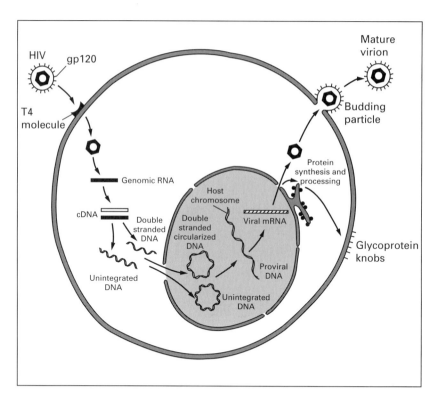

Fig. 2.4 HIV replication cycle. Entry of the virus through the T4 molecule, the formation of double-stranded DNA and integration of the DNA into the host chromosome. Activation of the cell leads to the formation of the mature virion released into the environment. Reproduced by permission of the author and the *New England Journal of Medicine* [15].

neutralized several HIV-1 isolates and complement did not affect the neutralization titres. The findings indicated that genetically diverse strains of HIV carried variable and widely conserved epitopes for neutralizing antibodies. Useful vaccines will depend on the identification of epitopes conserved among different isolates, providing the epitopes are neutralizing. Probably the major viral envelope glycoprotein in this respect is gp120.

Humoral immunity alone has not been protective in chimpanzees. Production of anti-HIV-1 antibodies does not prevent animals becoming infected when subsequently challenged with HIV-1. It is possible that, in humans, a strong antibody response to HIV-1 may delay the progression of disease without eliminating the virus.

2.3.2 Activation of the complement system

High levels of circulating immune complexes are found in patients infected with HIV, as well as antibodies that are cytotoxic *in vitro* to CD4 lymphocytes. The potential benefits of the complement system would be in the disposal of immune complexes, together with the killing of cells infected with virus, via the final phase of complement activation, leading to the 'membrane attack complex'. Levels of the intact components of the complement system, C4, factor B and C3, in patients with HIV disease are normal but the levels of their activation components, C4d, Ba and C3d, are elevated, as well as the ratio of activated to intact concentration [17]. The activation of the complement system was predominantly through the classical pathway, although there was evidence of involvement of the alternative route. Indices of the magnitude of complement activation were positively correlated with the clinical severity of disease and the levels of circulating immune complexes and β_2-microglobulin but were inversely correlated with the CD4 count.

2.3.3 Cell-mediated cytotoxicity

Perhaps the most appropriate immunological defence against a resident virus is cell-mediated cytotoxicity. CTLs recognize viral antigen processed endogenously in infected cells and presented on their surface as a binary complex of a peptide fragment and the human leucocyte antigen (HLA). In HIV-1-infected patients, circulating CTLs have been found which are specific for an envelope protein of the virus (usually gp120) and which are HLA class-I-restricted [18,19]. Class-II-restricted CTLs (CD4) have been detected in peripheral blood but only following repeated stimulation *in vitro*. Also, no HLA class-II-restricted CTLs have been detected in fresh tissues of infected patients, so their role in the immune response remains to be determined [19].

Studies of the cellular immune response have been made on patients with the primary acute, self-limited, symptomatic illness, which occurs before, at and after seroconversion. CTL precursors were found which were specific for cells expressing antigens of HIV-1 — Gag, Pol and Env [20,21]. The CTL precursors were detected within a few weeks, often before seroconversion, and were associated with the clearance of the viraemia. Delay in the appearance of these CTLs was associated with a prolongation of symptoms and a delay in the clearance of the viraemia. Neutralizing antibodies were first detected after the rise in CTLs and were not coincident with the clearance of viraemia. In these studies, provided the assay of neutralizing antibodies was sufficiently sensitive to detect any antibodies that were biologically active, the results suggest a dominant role for CD8 T lymphocytes in the initial immune control of the HIV-1 virus [20,21]. Development of a vaccine which stimulated HIV-1 CD8 CTLs might be a successful strategy for vaccine development.

Cell lysis which is not HLA-restricted has been shown to occur *in vitro*, the effector cells being NK cells [22].

2.3.4 CD8 cell anti-HIV activity without cytolysis

There is substantial evidence that CD8 cells *in vitro* can suppress viral replication in endogenous or exogenous infected CD4 cells. This action is not due to antigen-specific CTL activity or to the inhibition or killing of infected CD4 cells. Clinical studies have shown a highly significant correlation between the CD8 suppressive activity and clinical status, activity being highest in asymptomatic individuals. There was also a positive direct correlation between the CD8 cell-mediated anti-HIV activity and the patient's blood CD4 count but not the CD8 cell count [23]. CD8 T-cell anti-HIV activity (non-cytolytic) has been found in patients at seroconversion which has persisted in some for up to 2 years. This was associated with a fall in plasma viraemia which could not be attributed to neutralizing antibodies. Interestingly, this anti-HIV effect was found in some patients before seroconversion and raises the possibility of exposure to HIV without the establishment of infection [24].

CD8 cells were found to suppress HIV activity in the absence of direct cell-to-cell contact with the infected CD4 cells, although it was more efficient when contact was present. It has been proposed that CD8 cells produce a soluble factor acting as an anti-HIV lymphokine. It is likely that the suppression of HIV activity is due to more than one factor and that these are the β chemokines, RANTES, Macrophage inflammatory protein-1α (MIP-1α) and MIP-1β. They act through a newly identified co-receptor to the CD4 molecule for HIV infection of cells and this chemokine receptor is known as CC-CXR-5 (see [25] for review). However, CD8 suppression activity is more efficient when there is cell-to-cell contact and this has prompted investigation of cell-surface molecules involved in cellular adhesion. The evidence at present is that these molecules are not essential for the CD8 suppressor activity. However, the lymphocyte functional antigen 1 (LFA-1) is one of the molecules that regulates cell-to-cell adhesion, which could affect the efficiency of HIV infection of cells. In fact, the absence of LFA-1 from cells does not impair virus entry, HIV spreading and virus replication in cells *in vitro*. However, cell adhesion and syncytia formation, which are a feature of virus-infected cells *in vitro*, were not present in LFA-1-deficient cells. Syncytia formation leads to the death of cells (both infected and uninfected), so that LFA-1, and possibly other adhesion molecules, may be a component of one of the mechanisms for CD4 depletion in HIV disease [26].

2.4 The paradox of HIV infection

It will be apparent from the preceding sections that infection by HIV-1 leads to the immunological response characteristic of viral infections in humans. The central problem is to determine why this does not eliminate the infection or lead to a state of symbiosis between virus and host.

2.4.1 The cytopathic theory

The first and most obvious explanation is that the virus attacks, renders unresponsive and kills the cells (CD4) which are pivotal in cell-mediated and humoral immunity. Mechanisms that have been proposed for direct cell killing have included massive budding of HIV particles on the outer cell membrane, leading to loss of integrity of the membrane and high levels of unintegrated DNA in the cytoplasm, which impair cell viability and function. This cytopathic theory is certainly plausible but there remains doubt as to whether the virtual elimination of cellular immunity by HIV can be explained solely by this mechanism. Doubt has been raised on account of the apparent paucity of infected cells (originally 1 in 10 000) found in the peripheral blood of patients in the asymptomatic period of their infection in spite of the cell tropism of the virus for the CD4 cell observed *in vitro*.

More recent studies suggest a much higher frequency of infection of CD4 cells than was originally found. In the peripheral blood of patients with AIDS, it can be anticipated that about 1/1000 CD4 cells will be infected and expressing virus. By using the technique of the polymerase chain reaction (PCR), it is possible to determine in addition those cells that are latently infected but not expressing viral RNA or protein. It was found that in patients with AIDS about 1/100 cells contained HIV-1 DNA while in asymptomatic patients this frequency was much less, at 1/10 000 [27]. Support for a higher rate of infection of cells comes from culture of HIV from the peripheral blood of patients with AIDS, which points to 1 in 40 CD4 cells harbouring the virus [28]. Can this frequency of cell infection account for the subsequent depletion of CD4 cells? One view is that a simple cytopathic model for AIDS pathogenesis is not credible on the basis that: (i) the numbers of infected cells are small in relation to the regenerative capacity of the immune system; and (ii) virus isolated from the plasma is usually non-culturable, suggesting that it is neutralized or defective.

Determination of the number of virus-infected cells in the peripheral blood is not a measure of viral replication, cell turnover or the extent of the involvement of the reticulolymphatic system by HIV. It has been studies of these characteristics of HIV infection that have made a major contribution to the unravelling of the paradox posed at the start of this section.

2.4.2 Does the AIDS virus hide away?

So far we have viewed the cellular tropism of the virus through the peripheral blood, which in the asymptomatic phase of HIV infection suggests that the virus is latent. Examination of lymph glands in infected patients suggests a very different picture. During the initial stages of HIV infection, there are 5–10 times more infected cells in lymphoid tissue than in blood and it is only in the late stages of the disease that a similar number of infected cells are seen in the two compartments [29,30]. Also, during the latent (asymptomatic) phase of the illness, there is active viral replication and accumulation in lymphoid tissues.

Histological examination of the lymph glands reveals virus, virus particles and immune complexes on the surfaces of the villous processes of the FDCs [31]. One report claims that some FDCs are actually infected with virus, even though these cells are CD4-negative [31]. Many lymphocytes, infected and uninfected, are seen in close contact with the processes of the FDC. Thus it is hypothesized that during the asymptomatic phase of the illness there is mechanical filtering and trapping of virions by the FDC network and the sequestration of infected CD4 cells. In addition, the close contact between lymphocytes and the FDCs provides a means and opportunity for the infection of uninfected CD4 cells. In the late stages of HIV disease, the architecture of the lymph nodes is disrupted, with the loss of virus trapping and hence an equality of infected cells in blood and lymphoid tissue [30].

The above findings do not establish whether the regenerative capacity of the T-cell population (thymopoiesis) is impaired; animal experiments suggest that it may be so affected, even in the early stages of the disease. The animal used is the mouse which is homozygous for severe combined immunodeficiency defect (SCID), into which human fetal liver and thymus are implanted. These organ implants support human haemopoiesis, which includes normal and functionally competent T cells. Infection of these organs leads to severe depletion of human CD4 cells within a few weeks of infection, accompanied by increasing viral load in the implants. Reduced thymopoiesis in HIV disease may be one of the mechanisms responsible for the falling CD4 count in the peripheral blood [32,33].

2.4.3 Viral replication, virus-specific immune responses and CD4 survival and turnover

Two recent studies show that the composite lifespan of plasma virus and virus-producing cells is remarkably short, with a half-life of approximately 2 days [34,35]. This was shown by the use of two highly potent antiviral drugs, one which inhibits reverse transcriptase and the other protease. With these new drugs, 99% inhibition of plasma viraemia was achieved. By measuring the day-to-day reduction of plasma viraemia, the rate of elimination of plasma virus and virus-producing cells could be estimated. In addition, by following the day-to-day rise in CD4 cell counts upon drug administration, an estimate of the production rate of these cells could be made. Extrapolation of these kinetic data to the steady state enabled the daily rate of viral replication and CD4 cell turnover to be calculated. The results were remarkable. Of the total virus population, 30% or more must have been replenished daily. The entire population of peripheral CD4 lymphocytes was turning over every 15 days in the steady state when production and destruction were balanced. Disappointingly, there was almost complete replacement of the wild-type virus in plasma by drug-resistant variants within 14 days (only one of the inhibitors was used at any one time, so that the emergence of resistance so rapidly might be avoided by the use of two drugs with different activities). These results indicate that there are continuous rounds of *de novo* virus infection, replication and rapid cell turnover and, in these two studies, the process was not overtly related to the stage of the disease. The cells lost were those contributing to the viral pool and therefore in them the virus was replicating, which of itself could have led directly to their death. It is unlikely that this is the sole cause, the other effective cause being the normal immune responses to infected cells, in particular that of CTLs.

The mutation of the virus, leading to drug resistance, rapidly dominates the plasma viral pool but it spreads only slowly to blood mononuclear cells, with little effect on their survival, presumably because in these cells there is minimal viral replication. However, mononuclear cells and macrophages may be a reservoir of virus, maintaining survival of the virus in the face of an active and vigorous immune response.

During the asymptomatic phase of the disease, viral replication is not latent but active, as indeed is the response of the immune system, which is initially efficient in containing the virus. However, the immune system is plainly not infinite and in spite of its activity some virus survives and CD4 cells decline, albeit slowly. CD4 cells are destroyed faster than the production of virus, so other mechanisms may contribute to their loss, and these are considered in subsequent sections of this chapter.

2.4.4 Varying cytopathicity among HIV strains

Variation in the cytopathicity of different strains of HIV will determine in part the rate of progression of HIV disease. The cytocidal activity of the virus is usually assessed in cell culture, and one classification categorizes strains into those that replicate rapidly to a high titre and those that replicate slowly to a low titre. Another means of assessment relies on the ability of some viruses to induce syncytial formation in cultured cells. This formation involves fusion between T lymphocytes through their cell-surface CD4 antigen, leading to the formation of multinucleated giant cells, which then die. While the process is initiated through virus-infected cells, it then involves fusion with uninfected CD4 lymphocytes and hence this may be one mechanism leading to the depletion of T lymphocytes [11]. *In vitro* the formation of syncytia may be regulated by the leucocyte adhesion molecule LFA-1 [26]. Central to this process is the virus envelope glycoprotein gp120, which has an affinity for the CD4 antigen. This glycoprotein on the surface of virus-infected cells binds to the CD4 antigen on uninfected cells, hence leading to syncytial formation. In addition, gp120 (protein or antigen) may be shed into the circulation as budding virions are released from the surface of infected cells and this glycoprotein may then attach itself to CD4 antigen on uninfected cells, thereby initiating syncytial formation. While this is a potential mechanism for the continuing depletion of CD4 lymphocytes, the magnitude and importance of syncytium formation *in vivo* remains to be established.

Isolates of HIV-1 have been divided into two groups according to their ability to replicate *in vitro*: namely, those that replicate rapidly with high reverse transcriptase activity (rapid/high) and cause syncytium formation (SI) and those that replicate slowly (slow/low) and do not form syncytia (NSI) [36]. There is evidence that in the asymptomatic phase virus isolates are of the slow/low and NSI phenotype and their target is preferentially monocyte-derived macrophages. In a proportion of persons progressing to AIDS, viral isolates are of the rapid/high and SI phenotype and their target is preferentially blood lymphocytes [37]. The two phenotypes have been shown to have different amino acid sequences in the V3 region of the HIV *env* gene. The macrophage-tropic viruses had either an acidic amino acid or alanine at position 25, in contrast to the T-cell-tropic viruses which usually had a non-acidic amino acid at this position [38].

The importance of these *in vitro* findings for viral 'pathogenicity' and disease progression has been questioned by an *in vivo* study using post-mortem tissue in patients who died of AIDS or for unrelated reasons while they were asymptomatic [39]. All patients were predominantly infected with variants of the NSI/macrophage-tropic phenotype, irrespective of the degree of disease progression. The amino acid sequences of the V3 loop were highly conserved, in contrast to the standard laboratory isolates of HIV-1 from the peripheral blood. Proviral sequences were detected in brain, spinal cord and lung only in those patients with AIDS. In these patients, the cells expressing viral antigen (p24) were macrophages and microglia, frequently forming syncytia with surrounding tissue damage, even though the virus isolates resembled the NSI phenotype. These findings show that lack of the ability to form syncytia in established T cells *in vitro* does not necessarily predict the ability to form syncytia *in vivo* [39].

HIV strains evolve within the host with time, which may be because the host is infected with more than one strain, as a result of antiretroviral treatment or because of mutation within the virus. Changing cytopathicity or cytocidal ability of the virus may be responsible for the change from the asymptomatic period of infection into the rapid downhill course into AIDS. The initial depletion of the immune system by a non-cytopathic strain may eventually lead to the emergence of a highly cytopathic variant and this may herald the onset of AIDS. At the moment, there is some difficulty in assessing this hypothesis because tests of cytopathicity in *in vitro* cell culture do not always relate directly to the *in vivo* situation in infected animals [40]. In addition, the phenotype of virus isolated from the blood may differ from that obtained from tissues such as brain, lung and bowel [39].

2.5 Immune suppression and lymphocyte destruction in the absence of viral infection of these cells

Evidence for this suppression and destruction comes from experiments *in vitro*. The assumption that this takes place *in vivo* is based on the premise that the envelope glycoprotein gp120 circulating freely (or bound as an immune complex) combines with the CD4 molecule on uninfected cells bearing this marker. The gp120 is presumed to be released from the budding virions or following the lysis of infected cells. When uninfected CD4 lymphocytes were coated with gp120, it was found that over 30% of the cells became susceptible to ADCC, which did not occur when the cells were not coated with the glycoprotein [41]. The normal immune response of CD4 cells coated with gp120 was tested in two ways. The first was to test their response to a toxin to which they had previously been sensitized and the second was to test their ability to lyse cells infected with a virus against which they had specific activity.

The effect of gp120 on the immune response of CD4 cells was tested using donor cells from a subject immunized with tetanus toxoid. These cells were activated (stimulated to proliferate) *in vitro* by tetanus toxoid in the presence of the appropriate APC (MHC class II). Purified gp120 inhibited this activation (i.e. a normal immune response to a known antigen) in a dose-dependent manner, achieving over 80% inhibition at saturation. It was also shown *in vitro* that CD4 CTLs, with anti-Epstein–Barr virus (anti-EBV) activity, when coated with gp120 had impaired ability to lyse target cells, which in this case were B lymphocytes transformed by EBV [41].

Thus it would appear that gp120 can render uninfected CD4 T lymphocytes susceptible to lysis by normal immune mechanisms. In addition, gp120 can impair the antigen-specific immune responses of these T lymphocytes *in vitro*. It remains to be shown whether these effects are operative *in vivo* and hence contribute to the immunosuppression seen in HIV disease.

2.5.1 Superantigen

Normally the variable elements of the α and β chains of the T-cell receptor are involved in the recognition of the antigen (peptide) in the groove of the MHC class II molecule (Fig. 2.1). Because this recognition is to a specific antigen, few T cells are involved. Superantigen binds only to the V_β region (Fig. 2.1), causing stimulation and expansion of a much larger number of T cells because it is less specific. These cells may be deleted, rendered anergic or made more susceptible to viral infection [42]. Lymphocytes with a V_β domain that react with superantigen are deleted from the mature thymocyte pool, leading to the eventual loss of these lymphocytes. Endogenous superantigens are the minor lymphocyte-stimulating antigens which are encoded outside the MHC. These antigens lead to incompatibility between lymphocytes (mixed leucocyte reactions) from MHC-identical strains of mice. Exogenous superantigens may arise from staphylococcal, streptococcal or mycoplasmic infection. Most important, in relation to HIV infection, is that superantigens may be encoded by retroviruses, as in the mouse mammary tumours. In HIV infection the superantigen could be gp120 or immune complexes with this glycoprotein. It has been found that T cells expressing certain V_β elements which are present in control subjects who are not infected with HIV are absent in patients with AIDS. The selective elimination of T cells expressing a defined set of V_β sequences may lead to a considerable loss of these cells *in vivo* [43].

2.5.2 Apoptosis

Programmed cell death (apoptosis) is a normal response of immature thymocytes to cellular activation. It is a mechanism for the elimination of autoreactive T cells and hence the establishment of tolerance and the avoidance of autoimmunity. An increase in apoptosis is a normal phenomenon of infection. It is the primary mechanism for the control and termination of antigen-specific immune responses by the elimination of unwanted effector cells during and after infection. Apoptosis is increased in HIV infection, so this increase may be a normal response to the activation of a large number of effector cells [44]. Alternatively the increase in apoptosis could be a direct result of infection of cells with virus. In fact, examination of lymph nodes from HIV-1-infected people showed that apoptosis very rarely occurs in infected cells but that it is increased in nearby cells, referred to as 'bystander cells'. It has therefore been proposed that virus-infected cells have an intracellular mechanism for inhibiting apoptosis while at the same time there is some other process which leads to apoptosis in nearby uninfected cells [45].

Apoptosis has been shown to occur *in vitro* in mature T cells when the CD4 molecule is blocked by antibodies and subsequently (but not simultaneously) activated through the α and β chains of the T-cell receptor [46]. It has been proposed that this form of apoptosis may occur in HIV disease, leading to depletion of CD4 lymphocytes [47]. The first step would be the binding of gp120, alone or as immune complexes, to the CD4 molecules on the surface of the T cell. Subsequently the cell could be activated through the T-cell receptor by the appropriate antigen or alternatively by superantigen, which would lead to apoptosis of the cell in the absence of infection of that cell by HIV.

2.5.3 Autoimmunity

The HIV envelope glycoprotein gp160 has two components, gp120 and gp41. The amino acids of these glycoproteins have been sequenced and they contain areas of homology to MHC class II molecules, namely HLA-DR, HLA-DP and HLA-DQ [13]. Furthermore, the binding site on the CD4 molecule (V_1 domain) for gp120 overlaps the site for binding of MHC class II molecules. This homology and overlap of gp120 points to a mechanism whereby the binding of this glycoprotein to the CD4 molecule could disrupt antigen presentation to the T-cell–CD4-receptor complex (Fig. 2.2), thereby impairing the normal immune response of the host.

The glycoprotein gp120 is immunogenic and will give rise to neutralizing antibodies in HIV infection or following vaccination with the glycoprotein. Because of the homology of gp120 to class II molecules, the possibility of an autoimmune reaction occurring in HIV infection has been postulated. Those areas of gp120 which bind to the CD4 molecule will resemble the invariant and conserved domains of the class II molecules and therefore be recognized as 'self'. These areas would not be immunogenic. However, there are areas of homology to class II molecules outside the binding site and antibodies to these areas might cross-react with the polymorphic (non-invariant) regions of the class II molecules. In this case, gp120 would be acting as an alloepitope (an antigen of another member of the same species) and might give rise to an autoimmune reaction similar to graft-versus-host disease, or, more correctly, chronic experimentally induced allogenic disease. This experimentally produced condition has many of the features of AIDS [48]. Antibodies that cross-react between gp41 and class II molecules have been found in some patients with AIDS. These antibodies were shown *in vitro* to impair the normal proliferative response to T cells to stimulation and also to interfere with ADCC [49]. In addition to these findings, another cytotoxic autoantibody has been found in sera from patients with HIV infection which reacts with antigen on stimulated CD4 T cells. It is different from the aforementioned autoantibodies in that it is not directed against virus or HLA antigens and only acts in the presence of complement. This anti-T-cell autoantibody selectively inhibited CD4 T-cell proliferation [50].

Thus there are theoretical reasons and laboratory investigations which support a potential role for autoimmunity in the pathogenesis of HIV infection, but whether this does exist *in vivo* remains to be established.

2.6 T-cell activation, viral replication and cytokines

The depletion of CD4 lymphocytes in the late stage of disease due to HIV might be expected to impair the production of the lymphokines in response to infection, bacterial or viral. In particular, a reduced or absent release of interleukin 2 (IL-2) would impair the activation and expression of CD4 and CD8 cells, with a corresponding failure in the production of interleukins, including gamma interferon (IFN-γ) and tumour necrosis factor beta (TNF-β). Initially, support for this prediction came from a study where stimulation of T lymphocytes of patients with AIDS *in vitro* did not generate an effective lymphokine response and in particular the production of IFN-γ was subnormal [51]. The antimicrobial activity of monocytes from the same patients was not impaired and, once stimulated by exogenous lymphokines, they showed effective intracellular antimicrobial activity.

More recent studies have shown that TNF in serum is raised in patients with AIDS and in most patients with AIDS-related complex (ARC) but is within the normal range for asymptomatic HIV-seropositive patients and most patients with persistent generalized lymphadenopathy (PGL) [52].

Monocytes grown on cell culture and then infected with HIV have been shown, on stimulation with lipopolysaccharide (LPS) or a combination of LPS and IFN-γ, to produce TNF-α and IL-1β acutely. This stimulation of infected cells increased virus production. Acutely HIV-infected cells produced more TNF-α and IL-1β than was found on stimulation of uninfected cells or chronically infected cells [53]. Peripheral-blood mononuclear cells (PBMCs), which include monocytes and lymphocytes, from patients with AIDS have been shown *in vitro* to have an increased capacity to lyse tumour cells and to release higher levels of TNF spontaneously than normal PBMCs [54]. The above experiments suggest that infection of monocytes with HIV leads to increased production of TNF and that monocytes from AIDS patients have been activated *in vivo*, as shown by their cytotoxicity and production of TNF. The relationship between cell activation and viral replication is well illustrated *in vitro* in cell culture. In order to isolate the HIV from infected cell culture, it is necessary to amplify viral replication by exposing the cells to activating factors, such as mitogen or phytohaemagglutinin. Activation of cells in culture in this way leads to enhanced spread of virus to uninfected cells.

The common denominator of T-cell activation and the induction of viral replication is the sharing of common mechanisms for the activation of mRNA in cell and virus. The best-known mechanism involves a specific component of the IL-2 and IL-2 receptor genes of the T cell referred to as kappa B (κB). These tandemly repeated κB elements are also part of the HIV LTR sequences (Fig. 2.5). Hence the common mechanism for activation and replication.

Activation of the T cell by antigen leads to the release of a DNA-binding protein, with binding sites in the viral enhancer, (NFκB) in the cytosol of the cell from its inhibitor (IκB) by phosphorylation of IκB by protein kinase C, permitting translocation of NFκB to the nucleus. The

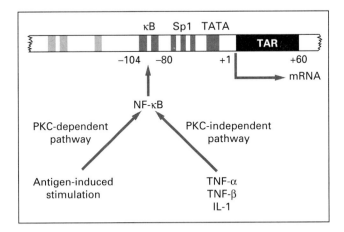

Fig. 2.5 Functional regulatory regions in the long terminal repeat of HIV-1 gene and pathways of transcriptional factor NFκB activation by immunological stimuli. The antigen-induced stimulation pathway is protein kinase C (PKC)-dependent. In contrast, stimulation by tumour necrosis factor (TNF)-α/β and interleukin (IL)-1 appears to be independent of the PKC pathway. κB, NFκB-binding site; Sp1, Sp1-binding site; TAR, tat-responsive element. Reproduced by permission of the authors and the journal *AIDS* [55].

same process may be initiated by TNF-α/β and IL-1 but by a protein-kinase-C-independent pathway (Fig. 2.5). Thus κB is a point of convergence for multiple cofactors which can enhance viral replication [55].

Several regulatory elements of cytokines share identical sequences with NFκB, as well as other promoter and enhancer regions of HIV. Examples of such cytokines are IL-2, TNF-α and IL-6. These cytokines are upregulated by herpesvirus infection of immune cells, which could form a positive-feedback loop between HIV-induced growth factor, cell proliferation and HIV replication [56]. The viral infections associated with HIV disease which could be part of this positive-feedback loop are EBV, cytomegalovirus (CMV), herpes simplex virus 1 and 2, varicella-zoster virus and human herpesvirus 6 [56]. Vyakarnam *et al.* [57] have shown that HIV-1 induces PBMC and CD4 T lymphocytes to secrete TNF-α and β and IFN-γ. These cytokines increase syncytium formation in PBMC and CD4 cells, TNF-α being the most potent. IFN-γ is the least potent, probably due to its antiviral activity [57]. The fact that this effect of HIV-1 on cytokine production occurs in freshly prepared PBMC and CD4 cells suggests that it may operate *in vivo* as well as *in vitro*. Two other cytokines may be important in supporting viral replication: granulocyte–macrophage colony-stimulating factor (GM-CSF) and IL-6. GM-CSF operates through the HIV LTR at a binding site other than NFκB for the induction of enhanced replication in infected macrophages, while IL-6 is presumed to act at a post-transcriptional level [55].

On the basis of the above findings *in vitro*, T-cell activation and cytokine production, which are the normal protective immune response to infection, result in enhancement of HIV replication in HIV-producing cells, activation of HIV expression in latently infected cells and spread of HIV infection to newly activated CD4 cells [58]. Infection of monocytes/macrophages by HIV leads to the production of IL-1, TNF-α and IL-6 and hence activation of HIV. IL-1 activates T cells to produce IL-2 and activated T cells increase the production of TNF-α and β, as well as adding IL-3, IL-4, GM-CSF and IL-6. The final result is acceleration of HIV replication in lymphocytes and macrophages. The persistent increase in TNF-α might be responsible for some of the clinical findings in AIDS, such as fever and weight loss. Indeed, it has been suggested that AIDS is a TNF disease [55]. The foregoing description centres on T-cell activation as the main initial event leading to viral replication and destruction of CD4 cells. However, this may be putting the cart before the horse. Thus viral replication may be the primary and dominant factor in disease progression, with T-cell activation being the secondary event. 'The question of whether activation drives disease progression or whether it is merely the result of virus replication' has yet to be answered [59].

2.7 Changes in T-helper-cell phenotypes and T-cell function with disease progression

2.7.1 Change in cytokine production with disease progression

Progression of HIV disease to the clinical condition of AIDS is associated with progressive loss and change in T-cell function, as tested *in vitro*. One of the first functions to go is loss of response to recall antigens, such as influenza A, tetanus toxoid and HIV peptides. Later the response to alloantigens (HLA) and phytohaemagglutinin is lost.

The phenotypes of Th cells have been classified into three groups, each with a different function and cytokine expression. Th1 refers to a subset which produce IL-2, IFN-γ and TNF-β when activated and is closely related to cell-mediated immunity. The Th2 subset is made up of a group of cells which produces predominantly IL-4 and IL-10 but also includes IL-6, IL-9 and IL-13. These cytokines enhance antibody production. The third subset (Th0) of Th cells produces a range of cytokines common to both Th1 and Th2 subsets [60].

Clerici and Shearer [61] have produced experimental results showing a loss of IL-2 and IFN-γ production with progression to AIDS, combined with increases in IL-4 and IL-10. These findings led to the hypothesis that HIV disease progression is associated with a change in T-cell subsets from Th1 to Th2, leading to an impairment of the cell-mediated immunity needed for the suppression of HIV replication and other infections which require this type of immunological response for protection [61]. Results from other laboratories have not found evidence of a change from a Th1 to a Th2 cytokine phenotype during the course of HIV infection. In one study, production of both IFN-γ and IL-10 from monocytes isolated from peripheral blood was increased in HIV-infected patients compared with controls, and this was also true of cells derived from lymph nodes. Production of IL-2 and IL-4 was very low in both patients and healthy control subjects. No change in this pattern of cytokine expression occurred with disease progression. The increased production of IFN-γ and IL-10 was mainly from CD8 cells, with very low levels of cytokine production from CD4 cells. This was in spite of evidence of activation *in vivo* of both CD4 and CD8 cells derived from lymph nodes, as shown by the marker of activation, HLA-DR. This discrepancy in the response of cytokine production between the two cells indicates an impairment of function of CD4 cells *in vivo*, in spite of the fact that these same cells will express cytokines normally when stimulated *in vitro* [62].

In another study of T cells in HIV disease, an enhanced number of T-cell clones producing cytokines typical of the Th0 subset was found in seropositive patients. These clones were derived from activated T cells from the skin and in T cells derived from the peripheral blood and stimulated with antigen. It was also found that infection of T cells with HIV *in vitro* led to replication of the virus preferentially in clones of the Th0 and Th2 subsets, with no evidence of replication in the Th1 subset [63].

2.7.2 Intracellular signal transduction by inositol polyphosphate and calcium regulation in lymphocytes

Another change in T-cell function in HIV disease is a disturbance of intracellular calcium (Ca) and inositol polyphosphate metabolism. The hydrolysis of phosphatidylinositol-4,5-biphosphate by phosphoinositidase C produces two second messengers within the cell, 1,2-diacylglycerol and inositol-1,4,5-triphosphate ($Ins(1,4,5)P_3$). These second messages activate protein kinase C and release Ca from intracellular stores. The sequence of events is shown in Fig. 2.6. It is the balance between $Ins(1,4,5)P_3$ and $Ins(1,3,4,5)P_4$ which regulates intracellular Ca levels and

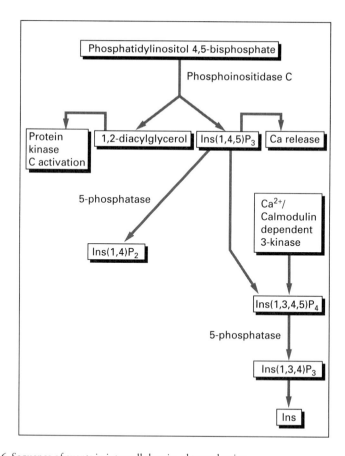

Fig. 2.6 Sequence of events in intracellular signal transduction.

hence cell activation. Activation of the normal lymphocyte leads to a rapid rise in intracellular $Ins(1,4,5)P_3$ and Ca, followed by a slower and later rise in $Ins(1,3,4,5)P_4$. In contrast, lymphocytes from patients with HIV disease have higher resting intracellular Ca concentrations, as well as detectable levels of $Ins(1,4,5)P_3$ and $Ins(1,3,4,5)P_4$, the latter two polyphosphates being undetectable in normal resting lymphocytes [64]. Thus the lymphocytes in HIV patients appear to be partially activated at rest. Further, these lymphocytes when activated produce only small rises in Ca and $Ins(1,4,5)P_3$. The defective inositol polyphosphate metabolism correlates well with the severity of the HIV disease and, after 12 weeks of treatment with zidovudine, the disturbance of metabolism approximates to that seen in HIV-infected asymptomatic subjects. Thus the authors of this research suggested that the assessment of inositol polyphosphate metabolism within the lymphocytes may make the assessment of the immunological status of the patient more precise and direct than surrogate markers.

The change in inositol polyphosphate metabolism is likely to be due to inhibition of 5-phosphatase (Fig. 2.6), which is reversible if HIV replication is reduced, as by zidovudine therapy. Only a minority of the cells studied were likely to have been infected by HIV and it is possible that the disorder of metabolism in uninfected cells could have been induced by the binding of gp120 to those cells [64].

2.8 HIV infection and the lung

2.8.1 Bronchoalveolar lavage

Bronchoalveolar lavage (BAL) has provided a unique opportunity to study the result and course of infection of the lung by HIV, together with the immunological response to that infection, which cannot be so readily achieved in other organs.

There are several reports in the literature on the cellular content of BAL in HIV disease but comparison is difficult when comparing cell numbers because of different methods used to obtain BAL. However, a universal finding has been a relative percentage increase in lymphocytes and decrease in macrophages compared with normal controls. Table 2.1 shows the results of lavage in normal controls compared with patients with a broad spectrum of manifestations of HIV disease, namely constitutional disease, neurological disorders and full-blown AIDS, the last group being 13 patients with *Pneumocystis carinii* pneumonia (PCP). BAL was carried out in a segment of the right lobe or lingula, using four aliquots of 25 ml of saline with aspiration after each aliquot [65].

The results shown in Table 2.1 show a significant increase in lympho-

Table 2.1 Cellular content of BAL in patients with HIV compared with normal control subjects. Mean (standard error (SEM)). Counts are expressed as cells × 10³/ml.

Group	n	Cell total	Lymphocytes %	Cells	Macrophages %	Cells	Neutrophils %	Cells	Eosinophils %	Cells
Patients with HIV	24	283.9 (42.0)	10.7 (1.6)	30.2* (7.1)	86.3 (3.9)	249.3 (35.2)	4.5* (3.9)	9.2* (4.1)	0.5 (0.1)	1.9 (0.7)
Control subjects	8	154.4 (33.2)	6.7 (0.5)	10.4 (3.5)	90.6 (6.2)	140.3 (28.3)	0.6 (0.2)	1.1 (1.1)	0.5 (0.3)	1.4 (0.5)

* Statistically significant difference from controls [65].

cyte and neutrophil count in the patients compared with controls and a non-significant drop in the percentage of macrophages but an increase in the absolute cell count. There were no differences in the cellular content of BAL depending on whether the patients were suffering from constitutional disease, neurological disease or full-blown AIDS, except for the rise in neutrophil count, which was confined to patients with full-blown AIDS. The relative increase in lymphocytosis in BAL contrasts with the lymphopenia usually observed in the peripheral blood. Analysis of T-cell subsets showed a significant decrease in the percentage of CD4 cells, but the absolute number of these cells was only decreased significantly in patients with full-blown AIDS. Pulmonary CD8 cells were significantly increased in percentage and absolute terms, with a marked decrease in the CD4/CD8 ratio [65].

2.8.2 Isolation of HIV-1 and HIV-1 proviral deoxyribonucleic acid from the lung and peripheral blood

HIV can be cultured from cells obtained at BAL in patients with AIDS, as well as in patients with lymphocytic interstitial pneumonitis [66–68]. In one study, all 10 BAL samples in nine patients were positive for HIV in culture [68], while in another study only two out of 23 samples was culture-positive [67]. Antibodies directed specifically at the HIV proteins p24 and gp41 have also been detected in BAL fluid [66,68]. In two patients with lymphocytic interstitial pneumonitis, the rate of IgG specific for HIV to total IgG was higher in BAL than in the peripheral blood, which suggests a humoral response occurring locally within the lung [66]. In these early studies, there was no specific clinical, radiological or histological pattern associated with patients in whom virus was cultured compared with those in whom virus was not detected.

Viral RNA has been detected in frozen sections from lungs in patients with AIDS and respiratory disorders by the *in situ* hybridization technique but at a low level and not consistently in all lungs tested. This technique may underestimate the number of infected cells because a proportion of such cells may not express viral RNA [69]. That this is likely to be the case is shown by the higher frequency with which HIV proviral DNA can be detected in cells from BAL by PCR.

In an investigation of 63 seropositive patients, HIV-1 proviral DNA was detected in leucocytes from the peripheral blood of all patients, while the simultaneous detection rate in BAL was 72%. Virus was cultured from the peripheral blood and BAL in 50% and 59% of the patients, respectively. Isolates of HIV were more readily achieved in patients suffering from PCP but were unaffected by concomitant infection of lung cells with CMV and were also unaffected by zidovudine therapy [70]. In another investigation, which looked specifically at lung monocytes/macrophages in BAL, HIV-1 proviral DNA was detected in 47% of patients tested [71]. In a study of HIV-infected persons with respiratory symptoms, HIV DNA was detected in 0.001–0.075% of peripheral-blood leucocytes and in 0.01–1% of BAL cells. Higher levels of HIV DNA were detected in monocyte/macrophage-enriched cell populations compared with leucocytes [72]. The ability to detect proviral DNA and to coculture HIV from cells derived from BAL increases with time in seropositive patients; it is also inversely correlated with the CD4 cell count and is more frequently detected in smokers [73].

On the basis of the phenotype of HIV-1 isolated from the lungs and peripheral blood of patients with AIDS, as well as on the genetic analysis of proviral DNA, it has been shown that there are differences in the strains of virus obtained simultaneously from these two sites [74,75]. The genetic analysis is based on the amino acid sequences of the V_3 domain of the envelope of the HIV. This analysis suggests that, as disease progresses, HIV-1 strains (within the same cell lineage) evolve differently and independently in lung and blood. Thus, after the initial lung infection from the blood, the virus evolves and replicates independently in an extracirculatory microenvironment. The strains isolated from BAL, unlike those from blood, had a degree of homogeneity of nucleotide sequences and a relatively conserved amino acid sequence compared with blood. This suggests that these strains were 'selected' during the evolution of the disease, perhaps because of their ability to infect and survive in AMs [74].

2.9 The alveolar macrophage

Macrophages and monocytes within the lung parenchyma and dendritic cells within the airway epithelium [76] are potential APCs, which, together with T lymphocytes, provide the lung with its defence against certain opportunistic and non-opportunistic infections. Impairment of this defence is largely due to malfunction and depletion of the CD4 cells, but infection of AMs with HIV-1 may also be relevant to the inability of the lung to counter viral, bacterial and parasitic attack.

2.9.1 Infection of alveolar macrophages with HIV-1

AMs are a major target for HIV-1 in lung tissue. Their infection is through the CD4-binding domain of gp120, as in T lymphocytes, but, in addition, HIV-1 tropism for mononuclear phagocytes can be determined by another region of gp120 upstream from the CD4-binding domain [77]. Primary cultures of AMs spontaneously produce virus, suggesting that these cells were infected *in vivo*. Pulmonary macrophages infected with HIV *in vitro* continue to produce virus and this is not dependent on host-cell proliferation. Virus isolates from lung- and brain-derived macrophages have a significantly higher ability to infect macrophages other than T cells *in vitro*. In contrast, some virus isolates infect T cells more readily than macrophages. Macrophages are more resistant to the cytocidal effects of HIV than T cells, and persistence of infection in these cells may act as a reservoir of virus [78,79]. This reservoir could be an agent for virus dissemination—the 'Trojan Horse' effect.

2.9.2 Transfer of HIV infection from macrophage to T cell

Although AMs appear to be resistant to the cytopathological effects of infection with HIV-1, they may still be responsible for infecting T cells, leading to depletion of the latter. There is evidence *in vitro* of enhanced accessory cell function (antigen-presenting capacity) in AMs infected with HIV-1 [80], which could stimulate lymphocyte proliferation, leading to increased susceptibility of T cells to infection with HIV. In addition, HIV-infected AMs secrete more cytokines (IL-1 and IL-6) than normal AMs, leading to a greater and more widespread stimulation of T cells. During antigen presentation, some T cells become adherent to AMs, which is dependent on β_2-integrins and the intercellular adhesion molecule I (ICAM-I). This cell-to-cell contact may facilitate the transmission of virus from AM to lymphocyte [81]. This proposed mechanism for T-cell depletion is derived from *in vitro* observations and it has yet to be established that it occurs *in vivo*. Antigen presentation is a necessary component of the process and this would presumably be dependent on viral replication within the AMs. Although in early studies viral RNA was detected in lung tissue, more recent work on AMs from BAL has been unable to identify viral RNA, p24 or gp120 antigens by immunocytochemistry. However, proviral DNA was detected in AMs by PCR, suggesting that the virus was latent. Viral replication could be induced in AMs derived from BAL *in vitro* by stimulation with GM-CSF or TNF-α. Thus it is possible that within the lung there is either inadequate stimulation of viral replication or there is some mechanism for its suppression in AMs [82]. The uncertainty that remains is whether inadequate stimulation or suppression of AMs is operative throughout all stages of HIV disease and in all patients with lung involvement.

2.9.3 The ability of alveolar macrophages to phagocytose and kill pathogens which infect the lung in patients who are HIV-infected

Information on this vital function of AMs is surprisingly scant and what there is is derived from *in vitro* experiments. AMs from subjects with AIDS and normal controls were tested for their ability to produce hydrogen peroxide (H_2O_2) and inhibit the replication of *Toxoplasma gondii* and *Chlamydia psittaci* (intracellular pathogens). Little of this activity in AMs was demonstrated unless they were stimulated with IFN-γ, when there was a two- to threefold increase in H_2O_2 production and ready inhibition of the two pathogens. There was no difference between the subjects with AIDS and the normal controls [83]. Similar results were found when AMs from HIV-infected subjects were tested for their ability to phagocytose and kill *Staphylococcus aureus*. In these experiments, the ability to kill the pathogen was greater in HIV-infected subjects than in controls, providing there was no infection of the lung when the cells were obtained. This antimicrobial activity of AMs was not dependent on *in vitro* stimulation with cytokines. In addition, there were changes seen on microscopy of the AMs which were consistent with their being activated *in vivo* by retroviral infection. This activation could be a direct effect of the virus on AMs or indirect via secretion of cytokines by T lymphocytes. Whatever the mechanism, AMs from HIV-infected subjects had an enhanced capacity to kill pathogens. This enhanced capacity was lost in AIDS patients with pneumonia, especially smokers, where the number, viability and phagocytic capacity of AMs were significantly decreased. Whether this effect was due to HIV or a secondary effect of the pneumonia could not be determined from these experimental results [84].

2.9.4 Are alveolar macrophages activated *in vivo* in HIV-infected subjects?

AMs obtained from BAL in HIV-infected patients and normal controls have been assessed for their ability to produce TNF *in vitro* during a standard cell lysis test [85]. In this reaction, the target cells for lysis by the AMs were a human cell line known to be sensitive to lysis by TNF. The spontaneous production of TNF by AMs were greater in patients than in

47

controls and the AMs responded normally to stimulation with IFN-γ *in vitro* with an increase in TNF production. AMs obtained from patients with opportunistic lung infections produced more TNF than those cells derived from patients without such infection. AMs from patients could be divided into those cells in which there was evidence of viral replication, because they expressed the core protein p24 of the HIV, and those AMs in which there was no expression of p24. Those AMs expressing p24 produced more TNF than those that did not, but they were unable to respond to further stimulation by IFN-γ. Those AMs without evidence of viral replication responded vigorously to exogenous IFN-γ. Thus, in two conditions, opportunistic infection of the lung and infection of AMs themselves by HIV, there is evidence of activation of AMs, as shown by the increased TNF production. This enhanced production was similar quantitatively to that produced from AMs from seronegative controls when these cells were stimulated by IFN-γ. This state of activation of AMs from patients was present without activation *in vitro* and therefore may represent their condition *in vivo* [85]. The increase in TNF production may not be beneficial in that it could lead to activation of viral replication in AMs latently infected with the virus, thereby leading to propagation of the virus within the lung. In addition, as AMs that are activated by retroviral infection are refractory to further stimulation, this population of cells will be unable to respond to opportunistic and other infections.

Are AMs activated *in vivo* in HIV-infected patients? Plainly the experimental data presented here are conflicting. Studies on TNF secretion by AMs and assessment of their ability to phagocytose and kill pathogens support the view that the cells are indeed activated by retroviral infection and/or opportunistic infection [83,84]. However, it has not always been possible to identify viral RNA or viral proteins in AMs from BAL, although it does appear that there is a population of AMs which are infected with HIV-1 but that this infection is latent [82]. The conflict of data on whether AMs are activated *in vivo* might be due to studies on BAL being carried out at different stages of disease progression — activation being a late development. While this may be the case, the investigation of TNF secretion by AMs from seropositive subjects does not suggest this explanation because the extent of TNF release was not related to the clinical course or CD4 count of the patients [85].

2.10 Lymphocytic alveolitis

2.10.1 CD8 T lymphocytes

Evidence for lymphocytic alveolitis usually depends on the finding of a lymphocytosis in BAL which is predominantly comprised of CD8 T lymphocytes [86–88]. This lymphocytosis has been observed in 78% (154 patients) of patients with lung infection or tumour. In a group of 122 HIV-infected patients without infection or tumour in the lung, a lymphocytosis was found in 72% of patients, and in 27 patients (59%) there were no respiratory symptoms or abnormalities of the chest radiograph [86]. In a small number of patients, the alveolitis was confirmed at open lung biopsy and the phenotype of the cells seen was the same as in BAL [86]. The phenotypes of the alveolar lymphocytes were CD3, CD8 and D44, which were partially activated *in vivo* because the cells expressed the HLA-DR antigen. There was a large discrepancy between BAL cells and those obtained from peripheral blood, suggesting a local pulmonary recruitment. The lymphocytes were considered to be functional CTLs since they lysed autologous AMs in an *in vitro* assay. The cytotoxicity was specific for HIV and was HLA class-I-restricted [89].

The phenotype and function of the CD8 cells has been found to vary during the progression of HIV infection. The CTLs (CD8, CD44), which are predominant in BAL during the early stages of HIV infection, decline in number as the patient progresses to AIDS and this is associated with an expansion of CD8 cells bearing the CD57 marker. This change in phenotype is associated with a fall in HIV-specific cytotoxic T-cell activity. The CD8, CD57 alveolar cells inhibit both HIV-specific CTLs and the non-specific killer-cell activity of NK cells and lymphokine-activated killer (LAK) cells. This inhibition is due to the release by CD8, CD57 CTLs of a soluble inhibitor (glycoprotein), which can be recovered in the cell-free supernatant of BAL. The inhibitor is not one of the well-known cytokines or prostaglandins and is not dependent for its action on cell-to-cell contact [90]. An inhibition of the killer-cell activity of lymphocytes might favour the spread of HIV infection of cells within the lung, as well as impairing the immune response to opportunistic and non-opportunistic infection.

2.10.2 Cytotoxic activity of lymphocytes which are not MHC-restricted

Cytotoxic lymphocytes which are not MHC-restricted and which can lyse certain tumour and virus-infected cells can be divided into three groups. The largest number of these cells are NK cells and are granular lymphocytes which are CD3-negative. The second group are a minority of T lymphocytes which are CD3-positive and express the NK markers CD56 and CD57. They can kill some cells without previous sensitization. Finally, there are LAK cells, which exhibit cytotoxic properties, are not MHC-restricted and have the ability to lyse a wider range of targets than NK cells. It is probable the LAK cells are derived from the first two groups of lymphocytes upon activation by IL-2.

The cytotoxicity of cells derived from BAL which are not MHC-restricted is normal or enhanced in the early stages of HIV infection, whereas in patients with AIDS it is profoundly depressed. Surprisingly, T-lymphocytes which were CD3-positive and expressed the CD56 or CD57 markers of NK activity were increased in patients with AIDS and could bind to their targets, but they were unable to release the cytotoxic factor that spontaneously kills. Cells which were CD3-negative but CD56-positive were detected in patients with AIDS but were small in number. Stimulation of the lymphocyte population from patients with AIDS by recombinant IL-2 enhanced the lytic capacity of these cells and also produced cells with LAK characteristics [91]. This raises the possibility that in the late stages of HIV disease there is a reduction or loss of IL-2 production, because of depletion of CD4 cells, and this in turn leads to a loss of the non-MHC-restricted killing capacity of pulmonary cells.

2.11 Cytokine activity in the lung in HIV infection

The release of cytokines in response to infection is a normal and protective mechanism, provided the pattern of release, the magnitude, the timing and the cessation are appropriate to the invading pathogen. There is experimental evidence that cytokines are released in the lung in response to HIV infection and other pathogens. The uncertainty is whether this cytokine response *in vivo* is beneficial, unimportant or pathogenic [92]. From the known biological effects of cytokines, it can be anticipated that an inappropriate and prolonged release of cytokines could be detrimental and lead to prolonged fever, fatigue, weight loss, lymphadenopathy, B-cell activation, hypergammaglobulinaemia, lymphocytic alveolitis, alveolar damage and enhanced viral replication. The particular adverse effect produced will depend on which cytokine(s) are released.

2.11.1 Interleukins 1, 2 and 4

These proinflammatory cytokines are central to T- and B-cell proliferation. IL-1 and IL-2 could be responsible for the expansion and activation of T cells from pre-existing cells within the lung and hence support and maintain an alveolitis. Circumstantial support for this concept comes from the demonstration of a functional IL-2 receptor on CD8 cells obtained at BAL from HIV-infected patients [93], which is a receptor not expressed by resting T cells. IL-2 stimulation of lymphocytes led to T-cell proliferation in a dose-dependent manner. It is possible that in the early stages of HIV infection IL-2 is in part responsible for maintaining the alveolitis, until later when, with disease progression and loss of CD4 cells,

IL-2 production declines. Examination of lymphocytes from BAL in HIV-
infected patients showed no expression of IL-4 receptors and the addition
of IL-4 to these cells had no effect on proliferation [93].

CHAPTER 2
*Pathogenesis of
infection with HIV*

2.11.2 Interleukin 6

Another cytokine of potential importance in HIV disease is IL-6, which
has a role in B-cell maturation and the development of fibrosis. The latter
may be important because some patients, following full clinical recovery
from PCP, have persistent radiological and physiological abnormalities.
In normal subjects there is no production *in vitro* from AMs of IL-6, stimulated or unstimulated. AMs freshly derived from BAL in HIV-positive
patients with pulmonary infection express IL-6 mRNA and produce high
amounts of IL-6 when cultured alone without stimulation. The production of IL-6 was further increased when the AMs were cultured with LPS,
a product derived from pathogens such as *P. carinii*. IL-6 can also be
recovered from cell-free BAL fluid [94]. This increased production of IL-6
has the potential for enhancing viral replication, which may be amplified
by other cytokines, particularly TNF-α. It is likely that the increased production of IL-6 can arise from HIV infection alone without opportunistic
infection. HIV infection of monocyte-derived macrophages from peripheral blood leads to the sustained release of IL-1α and IL-6 *in vitro* from
these cells without further stimulation [95]. Prolonged release of these
cytokines *in vivo* might impair the normal immune response to infection
and lead to some of the undesirable effects of inappropriate cytokine
secretion outlined at the beginning of this section. The increase in IL-6
production may be induced by the product of the HIV-1 *tat* gene, which is
required for HIV-1 production. Monocytes–macrophages transfected
with the HIV-1 *tat* gene led to increased levels of IL-6 secretion and
enhanced accessory cell function (antigen presentation, leading to T-cell
proliferation) compared with monocytes without transfection [96].

2.11.3 Interferon and tumour necrosis factor

The activity of these two lymphokines was reviewed in sections 2.6 and
2.7.1, with special reference to activation of AMs by infection with HIV-
1. This section reviews their activity in more general terms, albeit with
some repetition.

IFN and TNF can induce lysis of tumour cells and virus-infected cells
and therefore are potentially beneficial in HIV-infected patients, especially
IFN-γ. AMs from patients with AIDS respond to IFN-γ *in vitro* with
enhanced oxidative and antimicrobial activity which is indistinguishable
from the response of activated cells from healthy volunteers or from

patients without a diagnosis of AIDS [83,97]. The administration of aerosolized human recombinant IFN-γ or TNF-α to rats *in vivo* increased IL-1 production by AMs as well as blood monocyte-mediated tumour lysis. The combination of the two cytokines led to the activation of AMs as well as mild inflammatory changes seen on histology. The plasma TNF-α levels were several thousand-fold less than when given intravenously, although the lung levels of the cytokine were comparable in the two routes of administration [98]. These experiments suggest that cytokine(s) could be given by aerosol to the lung without the disadvantage of unwanted systemic side-effects.

It has been shown that AMs from HIV-infected patients with no current bacterial or opportunistic infection spontaneously produce more TNF in culture than controls. IFN-γ was able to induce a significant increase in TNF in these patients. The mean spontaneous release of TNF was the same in AMs and peripheral-blood monocytes, suggesting that there was no compartmentalization of monocyte/macrophages within the lung. The spontaneous release of TNF was not related to disease severity, as judged by clinical markers, such as the CD4 count, but was in part related to the presence of an alveolitis. During lung opportunistic infection, there was a marked increase in spontaneous production of TNF by AMs but not blood monocytes, suggesting compartmentalization of macrophages within the lung. Following opportunistic infection, AMs were then refractory to further stimulation by IFN-γ [85,99].

HIV infection of AMs affects their production of TNF in that infection leads to a higher production of TNF than in uninfected cells, the latter being little different from those obtained from control subjects. More importantly, infected cells were unable to produce more TNF on stimulation by IFN-γ, whereas a normal response was obtained from uninfected cells [85]. From these experiments, it would appear that, in the absence of opportunistic infection, AMs in culture produce more TNF, this being derived from cells infected with HIV. IFN-γ stimulation *in vitro* or opportunistic infection *in vivo* produces an increase in TNF production of AMs in cell culture, presumably through its effect on cells not infected with HIV, the infected cells being already maximally stimulated.

It is likely that the increased production of IFN-γ and TNF in HIV-1-seropositive patients is protective initially against opportunistic and non-opportunistic infection of the lung, as well as viral dissemination. That this protective mechanism eventually fails is evident from the clinical course of patients with HIV infection. Excessive and prolonged production of TNF may be pathogenic, leading to changed endothelial and polymorphonuclear function, granuloma formation and the induction of fibrosis and unwanted inflammation.

2.11.4 Granulocyte–macrophage colony-stimulating factor

GM-CSF is released by activated macrophages and T cells and modulates production of human monocyte–macrophage cells and enhances antigen presentation. GM-CSF will induce growth and differentiation of monocyte–macrophage cells as well as regulating neutrophil accumulation and activation in infected tissues, such as the lung. This action of GM-CSF could account for macrophage and neutrophil accumulation within the lung of HIV-infected patients.

GM-CSF is present in the cell-free supernatant of BAL of HIV-1-infected patients, suggesting it is released *in vivo*. A significant positive correlation has been found between the concentration of GM-CSF and the number of AMs and neutrophils in BAL. The supernatant of cultures of AMs from patients also contained GM-CSF, which was significantly increased when cells were stimulated by LPS and this increase was 10-fold greater in patients than in healthy subjects. AMs from patients have been shown to express the receptor for GM-CSF and also to release its mRNA on stimulation by LPS. No detectable levels of mRNA were found in stimulated cells in cell culture *in vitro* and the reason for this absence is unknown. However, it raises the possibility that HIV infection of AMs itself leads to an increase in GM-CSF production [100].

Are the accumulation and activation of AMs and neutrophils within the lung beneficial or pathogenic? There is no clear answer to this question. Activated AMs will secrete TNF-α and IL-6 in the normal immune response of the lung but their release may be inappropriate in the absence of bacterial or opportunistic infection. In addition, activation of AMs may enhance viral replication. Whether appropriate or inappropriate, the accumulation of AMs does not ultimately protect the lung from infection and often respiratory failure. The accumulation of neutrophils in the lung will help in the clearance of pathogens, which is plainly beneficial. However, these cells may release enzymes and oxygen intermediates which cause unwanted local damage.

2.11.5 Interleukin 8 and macrophage inflammatory protein 1α

IL-8 is a cytokine with chemotactic and activation properties for neutrophils. The role of this cytokine could be important in patients with PCP, for a neutrophilia in BAL is a poor prognostic sign in this pneumonia. In fact, a positive correlation has been found between IL-8 levels and the percentage of neutrophils in BAL of patients with PCP [101] and therefore this cytokine could in part be responsible for the inflammatory response. It has been suggested that the beneficial effect of steroids in PCP could be in the reduction of this inflammatory process. If this is correct, there may be a case for finding means of reducing IL-8 in some patients with PCP where there is an indication for the use of steroids.

Another more recently identified pro-inflammatory cytokine is MIP-1α. MIP-1α is a chemoattractant for CD8 cells and activates neutrophils and monocytes. AMs from HIV-infected subjects, with increased CD8 cells in BAL, have been shown to express MIP-1α spontaneously and in response to LPS, which was not the finding in normal subjects. The supernatant of BAL was chemoattractant for CD8 cells and this was inhibited by neutralizing MIP-1α [102].

2.11.6 Interleukin 10 and transforming growth factor β

Unlike most of the preceding cytokines, an increased expression of IL-10 and transforming growth factor β (TGF-β) would be likely to reduce viral replication and damp down any inflammatory response to infection. The role of IL-10 and TGF-β in HIV infection has been assessed so far in monocyte-derived macrophages, so their precise role in the lung remains to be determined.

IL-10 inhibits viral replication in monocyte-derived macrophages *in vitro*, which was correlated with an inhibition of endogenous secretion of TNF-α and IL-6 [103]. Elevated levels of IL-10 have been reported in HIV disease and the importance of this observation is that IL-10 not only affects cytokine production but also has inhibitory and stimulatory effects on cells of the immune system; in particular, it is a chemotactic factor for CD8 CTLs (see [103] for discussion).

TGF-β is a chemotactic factor for monocytes. It suppresses virus expression in chronically infected monocyte–macrophage cell lines as well as in monocyte-derived macrophages acutely infected with HIV. The growth factor also suppresses the ability of IL-6 and GM-CSF to upregulate synthesis of viral proteins. No such effect has been observed in chronically infected T-cell lines [94]. At first sight, these effects could be viewed as beneficial to the host. However, TGF-β suppresses T- and B-lymphocyte proliferation, NK-cell activity, macrophage activation and the production of specific cytotoxic T cells (see [104] for discussion).

2.12 Alveolitis and lung epithelial permeability

There is indirect evidence that the alveolitis seen in HIV-infected patients may lead to lung damage. This rests on studies measuring the clearance of inhaled technetium-99m-labelled diethylenetriamine penta-acetate (DTPA) in patients with evidence of an alveolitis determined on the basis of the cellular content of BAL (i.e. more than 15% lymphocytes and a minimum of 25 lymphocytes/mm³). Of 22 patients studied, 13 had an abnormally raised DTPA clearance with a high number of lymphocytes, mainly expressing the marker CD8 and which spontaneously lysed autologous AMs in a chromium release assay. In the 11 patients with a normal DTPA clearance, there were few or no CD8, D44 lymphocytes and the lymphocytes exhibited no significant cytolytic activity [105]. It is claimed that an increased DTPA clearance is associated with increased lung epithelial permeability and there is some indirect support for this concept in this study, in that other lung-function tests were significantly more abnormal in those with an increased clearance. Thus the patients with an increased clearance had, on average, a lower arterial partial pressure of oxygen (Pa,o_2), a higher alveolar to arterial Po_2 difference, a lower carbon monoxide transfer factor and a reduced lung diffusion coefficient for carbon monoxide (Kco) [105].

2.13 Lung-function abnormalities in patients infected with HIV

In view of the many infections and immunological changes within the lung of patients infected with the HIV, changes in lung function would be likely and this is indeed the case. The test of function most likely to be abnormal is the carbon monoxide transfer factor (carbon monoxide diffusing capacity, $D_L$co). In a study of 474 patients, at varying stages of their illness, it was found that even in the asymptomatic group (126 persons) the $D_L$co and Kco (diffusion coefficient) were slightly reduced, being 88% and 92% of predicted normal, respectively [106]. The remaining patients were classified clinically into groups and their lung function results compared with the *asymptomatic* HIV-seropositive group. The results are tabulated in Table 2.2.

Tests of airway function, in contrast to the $D_L$co and vital capacity, were normal or near normal in most groups of patients, the exception being those patients with PCP, where the peak expiratory flow rate (PEFR) and forced expiratory volume in 1 second (FEV_1) were reduced [106]. The preservation of airway function, with a decline in the uptake of carbon monoxide, is compatible with the assumption that involvement of the lung in HIV-seropositive patients is mainly at the alveolar level. This would also be consistent with the immunological changes within the lung described in the preceding sections.

Serial measurement of lung function over 18 months revealed no change in $D_L$co in HIV-seropositive patients, provided they remained clinically stable within the same group (i.e. asymptomatic, PGL, ARC, etc.). Clinical deterioration, such as an attack of PCP, was the determining factor in the decline in lung function. The fall in $D_L$co following PCP was in part reversible, which occurred over the 3 months following the

Table 2.2 Reductions in D_LCO and forced vital capacity (FVC) observed in HIV-seropositive patients grouped according to clinical status [106]. The mean D_LCO results are expressed as a percentage of the mean D_LCO obtained in HIV-seropositive patients who were asymptomatic. In all groups the KCO was reduced in line with the D_LCO. The reductions in D_LCO, KCO and FVC were statistically significant when compared with the asymptomatic group.

Clinical grouping of patients	D_LCO (%)	FVC
PGL	82	Normal
ARC	73	Reduced
AIDS	73	Reduced
AIDS (no pulmonary complications)	73	Reduced
Kaposi's sarcoma (no pulmonary complications)	72	Reduced
Pulmonary Kaposi's sarcoma	63	Reduced
Acute PCP	49	Reduced
Pyogenic infection	70	Normal

PGL, persistent generalized lymphadenopathy; ARC, AIDS-related complex; PCP, *Pneumocystis carinii* pneumonia.

pneumonia. Cigarette smoking was associated with greater reductions in D_LCO than in non-smokers, as well as impaired recovery of the D_LCO following PCP. No beneficial effect of zidovudine therapy was found on tests of lung function [106].

The conclusion from the serial study of lung function is that there is no gradual decline in lung function providing the patient is clinically stable [106]. Progression of HIV disease is associated with a deterioration in lung function. Pulmonary infection is one of the events leading to progression, which suggests that prophylaxis against infection in the lung may avoid or delay the deterioration in pulmonary function.

The foregoing description of the serial changes in lung function found no significant fall in expiratory rates of airflow except in patients with PCP. In contrast, in another study of 105 patients with AIDS, evidence of abnormal airway function was found in 44 (42%), the abnormality being either a reduced expiratory rate of airflow or a significant response to inhaled bronchodilator or both [107]. Eleven of the patients had a significant response to a bronchodilator with normal baseline flow rates. These changes could not be ascribed to smoking and occurred in the absence of PCP and Kaposi's sarcoma (KS). There was a significant association between cough, wheeze and chest tightness and abnormal tests of airway function [107].

The use of lung-function tests in patients who are HIV antibody-positive requires modification of apparatus to prevent cross-infection between patients, especially in relation to microbial disease. The modifications are simple and inexpensive and include one-way valves for spirometry and a filter distal to the mouthpiece in D_LCO measurement.

2.14 Summary and speculation

Following infection with HIV-1, there is a viraemia, followed after a few weeks by seroconversion. Subjects are often unable to identify an illness associated with infection and seroconversion and, if there are symptoms, they are likely to be shrugged off as a 'cold' or 'influenza'. The classic seroconversion illness is described as being like infectious mononucleosis, with malaise, fever, sore throat (with or without oral ulceration) and lymphadenopathy. In addition, there may be arthralgia, a maculopapular rash and lymphocytic meningitis. Occasionally, there is profound immunosuppression, with a fall in CD4 T lymphocytes, which renders the subject liable to opportunistic infections, such as candidiasis and PCP.

The first, and probably the most effective, immunological response in defence of the subject is the appearance of CTLs, which are HIV-1- and HLA class-I-specific. There is evidence for other immunological responses to infection, including neutralizing antibodies, ADCC, activation of the complement system and involvement of NK cells.

The next stage in the response to HIV infection is the asymptomatic phase, where the patient remains well, and this may usually last about 10 years, although the duration is highly variable. Studies in the blood initially supported a view that the virus was quiescent during this stage, remaining predominantly in its proviral form, with little replication. Virions were difficult to culture from the blood and the number of lymphocytes infected would probably present no difficulty in control by the immune system. In fact, this postulated quiescence of viral activity has turned out not to be the case, as studies of virus and cell dynamics have shown continuous rounds of *de novo* virus infection, replication and rapid cell turnover. Thirty per cent of the virus population is replaced daily and the entire population of peripheral CD4 lymphocytes is replaced every 15 days. The loss of cells is due not only to direct killing by the virus but also to elimination by an efficient and effective immune system. Examination of the lymph glands during the asymptomatic period reveals virus, virus particles and immune complexes in the villous processes of the FDCs, providing a ready source of virus for the uninfected lymphocytes tracking through the lymphatic system. There are 5–10 times more infected cells in lymphoid tissue than in the blood.

Most of the virus isolated from the plasma comes from an actively replicating short-lived population of cells, namely the CD4 lymphocytes. However, the monocyte–macrophage group of cells are outside this rapid turnover of cells and yet they are infected with virus without any apparent effect on their viability. Such cells provide a large reservoir of virus, maintaining survival of the virus in the face of an active and vigorous immune system.

Is the depletion of the CD4 T lymphocytes and the progression to AIDS due to viral replication just exceeding T-lymphocyte production, leading slowly but relentlessly to destruction of the immune system? This seems likely to be the case, but other causes for CD4 cell depletion include: emergence of more pathogenic strains of virus, increased apoptosis, superantigen formation, autoimmunity and immune suppression and cell cytolysis of CD4 cells (infected or uninfected) coated with gp120.

The mode of entry of the virus into the lung is not known but it could be from infected cells migrating from the blood. Infected monocytes could enter the lung and there mature into macrophages or the transfer could occur through HIV-infected CD4 lymphocytes accumulating in the lung in response to opportunistic or non-opportunistic infection.

AMs, even if infected with HIV, have been found on testing *in vitro* to be able to phagocytose and kill pathogens. Their lifespan and viability do not appear to be compromised by HIV-1. However, although infected AMs have been shown to spontaneously produce more TNF than seronegative controls, these cells are refractory to further stimulation with IFN-γ and therefore *in vivo* may be unable to provide a defence against additional pulmonary infections. Such defence would therefore rely on AMs uninfected by HIV. Are AMs activated *in vivo* by infection with HIV and/or opportunistic infection and if so is this important? The evidence here is conflicting, with some studies supporting activation and others in favour of the virus being latent in its proviral form. It is possible that both observations are correct and the state of activation of AMs is determined by the stage of disease progression and the frequency and nature of any other infection of the lung. AMs which are activated by HIV may, during antigen presentation, become adherent to T cells and this cell-to-cell contact may facilitate transmission of the virus and hence viral spread within the lung. Activation of AMs also leads to the release of several cytokines, of which TNF-α and β are the best known. This leads to increased viral replication by their induction of the DNA-binding protein NFκB, with binding sites on the viral enhancer in the LTR of HIV. Other cytokines and factors that accelerate viral replication are IL-1, IL-6, GM-CSF and infection with the herpesviruses and CMV. Activated T cells also produce TNF-α, TNF-β, IL-6 and GM-CSF, which will further accelerate replication of virus in T lymphocytes and macrophages (Fig. 2.7) [108]. Thus any protective effect of activation of AMs, whether by HIV or by other pathogens, in combating infection may be lost by the subsequent dissemination of virus and the enhancement of its replication.

The lymphatic alveolitis seen in patients with HIV infection is predominantly composed of CD8 T lymphocytes which are specific for HIV and are HLA class-I-restricted. They express the CD3, CD8 and CD44 markers. The alveolitis may well be maintained by increased pro-inflammatory cytokine expression, in particular IL-2. However, IL-2, TNF-α and IL-6 affect genes that regulate cell proliferation and differentiation through activation of such factors as NFκB, so it is likely that more than one cytokine is responsible.

Thus the lung is the site of a vigorous inflammatory reaction, which in some subjects is asymptomatic while in others it leads to impairment of lung function. The cells involved and the cytokines released are illustrated pictorially in Fig. 2.7 [108]. Progression of disease leads to a change in phenotype of T lymphocytes, which are CD8, CD57 and inhibit CTLs and NK cells. Viral replication leads to depletion of CD4 cells and the collapse of the immune system within the lung, heralding the onset of opportunistic infections.

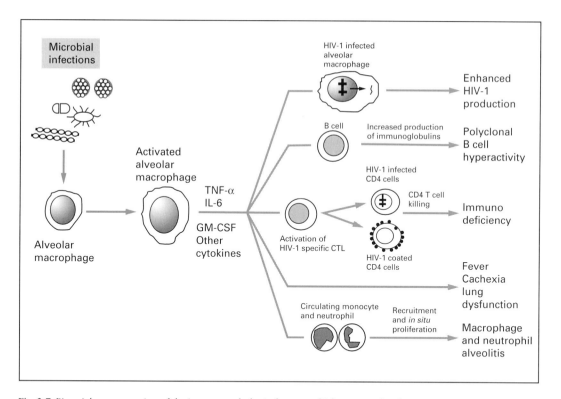

Fig. 2.7 Pictorial representation of the immunopathological events which are postulated to occur in the lung parenchyma during HIV-1 infection. IL-6, interleukin 6; GM-CSF, granulocyte–macrophage colony-stimulating factor; TNF-α, tumour necrosis factor α. Reproduced by permission of the authors and the *American Review of Respiratory Disease* [108].

References

1 Semenzato G. (ed.). *AIDS and the Lung*. Sheffield, UK: European Respiratory Society Journals, 1995.

2 Brodine S.K., Mascola J.R., Weiss P.J. *et al*. Detection of diverse HIV-I genetic subtypes in the USA. *Lancet* 1995; **346**: 1198–1199.

3 Artenstein A.W., Coppola J., Brown A.E. *et al*. Multiple introductions of HIV-1 subtype E into the Western hemisphere. *Lancet* 1995; **346**: 1197–1198.

4 Mascola J.R., Louwagie J., McCutchan F.E. *et al*. Two antigenically distinct subtypes of human immunodeficiency virus type 1: viral genotype predicts neutralisation serotype. *Journal of Infectious Diseases* 1994; **169**: 48–54.

5 Trkola A., Pomalis A.B., Yuan H. *et al*. Cross-clade neutralisation of primary isolates of human immunodeficiency virus type I by human monoclonal antibodies and tetrameric CD4-IgG. *Journal of Virology* 1995; **69**: 6609–6617.

6 Phillips D.M., Bourinbaiar A.S. Mechanism of HIV spread from lymphocytes to epithelia. *Virology* 1992; **186**: 261–273.

7 Klatzmann D., Barré-Sinoussi F., Nugeyre M.T. *et al*. Selective tropism of lymphadenopathy associated virus (LAV) for helper-inducer T lymphocytes. *Science* 1984; **225**: 59–63.

8 Dalgleish A.G., Beverley P.C.L., Clapham P.R., Crawford D.H., Greaves M.F., Weiss R.A. The CD4 (T4) antigen is an essential component of the receptor for the AIDS retrovirus. *Nature* 1984; **312**: 763–767.

9 Klatzmann D., Champagne E., Chamaret S. *et al*. T-lymphocytes T4 molecule behaves as the receptor for human retrovirus LAV. *Nature* 1984; **312**: 767–768.

10 McDougal J.S., Mawle A., Cort S.P. *et al*. Cellular tropism of the human retrovirus HTLV-III/LAV. I. Role of T cell activation and expression of the T4 antigen. *Journal of Immunology* 1985; **135**: 3151–3162.

11 Lifson J.D., Reyes G.R., McGrath M.S., Stein B.S., Engleman E.G. AIDS retrovirus induced cytopathology: giant cell formation and involvement of CD4 antigen. *Science* 1986; **232**: 1123–1127.

12 McDougal J.S., Kennedy M.S., Sligh J.M., Cort S.P., Macole A., Nicholson J.K.A. Binding of HTLV-III/LAV to T4+ T cells by a complex of the 110K viral protein and the T4 molecule. *Science* 1986; **231**: 382–385.

13 Habeshaw J.A., Dalgleish A.G., Bountiff L. *et al*. AIDS pathogenesis: HIV envelope and its interaction with cell proteins. *Immunology Today* 1990; **11**: 418–424.

14 Eiden L.E., Lifson J.D. View points on HIV T-cell interactions. *Immunology Today* 1992; **13**: 201–206.

15 Ho D.D., Pomerantz R.J., Kaplan J.C. Pathogenesis of infection with human immunodeficiency virus. *New England Journal of Medicine* 1987; **317**: 278–286.

16 Weiss R.A., Clapham P.R., Weber J.N., Dalgleish A.G., Lasky L.A., Berman P.W. Variable and conserved neutralization antigens of human immunodeficiency virus. *Nature* 1986; **324**: 572–575.

17 Senaldi G., Peakman M., McManus T., Davies E.T., Tee D.E.H., Vergani D. Activation of the complement system in human immunodeficiency virus infection: relevance of the classical pathway to pathogenesis and disease severity. *Journal of Infectious Diseases* 1990; **162**: 1227–1232.

18 Nixon D.F., Townsend A.R.M., Elvin J.G., Rizzi C.R., Gallway J., McMichael A.J. HIV-1 gag-specific cytotoxic T-lymphocytes defined with recombinant vaccinia virus and synthetic peptides. *Nature* 1988; **336**: 484–487.

19 Walker B.D., Plato F. Cytotoxic T lymphocytes against HIV. *AIDS* 1990; **4**: 177–184.

20 Borrow P., Lewicki H., Hahn B.H., Shaw G.M., Oldstone M.R.A. Virus-specific CD8+ cytolytic T-lymphocyte activity associated with control of viraemia in primary human immunodeficiency virus type 1 infection. *Journal of Virology* 1994; **68**: 6103–6110.

21 Koup R.A., Safrit J.T., Cao Y. *et al.* Temporal association of cellular immune responses with the initial control of viraemia in primary human immunodeficiency virus type 1 syndrome. *Journal of Virology* 1994; **68**: 4650–4655.

22 Weinhold K.J., Lyerly H.K., Matthews T.J., Tyler D.S., Nastala C.L., Bolognesi D.P. Specific cell-mediated cytotoxicity against HIV-1 envelope glycoprotein coated CD4 cells. In: L'Etang H. (ed.) *Autoimmune Aspects of HIV Infection.* London, New York: Royal Society of Medicine Services, 1988: 143–151.

23 Mackewcz C.E., Levy J.A. CD8 cell anti-HIV activity: nonlytic suppression of virus replication. *AIDS Research and Human Retroviruses* 1992; **8**: 1039–1050.

24 Mackewcz C.E., Yang L.C., Levy J.A. Non-cytolytic CD8 T-cell anti-HIV responses in primary HIV-1 infection. *Lancet* 1994; **344**: 1671–1673.

25 Weiss R.A., Clapham P.R. Hot fusion of HIV. *Nature* 1996; **381**: 647–648.

26 Pantaleo G., Butini L., Graziosi C. *et al.* Human immunodeficiency virus (HIV) infection in CD4 T lymphocytes genetically deficient in LFA-1: LFA-1 is required for HIV-mediated cell fusion but not for viral transmission. *Journal of Experimental Medicine* 1991; **173**: 511–514.

27 Schnittman S.M., Psallidopoulos M.C., Lane H.C. *et al.* The reservoir for HIV-1 in human peripheral blood is a T cell that maintains expression of CD4. *Science* 1989; **245**: 305–308.

28 Ho D.D., Moudgil T., Alum M. Quantitation of human immunodeficiency virus type 1 in the blood of infected persons. *New England Journal of Medicine* 1989; **321**: 1621–1625.

29 Embretson J., Zupancic M., Ribas J.L. *et al.* Massive covert infection of helper T lymphocytes and macrophages by HIV during the incubation period of AIDS. *Nature* 1993; **362**: 359–362.

30 Pantaleo G., Graziosi C., Demarest J.F. *et al.* HIV infection is active and progressive in lymphoid tissue during the clinically latent stage of disease. *Nature* 1993; **362**: 355–358.

31 Spiegel H., Herbst H., Niedobitek G., Foss H.-D., Stein H. Follicular dendritic cells are a major reservoir for human immunodeficiency virus type 1 in lymphoid tissues facilitating infection of CD4 T-helper cells. *American Journal of Pathology* 1992; **140**: 15–22.

32 Bouyhadi M.L., Rabin L., Sabimi S. *et al.* HIV induces thymus depletion *in vivo*. *Nature* 1993; **363**: 728–732.

33 Aldrovandi G.M., Feuer G., Gao L. *et al.* The SCID-hu mouse as a model for HIV infection. *Nature* 1993; **363**: 733–736.

34 Wei X., Ghosh S.K., Taylor M.E. *et al.* Viral dynamics in human immunodeficiency virus type 1 infection. *Nature* 1995; **373**: 117–122.

35 Ho D.D., Neumann A.U., Perelson A.S., Chen W., Leonard J.M., Markowitz M. Rapid turnover of plasma virions and CD4 lymphocytes in HIV-1 infection. *Nature* 1995; **373**: 123–126.

36 Fenyo E.M., Morfeldt-Manson L., Chiodi F. *et al.* Distinct replicative and cytopathic characteristics of immunodeficiency virus isolates. *Journal of Virology* 1988; **62**: 4414–4419.

37 Shuitemaker H., Koot M., Koostra N.A. *et al.* Biological phenotype of human immunodeficiency virus type 1 clones at different stages of infection: progression of disease is associated with a shift from monocytotropic to T-cell-tropic virus populations. *Journal of Virology* 1992; **66**: 1354–1360.

38 Milich L., Margolin B., Swanstrom B. V3 loop of the human immunodeficiency virus type 1 env proteins: interpreting sequence variability. *Journal of Virology* 1993; **67**: 5623–5634.

39 Donaldson Y.K., Bell J.E., Holmes E.C., Hughes E.S., Brown H.K., Simmonds P. *In vivo* distribution and cytopathology of variants of human immunodeficiency virus type 1 showing restricted sequence variability in the V3 loop. *Journal of Virology* 1994; **68**: 5991–6005.

40 Mosier D.E., Gulizia R.J., Macisaac P.D., Torbett B.E., Levy J.A. Rapid loss of CD4+ T cells in human-PBL-SCID mice by non-cytopathic isolates. *Science* 1994; **260**: 689–692.

41 Weinhold K.J., Lyerby H.K., Stanley S.D., Austin A.A., Mathews T.J., Bolognes D.P. HIV-1 gp120-mediated immune suppression and lymphocyte destruction in the absence of viral infection. *Journal of Immunology* 1989; **142**: 3091–3097.

42 Pantaleo G., Graziosi C., Fauci A.S. The immunopathogenesis of human immunodeficiency virus infection. *New England Journal of Medicine* 1993; **328**: 327–334.

43 Imberti L., Sottini A., Bettinardi A., Puoti M., Primi D. Selective depletion of HIV infection of T cells that bear specific T cell receptor Vβ sequences. *Science* 1991; **254**: 860–862.

44 Pantaleo G., Fauci A.S. Apoptosis in HIV infection. *Nature Medicine* 1995; **1**: 118–120.

45 Finkel T.H., Tudor-Williams G., Banda N.K. *et al.* Apoptosis occurs predominantly in bystander cells and not in productively infected cells of HIV- and SIV-injected lymph nodes. *Nature Medicine* 1995; **1**: 129–134.

46 Newell M.K., Haughn L.J., Maroun C.R., Julius M.H. Death of mature T cells by separate ligation of CD4 and the T-cell receptor for antigen. *Nature* 1990; **347**: 286–288.

47 Ameisen J.C., Caprion A. Cell dysfunction and depletion in AIDS: the programmed cell death hypothesis. *Immunology Today* 1991; **12**: 102–105.

48 Habeshaw J., Hounsell E., Dalgleish A. Does the HIV envelope induce a chronic graft-versus-host-like disease? *Immunology Today* 1992; **13**: 207–210.

49 Golding H., Shearer G.M., Hillman K. *et al.* Common epitope in human immunodeficiency virus (HIV) 1-GP41 and HLA class II elicits immunosuppressive autoantibodies capable of contributing to immune dysfunction in HIV 1-infected individuals. *Journal of Clinical Investigation* 1989; **83**: 1430–1435.

50 Stricker R.B., McHugh T.M., Moody D.J. *et al.* An AIDS-related cytotoxic autoantibody reacts with specific antigen on stimulated CD4 T cells. *Nature* 1987; **327**: 710–713.

51 Murray H.W., Rubin B.Y., Masur H., Roberts R.B. Impaired production of lymphokines and immuno(gamma) interferon in the acquired immunodeficiency syndrome. *New England Journal of Medicine* 1984; **310**: 883–888.

52 Lähdevirta J., Maury C.P.J., Teppo A.-M., Repo H. Elevated levels of circulating cachectin/tumor necrosis factor in patients with acquired immunodeficiency syndrome. *American Journal of Medicine* 1989; **85**: 289.

53 Molina J.-M., Scadden D.T., Byrn R., Dinarello C.A., Groopman J.E. Production of tumor necrosis factor alpha and interleukin 1 beta by monocytic cells infected with human immunodeficiency virus. *Journal of Clinical Investigation* 1989; **84**: 733–737.

54 Wright S.C., Jewett A., Mitsuyasu R., Bonavida B. Spontaneous cytotoxicity and tumor necrosis factor production by peripheral blood monocytes from AIDS patients. *Journal of Immunology* 1988; **141**: 99–104.

55 Matsuyama T., Kobayashi N., Yamamoto N. Cytokines and HIV infection: is AIDS a tumour necrosis factor disease? *AIDS* 1991; **5**: 1405–1417.

56 Lawrence J. Molecular interactions among herpes viruses and human immunodeficiency viruses. *Journal of Infectious Diseases* 1990; **162**: 338–346.

57 Vyakarnam A., McKeating J., Meager A., Beverley P.C. Tumor necrosis factor (α,β) induced by HIV-1 in peripheral blood mononuclear cells potentiate virus replication. *AIDS* 1990; **4**: 21–27.

58 Rosenberg Z.F., Fauci A.S. Immunopathogenic mechanisms of HIV infection: cytokine induction of HIV expression. *Immunology Today* 1990; **11**: 176–180.

59 Dalgleish A.G. Viral burden in AIDS. *Nature* 1993; **366**: 22.

60 Street N.E., Schumacher J.H., Fong A.T. *et al.* Heterogeneity of mouse helper T cells. *Journal of Immunology* 1990; **144**: 1629–1639.

61 Clerici M., Shearer G.M. A TH1→TH2 switch is a critical step in the etiology of HIV infection. *Immunology Today* 1993; **14**: 107–111.

62 Graziosi C., Pantaleos G., Gantt K.R. *et al.* Lack of evidence of the dichotomy of TH1 and TH2 predominance in HIV-infected individuals. *Science* 1994; **265**: 248–252.

63 Maggi E., Mazzetti M., Ravina A. *et al.* Ability of HIV to promote a TH1 to TH0 shift and to replicate preferentially in TH2 and TH0 cells. *Science* 1994; **265**: 244–247.

64 Nye K.E., Knox K.A., Pinching A.J. Lymphocytes from HIV-infected individuals show aberrant inositol polyphosphate metabolism which reverses after zidovudine therapy. *AIDS* 1991; **5**: 413–417.

65 Agostini C., Pletti V., Zambello R. *et al.* Phenotypical and functional analysis of bronchoalveolar lavage lymphocytes in patients with HIV infection. *American Review of Respiratory Disease* 1988; **138**: 1609–1695.

66 Resnick L., Fisher E., Croney R. Detection of HTLV-III/LAV-specific IgG and antigen in bronchoalveolar lavage fluid from two patients with lymphocytic interstitial pneumonitis associated with AIDS-related complex. *American Journal of Medicine* 1987; **82**: 553–556.

67 Dean N.C., Golden J.A., Evans L.A. *et al.* Human immunodeficiency virus recovery from bronchoalveolar lavage fluid in patients with AIDS. *Chest* 1988; **93**: 1176–1179.

68 Linnemann C.C., Baughman R.P., Frame P.T., Floyd R. Recovery of human immunodeficiency virus and detection of p24 antigen in bronchoalveolar lavage fluid from adult patients with AIDS. *Chest* 1989; **96**: 64–67.

69 Chayt K.J., Harper M.E., Marselle L.M. *et al.* Detection of HTLV-III RNA in lungs of patients with AIDS and pulmonary involvement. *Journal of the American Medical Association* 1986; **256**: 2356–2359.

70 Clark J.R., Williamson J.D., Mitchell D.M. Comparative study of the isolation of human immunodeficiency virus from the lung and peripheral blood of AIDS patients. *Journal of Medical Virology* 1993; **39**: 196–199.

71 Clarke J.R., Krishnan V., Bennett J., Mitchell D., Jeffries D.J. Detection of HIV-1 in human lung macrophages using the polymerase chain reaction. *AIDS* 1990; **4**: 1133–1136.

72 Clarke J.R., Gates A.J., Coker R.J., Douglass J.A., Williamson, J.D., Mitchell D.M. HIV-1 proviral DNA copy number in peripheral blood leucocytes and bronchoalveolar lavage cells of AIDS patients. *Clinical and Experimental Immunology* 1994; **96**: 183–186.

73 Clarke J.R., Taylor I.K., Fleming J., Nukuna A., Williamson J.R., Mitchell D.M. The epidemiology of HIV-1 infection of the lung in AIDS patients. *AIDS* 1993; **7**: 555–560.

74 Itescu S., Simonelli P.F., Winchester R.J., Ginsberg H.S. Human immunodeficiency virus type 1 strains in the lungs of infected individuals evolve independently from those in peripheral blood and are highly conserved in the C-terminal region of the envelope V3 loop. *Proceedings of the National Academy of Sciences of the USA* 1994; **91**: 11378–11382.

75 Clarke J.R., Robinson D.S., Coker R.J., Miller R.F., Mitchell D.M. Role of the human immunodeficiency virus within the lung. *Thorax* 1995; **50**: 567–576.

76 Holt P.G., Schon-Hegradl M.A., Phillips M.J., Mcmenamin P.G. Ia-positive dendritic cells form a tightly meshed network within the human airway epithelium. *Clinical and Experimental Allergy* 1989; **19**: 597–601.

77 O'Brien W.A., Koyanagi Y., Namazie A. *et al.* HIV tropism for mononuclear phagocytes can be determined by regions of gp120 outside the CD4-binding domain. *Nature* 1990; **348**: 69–73.

78 Gartner S., Markovitz P., Markovitz D.M., Kaplan M.H., Gallo R.C., Popovic M. The role of mononuclear phagocytes in HTLV-III/LAV infection. *Science* 1986; **233**: 215–219.

79 Salahuddin S.Z., Rose R.M., Groopman J.E., Markham P.D., Gallo R.C. Human T lymphotropic virus type III infection of human alveolar macrophages. *Blood* 1986; **68**: 281–284.

80 Twigg H.L., Lipscomb M.F., Yoffe B., Barbaro D.J., Weissler J.C. Enhanced accessory cell function by alveolar macrophages from patients infected with the human immuno-

deficiency virus: potential role for depletion of CD4+ cells in the lung. *American Journal of Respiratory Cell and Molecular Biology* 1989; **1**: 391–400.

81 Twigg H.L., Soliman D.M. Role of alveolar macrophage–T cell adherence in accessory cell function in human immunodeficiency virus-infected individuals. *American Journal of Respiratory Cell and Molecular Biology* 1994; **11**: 138–146.

82 Lebargy F., Branellec A., Deforges L., Bignon J., Bernaudin J.-F. HIV-1 in human alveolar macrophages from infected patients is latent *in vivo* but replicates after *in vitro* stimulation. *American Journal of Respiratory Cell and Molecular Biology* 1994; **10**: 72–78.

83 Murray H.W., Gellene R.A., Libby D.M., Rothermel C.D., Rubin B.H. Activation of tissue macrophages from AIDS patients: *in vitro* response of AIDS alveolar macrophage to lymphokines and interferon-γ. *Journal of Immunology* 1985; **135**: 2374–2377.

84 Musher D.M., Watson D.A., Nickeson D., Gyorkey F., Lahart C., Rossen R.D. The effect of HIV infection on phagocytosis and killing of *Staphylococcus aureus* by human pulmonary alveolar macrophages. *American Journal of Medical Science* 1990; **299**: 158–163.

85 Israël-Biet D., Cadranel J., Beldjord K., Andrieu J.-M., Jeffrey A., Even P. Tumour necrosis factor production in HIV-seropositive subjects: relationship with lung opportunistic infections and HIV expression in alveolar macrophages. *Journal of Immunology* 1991; **147**: 490–494.

86 Guillon J.-M., Autran B., Denis M. *et al.* Human immunodeficiency virus-related lymphocytic alveolitis. *Chest* 1988; **94**: 1264–1270.

87 Plata F., Autran B., Martins L.P. *et al.* AIDS virus-specific cytotoxic T lymphocytes in lung disorders. *Nature* 1987; **328**: 348–351.

88 Autran B., Mayaud C.M., Raphael M. *et al.* Evidence for a cytotoxic T-lymphocyte alveolitis in human immunodeficiency virus-infected patients. *AIDS* 1988; **2**: 179–183.

89 Autran B., Plata F., Guillon J.M., Joly P., Mayaud C., Debre P. HIV-specific cytotoxic T lymphocytes directed against alveolar macrophages in HIV-infected patients. *Respiratory Virology* 1990; **141**: 131–136.

90 Sadat-Sowti B., Parrot A., Quint L., Mayaud C., Debre P., Autran B. Alveolar CD8+ CD57+ lymphocytes in human immunodeficiency virus infection produce an inhibitor of cytotoxic functions. *American Journal of Respiratory and Critical Care Medicine* 1994; **149**: 972–980.

91 Agostini L., Zambello R., Trentin L. *et al.* Cytotoxic events taking place in the lung of patients with HIV-1 infection. *American Review of Respiratory Disease* 1990; **142**: 516–522.

92 Mayaud C.M., Cadranel J. HIV in the lung: guilty or not guilty? *Thorax* 1993; **48**: 1191–1195.

93 Zambello R., Trentin L., Benetti R. Expression of a functional p75 interleukin-2 receptor on lung lymphocytes from patients with human immunodeficiency virus type 1 (HIV-1) infection. *Journal of Clinical Immunology* 1992; **12**: 371–380.

94 Trentin L., Carbisa S., Zambello R. *et al.* Spontaneous production of interleukin-6 by alveolar macrophages from human immunodeficiency virus type 1-infected patients. *Journal of Infectious Diseases* 1992; **166**: 731–737.

95 Berman M.A., Zaldivar F., Imfeld K.L., Kenney J.S., Sandborg C.I. HIV-1 infection of macrophages promotes long-term survival and sustained release of interleukins 1α and β. *AIDS Research and Human Retroviruses* 1994; **10**: 529–539.

96 Iwamoto G.K., Konicek S.A., Twigg H.L. Modulation of accessory cell function and interleukin-6 production by the HIV-1 tat gene. *American Journal of Respiratory Cell and Molecular Biology* 1994; **10**: 580–585.

97 Black C.M., Catterall J.R., Remington J.S. *In vivo* and *in vitro* activation of alveolar macrophages by recombinant interferon-γ. *Journal of Immunology* 1987; **138**: 491–495.

98 Debs R.J., Fuchs H.J., Philip R. *et al.* Lung-specific delivery of cytokines induces sus-

tained pulmonary and systemic immunomodulation in rats. *Journal of Immunology* 1988; **140**: 3482–3488.

99 Millar A.B., Miller R.F., Foley N.M., Meager A., Semple S.J.G., Rook G. Production of tumour necrosis factor (TNF-alpha) by blood and lung mononuclear phagocytes from patients with HIV-related lung disease. *American Journal of Respiratory Cell and Molecular Biology* 1991; **5**: 144–148.

100 Agostini C., Trentin L., Zambello R. *et al*. Release of granulocyte–macrophage colony-stimulating factor by alveolar macrophages in the lung of HIV-1 infected patients: a mechanism accounting for macrophage and neutrophil accumulation. *Journal of Immunology* 1992; **149**: 3379–3385.

101 Dohn M.N., Baughman R.P., Keaton D.A. Interleukin-8 and neutrophilia in pneumocystis pneumonia. *American Journal of Respiratory and Critical Care Medicine* 1994; **149**: A290.

102 Denis M., Ghadirian E. Alveolar macrophages from subjects infected with HIV-1 express macrophage inflammatory protein-1α (MIP-1α): contribution to the CD8+ alveolitis. *Clinical and Experimental Immunology* 1994; **96**: 187–192.

103 Weisman D., Poli G., Fauci A.S. Interleukin 10 blocks HIV replication in macrophages by inhibiting the autocrine loop of tumour necrosis factor α and interleukin 6 induction of virus. *AIDS Research and Human Retroviruses* 1994; **10**: 1199–1206.

104 Poli G., Kinter A.L., Justement J.S., Bressler P., Kehrl J.H., Fauci A.S. Transforming growth factor β suppresses human immunodeficiency virus expression and replication in infected cells of the monocyte/macrophage lineage. *Journal of Experimental Medicine* 1991; **173**: 589–597.

105 Meignan M., Guillon J.-M., Denis M. *et al*. Increased lung epithelial permeability in HIV-infected patients with isolated cytotoxic T-lymphocyte alveolitis. *American Review of Respiratory Disease* 1990; **141**: 1241–1248.

106 Mitchell D.M., Fleming J., Pinching A.J. *et al*. Pulmonary function in human immunodeficiency virus infection: a prospective 18-month study of serial lung function in 474 patients. *American Review of Respiratory Disease* 1992; **146**: 745–751.

107 O'Donnell C.R., Bader M.B., Zibrak J.D., Jensen W.A., Rose R.M. Abnormal airway function in individuals with the acquired immunodeficiency syndrome. *Chest* 1988; **94**: 945–948.

108 Agostini C., Trentin L., Zambello R., Semenzato G. Infectivity, pathogenic mechanisms, and cellular immune responses taking place in the lower respiratory tract. *American Review of Respiratory Disease* 1993; **147**: 1038–1049.

3 Acute bacterial and viral pulmonary infections in HIV-1 infection

D.M. MITCHELL & R.J. COKER

3.0 Epidemiology

Over the last few years it has become apparent that acute bacterial pulmonary infection in association with HIV infection is much more common than was initially thought. In the early years of the AIDS epidemic interest focused mainly on the late pulmonary complications of HIV disease, in particular *Pneumocystis* pneumonia, on account of its severity, frequency and associated mortality. It is now clear that respiratory problems are common early in the natural history of HIV disease and account for considerable morbidity. A recent large cohort study of 1353 individuals, either HIV-1-seropositive or at high risk for HIV infection, was stratified according to peripheral CD4 lymphocyte count and was followed up for an 18-month period. The causes of respiratory disease in this group were similar to the causes in the general population but more frequent. During the 18-month period, 33.4% reported upper respiratory infection, 16% had an episode of acute bronchitis and 5.3% an episode of acute sinusitis and bacterial pneumonia occurred in 4.8%. *Pneumocystis* pneumonia occurred in 3.9%. The frequency of upper respiratory-tract illness was independent of CD4 lymphocyte count, whereas bacterial pneumonia and *Pneumocystis* pneumonia occurred more frequently in individuals with CD4 lymphocyte counts of less than 350 cells/mm^3. In addition, bacterial pneumonia was more common in intravenous drug users in this immunocompromised group. Tobacco smoking did not predispose to respiratory infection, apart from increasing the incidence of acute bronchitis among the female-partner group of individuals in this cohort [1]. Acute bacterial pneumonia may now be responsible for proportionately more acute severe pulmonary infections requiring hospital-ization as a result of widespread use of effective prophylaxis for *Pneumocystis* pneumonia. In a study from Toronto, 48% of admissions of patients with AIDS were for *Pneumocystis* pneumonia before the introduction of prophylaxis with nebulized pentamidine and this fell to 29% after its introduction [2]. In a similar study from London [3], hospital admissions of HIV-positive patients with respiratory episodes due to *Pneumocystis* pneumonia fell from 68% to 48% following the introduction of prophylaxis. During the 1986–87 period, prior to prophylaxis, 14% of patients had bacterial pneumonia or bronchitis and this increased to 23% for the period 1990–91 after the introduction of prophylaxis. In this review chapter, the clinical characteristics of acute bacterial and viral respiratory infections will be discussed.

3.1 Upper airway infections

3.1.1 Sinusitis

Sinusitis is common and is found in between 6 and 16% of HIV-seropositive individuals, depending on the clinical and radiological criteria employed [4–6]. Generally the clinical features resemble sinusitis seen in non-HIV-infected individuals. Symptoms of sinusitis in these patients include frontal headache, nasal congestion with fever, facial pain and postnasal drip. In HIV disease, sinusitis may be acute, chronic or recurrent and symptomatic or asymptomatic. In patients with CD4 lymphocyte counts of less than 200 cells/mm^3, chronic sinus disease is particularly common. The diagnosis may be confused with meningitis or encephalitis when headache is a major feature [7]. Purulent nasal discharge and lymphoid hypertrophy may be seen in the posterior oropharynx and, as a result of the underlying immune defect, disease tends to be diffuse, bilateral and chronic. Plain radiographs of the sinuses are helpful in diagnosis if opacification or air–fluid levels are seen in the sinuses. Computed tomographic (CT) scanning and nuclear magnetic resonance (NMR) imaging have greater diagnostic sensitivity; sinus mucosal thickening is a very common finding in HIV infection [5,8]. Nasal endoscopy and antral puncture may be required for definitive diagnosis.

Sinusitis is generally underdiagnosed and may present with nonspecific symptoms [6,7]. In one retrospective study [5], 75 patients were identified as having radiographic evidence of sinusitis. All had mucosal thickening, indicating chronic disease. Fifty patients (67%) had symptoms with fever, congestion, discharge and headache. Nineteen patients (25%) were asymptomatic and yet radiologically had active disease. Ten patients (13%) had acute sinusitis. The mean CD4 lymphocyte count for the group was 276 cells/mm^3; 32 (43%) had CD4 lymphocyte counts of less than 100 cells/mm^3. The authors conclude that sinusitis is a frequent occurrence in HIV disease but may be asymptomatic or may be recurrent, as well as being associated with a decline in immune status.

A further retrospective study identified sinusitis in 72 HIV-seropositive patients, most of whom had CD4 lymphocyte counts of less than 200 cells/mm^3. Many had a history of previous respiratory infection. Symptoms of sinusitis were often non-specific and the diagnosis was incidental in 28 patients (33%). CT and NMR imaging were more sensitive than plain sinus radiographs. It was noted that response was often incomplete following antibiotic therapy [6]. A further retrospective study identified 30 patients with radiological evidence of sinus disease, 13 of whom were initially diagnosed as having meningitis. In four, sinusitis was caused by *Pseudomonas*. All these patients had advanced HIV disease and all responded to appropriate antibiotics, but early relapse was common [7]. The same spectrum of bacteria that caused lower respiratory-tract disease caused sinusitis, with *Streptococcus pneumoniae* and *Haemophilus influenzae* being the most frequently isolated and *Pseudomonas* being frequent in the late stages of HIV disease, when the CD4 lymphocyte count is low [7]. Non-bacterial pathogens can cause sinusitis, including fungi, such as *Cryptococcus* and *Alternaria* [9,10], and cytomegalovirus (CMV). This normally responds to treatment with ganciclovir [11]. Treatment of sinusitis in HIV-positive patients is similar to treatment of sinusitis generally, with appropriate antibacterial agents, decongestants and expectorants. There is a tendency to relapse and for chronicity to develop and it may be necessary to prescribe antibiotics for several weeks; even so, response may be disappointing [6]. As *Strep. pneumoniae* and *H. influenzae* are the most common pathogens, broad-spectrum antibiotics, such as amoxycillin, co-trimoxazole, amoxycillin and clavulanic acid, or oral cephalosporin, should be considered. If *Staphylococcus aureus* is isolated, flucloxacillin is appropriate, whereas Gram-negative or anaerobic infections require appropriate specific treatment with, for example, clindamycin [12]. Surgical drainage may be required for antibiotic-resistant disease.

3.1.2 Bronchitis

Bacterial bronchitis, reminiscent in presentation of bacterial exacerbations of chronic obstructive lung disease, occurs with increased frequency in HIV-infected individuals [1], particularly in those who are more severely immunocompromised. Most patients present with a cough productive of purulent sputum and low-grade fever. As with bacterial pneumonia in HIV-positive patients, the most common pathogens are *Strep.*

pneumoniae and *H. influenzae*, followed by *Pseudomonas aeruginosa*. Patients respond to appropriate antibiotic therapy, although relapse is frequent.

3.1.3 Bronchiectasis

Bronchiectasis has recently been described in HIV infection, probably on the basis of recurrent bronchopulmonary infection, either bacterial or following *Pneumocystis* pneumonia [13,14]. Precise prevalence has not yet been determined nor has its clinical significance; it may be relatively underdiagnosed as high-resolution CT scanning is required to confirm the diagnosis [15]. In children, bronchiectasis may complicate lymphocytic interstitial pneumonitis (LIP). Bronchiectasis in HIV infection is seen in association with *Strep. pneumoniae*, *Staph. aureus*, *H. influenzae*, *Moraxella catarrhalis* and *Pseudomonas cepacia* [14].

3.2 Pneumonia

3.2.1 Clinical patterns

The spectrum of bacteria causing pneumonia in HIV-infected individuals is similar to that of community-acquired pneumonia in non-HIV-infected individuals. *Strep. pneumoniae* is the most common cause of bacterial pneumonia, the second most common cause being *H. influenzae*. Other bacterial causes are listed in Table 3.1. In HIV-infected individuals the incidence of severe pneumonia, often with bacteraemia, caused by *Strep. pneumoniae* is high; indeed, *Strep. pneumoniae* is one of the most frequently occurring invasive bacterial infections in HIV-infected patients and such infection may precede an AIDS-defining diagnosis. In one study from San Francisco, the estimated rate for pneumococcal bacteraemia

Table 3.1 Bacterial causes of pneumonia.

Streptococcus pneumoniae
Haemophilus influenzae
Moraxella catarrhalis
Streptococci group B
Pseudomonas aeruginosa
Klebsiella pneumoniae
Enterobacter cloacae
Staphylococcus aureus
Legionella species
Mycoplasma pneumoniae
Rhodococcus equi

CHAPTER 3
*Acute bacterial and
viral pulmonary
infections in HIV*

was 9.4 cases per 1000 patients with AIDS per year [16]. Community studies estimate a rate of 0.07 cases per 1000 per year in HIV-seronegative individuals [17], suggesting that bacteraemia rates are 100-fold greater in patients with AIDS. In another study, the incidence of pneumococcal pneumonia has been estimated to be between 5.5 and 17.5 times greater in patients with AIDS than in the general population [18,19]. More than half of the episodes of pneumococcal bacteraemia in HIV-infected persons occur in patients without AIDS [16]. The distribution of serotypes of pneumococci causing bacteraemia is similar in HIV-infected people and HIV-1-seronegative patients. Twenty-seven of 33 (82%) pneumococcal isolates from HIV-infected patients and 107 of 119 (90%) without HIV infection belong to the 23 serotypes currently used in polysaccharide vaccine [16]. HIV-infected children seem to be at particular risk of bacterial pneumonia and bacteraemia with *Strep. pneumoniae* [20] and the incidence of bacterial pneumonia in intravenous drug abusers with HIV infection is also particularly high [21]. Injecting drug users have a higher rate of pneumococcal disease, independent of HIV status [19]. The annual incidence of pneumococcal pneumonia in HIV-seropositive intravenous drug users can be as high as 10% and yet it is 2% in seronegative patients [22]. In a cohort study of risk factors for bacterial pneumonia in intravenous drug users, the incidence of bacterial pneumonia was 1.93 per 100 person-years in HIV-seropositive and 0.45 per 100 person-years in HIV-seronegative intravenous drug users. A CD4 lymphocyte count of less than 200 cells/μl, a previous episode of *Pneumocystis* pneumonia and smoking of drugs, such as cocaine, crack or marijuana, were associated with bacterial pneumonia, whereas cigarette smoking was not [23].

Staph. aureus and *P. aeruginosa* are seen in more severely immunosuppressed HIV-positive individuals with lower CD4 counts. *Pseudomonas* infection was originally thought to be unusual except when associated with severe neutropenia or following cytotoxic drug therapy in patients with AIDS. Presentation is usually with acute pneumonia and sepsis. However, *Pseudomonas* infection is common in the late stages of HIV disease and can produce bacteraemia, pneumonia and sinusitis, particularly when the CD4 count is less than 100 cells/mm^3. The majority of patients who develop *Pseudomonas* pneumonia frequently have cavities and pulmonary infiltrates and mortality is high, at about 20%. Mortality associated with bacteraemia is even higher, at approximately 40% [24]. An association with CMV infection has been described. Pulmonary infection probably accounts for up to 40% of *P. aeruginosa* bacteraemia and septicaemia in AIDS patients [25]. A more indolent and relapsing form of *Pseudomonas* bronchopulmonary infection, somewhat similar to that seen in cystic fibrosis, has recently been described in patients with AIDS and a low CD4 count (mean 25 cells/mm³), but without the other risk factors [26].

Staph. aureus is a common cause of HIV-related bacteraemia and may be acquired nosocomially [27]. Patients with HIV infection seem to have increased nasal carriage of *Staph. aureus*, which may relate to the increased incidence. In one study, *Staph. aureus* was isolated in 23% of respiratory infectious episodes and accounted for pneumonia in 6%. Even though the pneumonia was appropriately treated, in all cases mortality was high, at 38% [28].

Legionella pneumonia has infrequently been described in association with HIV infection, despite being a well-known pathogen for immuno-compromised patients. When it does occur, it appears to be associated with moderately severe immunosuppression (CD4 <100 cells/mm³) and often with other coexistent pulmonary infections. Response to treatment is good [29,30].

Hospital-acquired pneumonia in AIDS patients is frequently due to Gram-negative organisms or *Staph. aureus* [19,28]. The organism *Rhodococcus equi* is a rare cause of pneumonia in AIDS patients and the onset of symptoms is often gradual. The chest radiograph may show localized infiltrates, frequently in the upper lobes, and these may cavitate. *Rhodococcus* is a Gram-positive rod and responds to erythromycin, with or without rifampicin [31,32].

Other less common pathogens, for example *Nocardia*, may cause pulmonary disease, although the widespread use of trimethoprim–sulphamethoxazole as prophylaxis for *Pneumocystis* pneumonia may have reduced the incidence of clinical *Nocardia* infections [33]. Interest has recently focused on more unusual pathogens and their role in HIV-associated pulmonary disease [34]—for example, the red or violet polypoid angiomatous lesions seen endobronchially which resemble Kaposi's sarcoma, caused by bacillary angiomatosis.

A recent retrospective study from London analysed 49 episodes of community-acquired lobar pneumonia occurring in patients with AIDS. Definitive bacteriological diagnosis was made in 25 episodes (51%) and seven patients had more than one organism. The pathogens were *Strep. pneumoniae* (11), *Staph. aureus* (six), *Pneumocystis carinii* (three), *H. influenzae* (three) and *Pseudomonas* (two). Four patients died (8%). In 11 episodes cavity or abscess formation occurred, in three empyema was seen and 10 had pleural effusion [35]. This and other studies demonstrate that bacterial pneumonia in these patients gives a high complication rate and infections are often dual. Twenty-three of the patients had a prior AIDS diagnosis, of which 17 had had previous *Pneumocystis* pneumonia, 21 were taking anti-*Pneumocystis* prophylaxis, 29 (59%) had sputum production and 25 (51%) had pleural pain. All had fever, cough and

CHAPTER 3
*Acute bacterial and
viral pulmonary
infections in HIV*

dyspnoea. Six of 11 patients with *Strep. pneumoniae* had positive blood cultures. Chest radiographs showed lobar consolidation in 20 and segmental consolidation in 29. Other lobes were involved in nine and lower lobes in 36. The middle lobe was involved in 15. In 11 cases, interstitial shadowing was also present. In a recent series from North America [36], 27% of all patients with AIDS requiring hospital admission had a pleural effusion; in 66% infection was the cause (bacterial 31%, *Pneumocystis* pneumonia 15%, tuberculosis 8%, *Nocardia* 3%, *Cryptococcus* 2%, *Mycobacterium avium intracellulare* 2%). A further 31% non-infectious causes were determined, including hypoalbuminaemia 9%, congestive cardiac failure 5% and Kaposi's sarcoma 2%. The conclusions of the study were that the most common cause of a pleural effusion in AIDS was bacterial pneumonia. Large pleural effusions were caused by Kaposi's sarcoma or tuberculosis, and hypoalbuminaemia was a common cause of non-infectious pleural effusions [36].

3.2.2 Clinical presentations

The majority of HIV-infected persons with pneumococcal infection present with pneumonia with features similar to those seen in non-HIV-infected individuals, with fever, cough, rigors and dyspnoea and sometimes pleuritic pain. Occasionally meningitis, pericarditis or endocarditis occurs [37]. The onset of pneumonia is normally rapid and severe, with associated septicaemia being common.

Generally the complication rate is low but overwhelming fatal infection, often in bacteraemic cases, is seen. The tendency to recurrent disease is greater with HIV infection than in normal individuals. Mortality from pneumococcal infection is similar in HIV-infected and non-HIV-infected individuals [37].

3.2.3 Treatment of pneumonia in HIV

Response to appropriate antibiotic therapy is usually satisfactory. Treatment normally has to start before the causative organism and antibiotic sensitivities are known. As the spectrum of organisms causing pneumonia in these patients is similar to that causing community-acquired pneumonia, a similar therapeutic stategy is appropriate in terms of antibiotic choice. In view of the relatively high resistance to penicillin overall, empirical therapy is best commenced with a second- or third-generation cephalosporin (e.g. cefuroxime or cefotaxime), a macrolide (e.g. erythromycin or clarithromycin) or even trimethoprim/sulphamethoxazole. Patients being treated presumptively for *Pneumocystis* pneumonia with trimethoprim/sulphamethoxazole who have concomitant pneumococcal pneumonia or *H. influenzae* pneumonia will also improve, as the majority of organisms are sensitive to this antibiotic combination. However, in patients being treated for pneumococcal pneumonia who do not respond, a second diagnosis, such as *Pneumocystis* pneumonia, should be considered.

Treatment response to appropriate antibiotics is usually rapid and the clinical pattern resembles that seen in normal individuals. For pneumococcal pneumonia a 10–14-day course of antibiotics is normally sufficient.

3.2.4 Empyema

Empyema appears to be an unusual complication of adult HIV-related pneumonia and respiratory-tract infections. Most clinical reviews are notable for the lack of documentation on empyema. Immunological factors, such as cytokine production and interactions from monocyte/macrophages, dendritic cells, B lymphocytes and neutrophils, may be necessary for empyema formation. It may be that HIV infection of mononuclear cells affects their subsequent cytokine production and indirectly their impact on neutrophils, impairing the development of empyema [38].

3.3 Acute viral infections and treatment

Upper respiratory infections are more common in HIV-seropositive than in seronegative individuals [1,39]. Both herpes simplex and herpes zoster may cause pneumonitis in HIV-infected patients [29,30]. Herpes simplex also causes chronic mucocutaneous disease in HIV infection and it has been suggested that reactivation of mucocutaneous material aspirated into the tracheobronchial tree may result in a focal pneumonitis, whereas haematogenous spread of virus may result in a diffuse interstitial pneumonia [40]. The diagnosis is supported by finding appropriate inclusions or multinucleate giant cells in bronchoalveolar lavage (BAL) fluid or biopsy material, or by specific immunofluorescence staining for the virus. Response to aciclovir is usual, except in occasional cases of drug-resistant disease, often arising in patients who have been on aciclovir for prolonged periods of time to suppress chronic skin disease [41]. The Epstein–Barr virus (EBV) can infect HIV-infected patients, is implicated in the pathogenesis of non-Hodgkin's lymphoma and may be responsible for hairy cell leucoplakia; it has also been implicated in LIP, a chronic condition most commonly seen in children and individuals of Afro-Caribbean origin [42]. Respiratory syncytial virus (RSV) infection is occasionally seen in HIV-infected children and adults and may cause a diffuse

CHAPTER 3
*Acute bacterial and
viral pulmonary
infections in HIV*

interstitial pneumonitis. The virus may be isolated from BAL fluid or identified by immunofluorescent staining. Ribavirin via nebulizer is often effective in the treatment of RSV [42]. CMV chronically infects the majority of HIV-infected individuals and eventually causes clinical disease in 40% of HIV-infected patients, most commonly retinitis [43]. The role of the virus in causing pneumonitis remains controversial. It is frequently isolated from BAL fluid, being found in 30–50% of samples. However, it is also present in saliva. The clinical course of most episodes of pneumonitis in patients with AIDS does not seem to be related to the presence or absence of CMV where clinical resolution occurs following appropriate antimicrobial therapy that is not effective against this virus. However, occasionally, pneumonitis occurs either when the CD4 count is high or around the time of seroconversion following HIV infection [44]. Convincing evidence that CMV is causing the pneumonitis is demonstrated in lung biopsies where an interstitial infiltrate includes the typical intracytoplasmic inclusion bodies; CMV pneumonitis is nearly always seen in conjunction with *Pneumocystis* pneumonia, where the presence of CMV increases mortality. If CMV is causing the pneumonitis, response to ganciclovir or foscarnet therapy is usual. Recently, the presence of CMV in BAL has been related to mortality in HIV-positive patients with pneumonitis. Mortality was greater at 3 months and 6 months in individuals in which CMV was present [45].

3.4 Diagnosis of pulmonary disease in HIV infection

The chest radiograph is a useful and routine diagnostic tool but appearances must be interpreted with caution. *Pneumocystis* pneumonia typically produces diffuse bilateral infiltrates, although atypical changes may also be seen. An acute bacterial infection can produce similar appearances, mimicking *Pneumocystis* pneumonia. The presence of pleural effusions is very uncommon in *Pneumocystis* pneumonia and is more commonly seen in acute bacterial infection, mycobacterial infection or pulmonary malignancy [46]. As sputum production is frequently not present, preventing Gram stain and culture for diagnosis, and where blood cultures are negative, establishing a microbial diagnosis of pulmonary infection often requires semi-invasive or invasive techniques to acquire relevant clinical material for microscopy and culture. These techniques include induced sputum, fibre-optic bronchoscopy with BAL, fibre-optic transbronchial biopsy, percutaneous needle aspiration and open-lung biopsy [47–49]. Semiquantitative bacterial cultures from BAL fluid provide excellent sensitivity and specificity for diagnosis [50]. Generally speaking, the more invasive the procedure the greater the diagnostic yield, and indeed there may be a role for open-lung biopsy in chronic pulmonary illness refractory to other diagnostic modalities as valuable diagnostic information may be forthcoming [51].

In bacterial pneumonia a neutrophil leucocytosis is common and hypoxaemia relating to the degree of severity of the pneumonia is seen. In 75% of cases the chest radiograph shows straightforward lobar, multilobar or segmental shadows, whereas in 25% diffuse infiltrates suggestive of *Pneumocystis* pneumonia are seen [19,52]. Atypical appearances, resembling *Pneumocystis* pneumonia, with diffuse interstitial infiltrates are particularly common in *H. influenzae* pneumonia [19].

3.5 Prophylaxis and immunization

The predominant abnormality in HIV infection is reduction in number and functional failure of CD4 helper T lymphocytes, but many defects in immune function have now been identified in HIV disease. A number of these are thought to be important in accounting for the predisposition to bacterial infection in HIV disease, including a diminished ability to produce an effective antibody response during acute infection, both systemically and at the mucosal level (immunoglobulin A (IgA) antibody production) [53,54], and thus reduced effector cell activation and killing of bacteria. Mild neutropenia (less than 1500 cells/μl) is common in HIV disease in the absence of myelosuppressive drugs, but profound neutropenia (less than 100 cells/μl) is rare [55]. Generally, low neutrophil counts are relatively well tolerated by these patients and do not seem to predispose to increased bacterial infection until the neutrophil count is very low [55]. Defects in neutrophil and macrophage chemotaxis and phagocytosis, as well as defects of complement activation, may also contribute, but failure of adequate IgG$_2$ subclass antibody response to bacterial capsule-specific antigens may be particularly important [56].

In view of the importance and frequency of pneumococcal infection in HIV infection, prevention would be desirable. Immunization with standard 23-valent pneumococcal polysaccharide vaccine for HIV-infected persons over the age of 2 years is currently recommended in the USA by the Centers for Disease Control [57] and the American College of Physicians [58], as, in one study, 82% of pneumococcal isolates from HIV-seropositive patients belonged to the 23 pneumococcal serotypes included in currently available pneumococcal vaccines [16]. However, benefit in this group has not yet been fully demonstrated [59,60]. Several studies have reported failure [61–63]. There is evidence that HIV infection is associated with impaired antibody responses [59,64,65], but patients with early HIV disease may be able to mount adequate antibody responses to pneumococcal antigens [59,60]. Several studies have demonstrated the efficacy of pneumococcal vaccine in normal individuals and the Centers for Disease Control and the American College of Physicians made their recommendations on the basis of this. However, several studies have demonstrated suboptimal antipneumococcal antibody titres following standard immunization [60,63,64]. The ability to make an antibody response is related to the CD4 count; while HIV-positive individuals with a relatively well-preserved CD4 count make normal antibody responses, the antibody response is diminished in those with low CD4 counts [66]. It is of interest that patients with low CD4 cell counts who are also receiving zidovudine have relatively normal antibody responses to vaccination [67]. The IgG_2 subclass is important in defence against capsulated bacterial disease and IgG_2 antibodies are generated in response to polysaccharide antigen [68]. A recent study has shown that 50% of HIV-infected individuals receiving pneumococcal polysaccharide vaccine had inadequate IgG_2 antibody responses and this poor response was unrelated to CD4 [56]. The role of pneumococcal vaccine therefore remains to be determined by appropriate clinical studies [69].

An alternative to immunization is antibiotic prophylaxis; in splenectomized patients or those with sickle-cell disease, pneumococcal bacteraemia is effectively prevented by prophylactic penicillin [70]. However, formal studies have not been performed in HIV disease, but lower rates of bacterial infection have been observed in a *Pneumocystis* prophylaxis trial in the patients randomized to receive a trimethoprim/sulphamethoxazole combination compared with those randomized to receive aerosolized pentamidine [71].

References

1 Wallace J.M., Rao A.V., Glassroth J. *et al*. Respiratory illness in persons with HIV infection. *American Review of Respiratory Disease* 1993; **148**: 1523–1529.

2 Chien S.M., Ruwaji M., Mintz S., Rachlis A., Chan C.K. Changes in hospital admission patterns in patients with HIV infection in the era of pneumocystis prophylaxis. *Chest* 1992; **102**: 1035–1039.

3 Pitkin A.D., Grant A.D., Foley N.M., Miller R.F. Changing patterns of respiratory disease in HIV positive patients in a referral centre in the United Kingdom between 1986–7 and 1990–1. *Thorax* 1993; **48**: 204–207.

4 Semple S., Lenahan G.F., Secwonska M.H. Allergic diseases and sinusitis in acquired immune deficiency syndrome. *Journal of Allergy and Clinical Immunology* 1989; **83**: 190–192.

5 Zurco J.J., Feuerstein I., Lebovics R., Lane A.C. Sinusitis in HIV-1 infection. *American Journal of Medicine* 1992; **93**: 157–162.

6 Godofsky E.W., Zinreich J., Armstrong M., Leslie J.M., Wewibel C.S. Sinusitis in HIV-1 infected patients a clinical and radiographic review. *American Journal of Medicine* 1992; **93**: 163–170.

7 Grant A., Schoenberg M., Grant H.R., Miller R.F. Paranasal sinus disease in HIV antibody positive patients. *Genitourinary Medicine* 1993; **69**: 208–212.

8 Chong W.K., Hall-Craggs M.A., Wilkinson I.D. *et al*. The prevalence of paranasal

CHAPTER 3
*Acute bacterial and
viral pulmonary
infections in HIV*

disease in HIV infection and AIDS on cranial MR imaging. *Clinical Radiology* 1993; **47**: 166–169.

9 Choi S.S., Lawson W., Buttone N.A. Cryptococcal sinusitis: a case report and review of the literature. *Otolaryngology Head and Neck Surgery* 1988; **99**: 414–418.

10 Gonzalez M.M., Gould E., Dickinson G. Acquired immunodeficiency syndrome associated with *Acanthamoeba* infection and other opportunist organisms. *Archives of Pathology and Laboratory Medicine* 1986; **110**: 749–757.

11 Brillhart T., Gathe J., Piot D. Symptomatic cytomegalovirus rhinosinusitis in patients with AIDS. *Proceedings of the 7th International Conference on AIDS*, Florence, Italy, 1991: 227, abstract MB 2182.

12 Meiteles L.Z., Lucente F.E. Sinus and nasal manifestations of the acquired immunodeficiency syndrome. *Ear, Nose and Throat Journal* 1990; **69**: 454–459.

13 Holmes A.H., Trotman-Dickenson B., Edwards A., Peto T., Luzzi G.A. Bronchiectasis in HIV disease. *Quarterly Journal of Medicine* 1992; **85**: 875–882.

14 Verghese A., Al-Samman M., Nabham D., Naylor A.D., Rivera M. Bacterial bronchitis and bronchiectasis in HIV infection. *Archives of Internal Medicine* 1994; **154**: 2086–2089.

15 McGuinness G., Naidich D.P., Garay S., Leitman B.S., McCauley D.I. AIDS associated bronchiectasis: CT features. *Journal of Computer Assisted Tomography* 1993; **17**: 260–266.

16 Redd S.C., Rutherford G.W., Sande M.A. *et al.* The role of HIV infection in pneumococcal bacteremia in San Francisco residents. *Journal of Infectious Diseases* 1990; **162**: 1012–1017.

17 Brieman R.F., Spika J.S., Navarro V.J., Darden P.M., Darby C.P. Pneumococcal bacteremia in Charleston County, South Carolina: a decade later. *Archives of Internal Medicine* 1990; **150**: 1401–1405.

18 Witt D.J., Craven D.E., McCabe W.R. Bacterial infections in adult patients with the acquired immune deficiency syndrome (AIDS) and AIDS related complex. *American Journal of Medicine* 1987; **82**: 900–906.

19 Polsky B., Gold J.W., Whimbey E. *et al.* Bacterial pneumonia in patients with the acquired immunodeficiency syndrome. *Annals of Internal Medicine* 1986; **104**: 38–41.

20 Krasinski K., Borkowsky W., Bonk S., Lawrence R., Chandwani S. Bacterial infections in human immunodeficiency virus-infected children. *Pediatric Infectious Disease Journal* 1988; 7: 323–328.

21 Selwyn P.A., Feingold A.R., Harte D. Increased risk of bacterial pneumonia in HIV-infected intravenous drug users without AIDS. *AIDS* 1988; **2**: 267–272.

22 Chaisson R.E. Bacterial pneumonia in patients with human immunodeficiency virus infection. *Seminars on Respiratory Infection* 1989; **4**: 133–138.

23 Caiaffa W.T., Vlahov D., Graham M.H. *et al.* Drug smoking, *Pneumocystis carinii* pneumonia and immunosuppression increase risk of bacterial pneumonia in HIV-seropositive injection drug users. *American Journal of Respiratory and Critical Care Medicine* 1994; **150**: 1493–1498.

24 Mendelson M.H., Gurtman A., Szabo S. *et al. Pseudomonas aeruginosa* bacteremia in patients with AIDS. *Clinical Infectious Disease* 1994; **18**: 886–895.

25 Keilhofner M., Atmar R.L., Hamill R.J., Musher D.M. Life threatening *Pseudomonas aeruginosa* infections in patients with HIV infection. *Clinical Infectious Disease* 1992; **14**: 403–411.

26 Baron A.D., Hollander H. *Pseudomonas aeruginosa* bronchopulmonary infection in late human immunodeficiency virus disease. *American Review of Respiratory Disease* 1993; **148**: 992–996.

27 Jacobson M.A., Gellermann H., Chambers H. *Staphylococcus aureus* bacteremia and recurrent staphylococcal infection in patients with acquired immunodeficiency syndrome and AIDS-related complex. *American Journal of Medicine* 1985; **85**: 172–176.

28 Levine S.J., White D.A., Fels A.O.S. The incidence and significance of *Staphylococcus aureus* in respiratory cultures from patients infected with HIV. *American Review of Respiratory Disease* 1990; **141**: 89–93.

29 Murray J., Mills J. State of the art: pulmonary infections, complications of HIV. Part I. *American Review of Respiratory Disease* 1990; **141**: 1356–1372.

30 Murray J., Mills J. State of the art: pulmonary infections, complications of HIV. Part II. *American Review of Respiratory Disease* 1990; **141**: 1582–1598.

31 Prescott J.F. *Rhodococcus equi*: an animal and human pathogen. *Clinical and Microbiological Review* 1991; **4**: 20–34.

32 Weingarter J.S., Huang D.Y., Jackman J.D., Jr. *Rhodococcus equi* pneumonia: an unusual manifestation of the acquired immunodeficiency syndrome (AIDS). *Chest* 1988; **94**: 195–196.

33 Coker R.J., Bignardi G., Horner P. *et al*. *Nocardia* infection in AIDS: a clinical and microbiological challenge. *Journal of Clinical Pathology* 1992; **45**: 821–822.

34 Slater L.N., Min K.W. Polypoid endobronchial lesions: a manifestation of bacillary angiomatosis. *Chest* 1992; **102**: 972–974.

35 Miller R.F., Foley N.M., Kessel D., Jeffrey A.A. Community acquired lobar pneumonia in patients with HIV infection and AIDS. *Thorax* 1994; **49**: 367–368.

36 Joseph J., Strange C., Sahn S.A. Pleural effusions in hospitalised patients with AIDS. *Annals of Internal Medicine* 1993; **118**: 856–859.

37 Janoff E.N., Breiman R.F., Daley C.I., Hopewell P.C. Pneumococcal disease during HIV infection: epidemiologic, clinical and immunologic perspectives. *Annals of Internal Medicine* 1992; **117**: 314–324.

38 Coker R.J. Empyema thoracis in AIDS. *Journal of the Royal Society of Medicine* 1994; **87**: 65–67.

39 Hoover D.R., Graham N.M.H., Bacellar H. Epidemiologic patterns of upper respiratory illness and *Pneumocystis carinii* pneumonia in homosexual men. *American Review of Respiratory Disease* 1991; **83**: 604–605.

40 Corey L., Spear P.G. Infections with herpes simplex viruses (second of two parts). *New England Journal of Medicine* 1986; **314**: 749–757.

41 Englund J.A., Zimmerman M.E., Swierkosz E.M., Goodman J.L., School D.R., Balfour H.H., Jr. Herpes simplex virus resistant to acyclovir: a study in tertiary care center. *Annals of Internal Medicine* 1990; **112**: 416–422.

42 Wallace J.M. Pulmonary infections in human immunodeficiency disease: viral pulmonary infections. *Seminars on Respiratory Infection* 1989; **4**: 147–154.

43 Drew W.L. Cytomegalovirus infection in patients with AIDS. *Clinics in Infectious Diseases* 1992; **14**: 608–615.

44 Squire S.B., Lipman M.C., Bagdades E.K. *et al*. Severe cytomegalovirus pneumonitis in HIV infected patients with higher than average CD4 counts. *Thorax* 1992; **47**: 301–304.

45 Hayner C.E., Baughman R.P., Linnemann C.C., Dohn M.N. The relationships between cytomegalovirus retrieved by bronchoalveolar lavage and mortality in patients with HIV. *Chest* 1995; **107**: 735–740.

46 Mitchell D.M., Miller R.F. Recent developments in the management of the pulmonary complications of HIV disease: AIDS and the lung update 1992. *Thorax* 1992; **47**: 381–390.

47 Bigby T.D., Margolskee D., Curtis J.L. *et al*. The usefulness of induced sputum in the diagnosis of *P. carinii* pneumonia in patients with AIDS. *American Review of Respiratory Disease* 1986; **133**: 515–518.

48 Findley R., Kielt E., Thomson S. Bronchial brushing in the diagnosis of pulmonary disease in patients at risk for opportunist infection. *American Review of Respiratory Disease* 1974; **109**: 379–387.

49 Stover D.E., White D.A., Romano P.A., Gellene R.A. Diagnosis of pulmonary disease in AIDS: role of bronchoscopy and bronchoalveolar lavage. *American Review of Respiratory Disease* 1984; **130**: 659–662.

50 Magnenat J.L., Nicod L.P., Auckenthaler R., Junod A.F. Mode of presentation and diag-

nosis of bacterial pneumonia in HIV infected patients. *American Review of Respiratory Disease* 1991; **144**: 917–922.

51 Miller R.F., Pugsley W.B., Griffiths M.H. Open lung biopsy and negative bronchoscopic investigations. *Thorax* 1994; **49**: 432P.

52 Steinhart R., Reingold A.L., Taylor F., Anderson G., Wenger J.D. Invasive *Haemophilus influenzae* infections in men with HIV infections. *JAMA* 1992; **268**: 3350–3352.

53 Terpstra F.G., Al B.J., Roos M.T. *et al.* Longitudinal study of leukocyte functions in homosexual men seroconverted for HIV: rapid and persistent loss of B cell function after HIV infection. *European Journal of Immunology* 1989; **19**: 667–673.

54 Muller F.R., Freland S.S., Hyatum M., Radl J., Brandtzaeg P. Both IgA subclasses are reduced in parotid saliva from patients with AIDS. *Clinical and Experimental Immunology* 1991; **83**: 203–209.

55 Shaunak S., Bartlett J.A. Zidovudine-induced neutropenia: are we too cautious? *Lancet* 1989; ii: 91–92.

56 Unsworth D.J., Rowen D., Carne C., Sonnex C., Baglin T., Brown D.L. Defective IgG response to Pneumovax in HIV seropositive patients. *Genitourinary Medicine* 1993; **69**: 373–376.

57 Pneumococcal polysaccharide vaccine. *Morbidity and Mortality Weekly Report* 1989; **3**: 64–68, 73–76.

58 American College of Physicians. *Guide for Adult Immunization*. Philadelphia: ACP, 1990.

59 Huang K.L., Ruben F.L., Rinaldo C.R., Jr, Kingsley L., Lyter D.W., Ho M. Antibody response after influenza and pneumococcal immunization in HIV-infected homosexual men. *JAMA* 1986; **257**: 2047–2050.

60 Klein R.S., Selwyn P.A., Maude D., Pollard C., Freeman K., Schiffman G. Response to pneumococcal vaccine among asymptomatic heterosexual partners of persons with AIDS and intravenous drug users infected with human immunodeficiency virus. *Journal of Infectious Diseases* 1989; **160**: 826–831.

61 Yamaguchi E.P., Charache P., Chaisson R.E. Increasing incidence of pneumococcal infections (PI) associated with HIV infection in an inner city hospital, 1985–1989 [abstract]. *World Conference on Lung Health*, Boston, Massachusetts, 1990.

62 Janoff E.N., O'Brien J., Ehret J., Meiklejohn G., Duval G., Douglas J.M., Jr. Bacteremia, pharyngeal colonization and immune response to *Streptococcus pneumoniae* in persons with HIV [abstract]. *31st Annual Interscience Conference on Antimicrobial Agents and Chemotherapy*, Chicago, Illinois, 1991.

63 Simberkoff M.S., El Sadr W., Schiffman G., Rahal J.J., Jr. *Streptococcus pneumoniae* infections and bacteremia in patients with acquired immune deficiency syndrome, with a report of pneumococcal vaccine failure. *American Review of Respiratory Disease* 1984; **130**: 1174–1176.

64 Ammann A.J., Schiffman G., Abrams D., Volberding P., Ziegler J., Conant M. B-cell immunodeficiency in acquired immune deficiency syndrome. *JAMA* 1984; **251**: 1447–1449.

65 Steinhoff M.C., Auerbach B.S., Nelson K. *et al.* Antibody responses to *Haemophilus influenzae* type b vaccines in men with human immunodeficiency virus infection. *New England Journal of Medicine* 1991; **325**: 1837–1842.

66 Rodriguez-Barradas M.C., Mushar D.M., Lahart C. *et al.* Antibody to capsular polysaccharides of *Streptococcus pneumoniae* after vaccination of HIV infected subjects with 23-valent pneumococcal vaccine. *Journal of Infectious Diseases* 1992; **165**: 553–556.

67 Glaser J.B., Volpe S., Aguirre A., Simpkins H., Schiffman G. Zidovudine improves response to pneumococcal vaccine among persons with AIDS and AIDS related complex. *Journal of Infectious Diseases* 1991; **164**: 761–764.

68 Bremard-Oury C., Aucouturier P., Le Diest F., Debre M., Preund'homme J.L., Griscelli C. The spectrum of IgG2 deficiencies. In: Vossen J., Griscelli C., eds. *Progress in Immunodeficiency Research and Therapy*, Vol II. Amsterdam: Excerpta Medica, 1986: 235–239.

CHAPTER 3
*Acute bacterial and
viral pulmonary
infections in HIV*

69 Jain A., Jain S., Gant V. Should patients positive for HIV infection receive pneumococcal vaccine? *British Medical Journal* 1995; **310**: 1060–1062.

70 Gaston M.H., Verter J.I., Woods G. *et al.* Prophylaxis with oral penicillin in children with sickle cell anaemia: a randomized trial. *New England Journal of Medicine* 1986; **314**: 1593–1599.

71 Hardy W.D., Feinberg J., Finkelstein D.M. *et al.* A controlled trial of trimethoprim–sulphamethoxazole or aerosolized pentamidine for secondary prophylaxis of *Pneumocystis carinii* pneumonia in patients with the acquired immunodeficiency syndrome. *New England Journal of Medicine* 1992; **327**: 1842–1848.

4 *Pneumocystis carinii* infection

R.F. MILLER

4.0 Introduction

Pneumocystis carinii pneumonia was the first major opportunistic infection to be described in association with AIDS [1]. Despite effective primary and secondary prophylaxis (see below), *P. carinii* pneumonia remains a common cause of respiratory disease in HIV-infected individuals. This chapter reviews the molecular biology, pathology, clinical presentation, treatment and prevention of *P. carinii* infection.

4.1 History

P. carinii was described in 1911 by Chagas in guinea pigs and humans but was not recognized as a disease-causing organism until 40 years later, when it was identified as the causative agent of plasma-cell interstitial pneumonitis, a fulminant pneumonia of premature babies and malnourished infants. In the mid-1960s *P. carinii* pneumonia once again became clinically important in patients who were immunosuppressed by malignancy, the treatment thereof or organ transplantation. The majority of

81

infection was treated successfully with pentamidine or co-trimoxazole. It was not until the early 1980s, with the explosion of AIDS-associated infection, that attention focused on understanding the basic biology of the infection and on developing strategies for prevention and efficient diagnosis.

4.2 Pathology

Within the lung, *P. carinii* infection is characterized by an eosinophilic, foamy, intra-alveolar exudate, which is associated with a mild plasma-cell interstitial pneumonitis [2]. Morphologically, two forms of *P. carinii* may be identified. Thick-walled cysts (6–7 μm diameter, each containing between four and eight sporozoites), which lie freely within the alveolar exudate, are demonstrated by use of Grocott's methenamine silver, cresyl violet or *o*-toluidine blue stains [3]. The exudate consists largely of thin-walled, irregularly shaped, single-nucleated trophozoites (each 2–5 μm in size), which adhere to type 1 pneumocytes and are best shown by Giemsa staining or electron microscopy. Indirect immunofluorescence with monoclonal antibodies raised against *P. carinii* may also be used to identify both forms [3].

Unusually and atypically, diffuse alveolar damage, interstitial fibrosis, granulomatous inflammation, nodular or cavitating lesions and intrapulmonary cyst (pneumatocoele) formation may occur [2].

P. carinii infection rarely extends beyond the air spaces but extrapulmonary pneumocystosis involving other organs, such as the eye, liver, spleen and gut, may occur [4]. The occurrence of extrapulmonary pneumocystosis is strongly associated with use of nebulized pentamidine for prophylaxis or treatment (see below) [4].

4.3 Molecular biology

Until recently, *P. carinii* has been regarded taxonomically as a protozoan, based on the inability to culture the organism *in vitro*, its morphology and its response to antiprotozoal but not antifungal drugs. Use of molecular biological techniques has challenged this assignment and suggests that *P. carinii* is a fungus [5].

Comparison of many chromosomal and mitochondrial genes by cloning and sequencing from *P. carinii* and from a large number of different fungi representing all seven phyla clearly shows *P. carinii* to be a fungus [6–10]. There are antigenic [11,12] and genetic [13–15] differences in *P. carinii* isolated from different hosts and *P. carinii* from the lungs of one host species will not grow if they are placed in the lungs of another species, indicating host specificity.

There is genetic diversity within *P. carinii* derived from a single host; the lungs of rats and ferrets may be coinfected [13,16,17] with two types of *P. carinii*. Human-derived *P. carinii* shows lower levels of diversity [10,18–20]. As the majority of healthy children and adults have antibodies to *P. carinii* [21,22], it has been hypothesized that in an immunocompromised individual *P. carinii* pneumonia arises by reactivation of a latent childhood-acquired infection. However, studies of bronchoalveolar lavage fluid and autopsy lung tissue from immune-competent individuals, using monoclonal antibodies or deoxyribonucleic acid (DNA) amplification, have failed to demonstrate *P. carinii* [23–25]. Low levels of *P. carinii* have been identified in the lungs of only 20% of HIV-infected patients with respiratory symptoms and diagnoses other than *P. carinii* pneumonia [26].

Rats acquire *P. carinii* infection by the airborne route and human infection is thought to occur in the same way. Using air filters and spore traps, *P. carinii* DNA sequences have been identified in the air of rural locations [27], in laboratory facilities housing rats with *P. carinii* infection [28] and in the hospital rooms of AIDS patients with *P. carinii* pneumonia. There is a marked seasonal variation in incidence of *P. carinii* pneumonia in patients with AIDS, which may be due to changes in environmental temperature and humidity, factors that are important for growth of fungi and for dissemination of spores [29,30].

Recently, genetic diversity has been demonstrated among isolates of *P. carinii* from HIV-infected patients with repeat episodes of *P. carinii* pneumonia [20], suggesting that clinical pneumonia arises as a consequence of reinfection rather than reactivation of latent infection.

In summary, *P. carinii* is a fungus, with different types infecting different hosts. Human infection is not a zoonosis and clinical pneumonia in the majority of individuals arises by reinfection with airborne parasites rather than by reactivation of latent infection.

4.4 Clinical presentation

Typically, patients present with progressive exertional dysponea, a nonproductive cough and fever of several weeks' duration [31]. Many report a sensation of inability to take in a deep breath which is not due to pleural pain [32]. Purulent sputum, haemoptysis and pleural pain are atypical of *P. carinii* and suggest a bacterial or mycobacterial infection, or Kaposi's sarcoma, or that *P. carinii* pneumonia exists with a copathology [32]. On auscultation, the chest is usually clear; rarely, fine end-inspiratory crackles may be heard [31,32]. Typical and atypical features of *P. carinii* pneumonia are shown in Table 4.1.

Table 4.1 Presentation of *Pneumocystis carinii* pneumonia. From [31].

Typical presentation	Atypical presentation
General symptoms	
Progressive exertional dyspnoea over days or weeks	Sudden onset of dyspnoea over hours/days
Dry cough ± mucoid sputum	Cough productive of purulent sputum
Difficulty in taking a deep breath not due to pleuritic pain	Haemoptysis
Fevers ± sweats	Chest pain (pleuritic or crushing)
Tachypnoea	
Examination of the chest	
Normal breath sounds or fine end-inspiratory basal crackles	Wheeze, signs of focal consolidation or pleural effusion
Chest radiograph	
Normal	
or	
perihilar haze	Early
or	
bilateral interstitial shadowing or alveolar–interstitial changes or 'white-out' (marked alveolar consolidation with sparing of apices and costophrenic angles)	Late

Arterial blood gases

	Pa,O_2	Pa,CO_2
Early	Normal	Normal or ↓
Late	↓	Normal or ↓

Pa,O_2, arterial oxygen tension; Pa,CO_2, arterial carbon dioxide tension; ↓, reduced.

4.5 Investigations

4.5.1 Empirical therapy

Whether all HIV-infected patients with suspected *P. carinii* pneumonia require bronchoscopy to confirm a diagnosis remains a controversial issue. It has been suggested by some centres that it is not necessary to perform bronchoscopy in those with symptoms, radiographic abnormalities and hypoxaemia typical of *P. carinii* pneumonia and that such patients may be treated empirically, bronchoscopy being reserved with atypical presentations or those with typical *P. carinii* pneumonia who fail to respond by day 5 of therapy or who deteriorate on treatment [32,33]. In contrast, other centres have recommended that diagnosis is confirmed in every case. In practice, many centres treat patients with *P. carinii* pneumonia empirically. However, patients with *P. carinii* pneumonia treated with co-trimoxazole (or other therapy, see below) usually take between 4 and 7 days to show signs of clinical recovery, and improvements in the chest radiograph may take 2 weeks to be evident, so a bronchoscopically confirmed diagnosis ensures that the patient is receiving the correct therapy, particularly during the first week of treatment. Both strategies are equally effective in clinical practice [33].

Several tests help make a diagnosis of *P. carinii* pneumonia; these include non-invasive tests and invasive tests.

4.5.2 Non-invasive tests

These tests have moderate to high sensitivity but lack specificity. They are useful in determining the presence or absence of pulmonary disease, in assessment of disease severity, in deciding whether an invasive diagnostic test is needed (see below) and in monitoring response to therapy.

Chest radiology

The chest radiograph may be normal in early or mild pneumonia. With more severe disease or later presentation, diffuse perihilar interstitial infiltrates are seen (Fig. 4.1). These may progress to diffuse bilateral alveolar (air-space) consolidation, which mimics the appearance of pulmonary oedema (Fig. 4.2). In untreated severe disease, confluent alveolar shadowing, which tends to spare the lung apices and costophrenic angles, may occur (Fig. 4.3). Radiographic deterioration, from normal or near-normal appearances at presentation to being markedly abnormal, may occur over a period of 48 hours or less. With treatment and clinical recovery, some chest radiographs remain abnormal for many months in the absence of symptoms. Others show postinfectious bronchiectasis or residual fibrosis.

In up to 20% of patients with *P. carinii* pneumonia, the presenting chest radiograph shows atypical appearances, including upper-zone infiltrates resembling tuberculosis (TB) (Fig. 4.4), hilar and mediastinal lymphadenopathy, pleural effusion, lobar infiltrates (Fig. 4.5) or unilateral consolidation, nodules (Fig. 4.6a,b), cystic air spaces (Fig. 4.7) and pneumatocoele formation (Fig. 4.8). These typical and atypical radiographic appearances of *P. carinii* pneumonia may also be seen in pulmonary bacterial, mycobacterial and fungal infection, in non-specific pneumonitis and in pulmonary Kaposi's sarcoma.

Arterial blood gases

In mild *P. carinii* pneumonia, the arterial blood-gas tensions may be

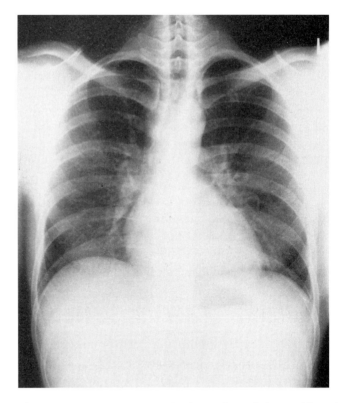

Fig. 4.1 Early *Pneumocystis carinii* pneumonia: chest radiograph showing bilateral perihilar infiltrates.

normal, but hypocarbia, indicating hyperventilation, with normal arterial oxygen tension may be the first detectable abnormality. With more severe pneumonia, hypoxaemia may occur. Hypercarbia together with hypoxaemia indicates severe respiratory compromise and is an ominous finding. Hypoxaemia and a widened alveolar–arterial oxygen gradient $(D(A–a)O_2)$ are present in over 70% of patients with *P. carinii* pneumonia; these abnormalities may also be found in patients with a bacterial infection, non-specific pneumonitis and pulmonary Kaposi's sarcoma.

Transcutaneous oximetry

Exercise-induced arterial desaturation, measured with a transcutaneous pulse oximeter, is a sensitive and specific method for diagnosis of *P. carinii* pneumonia in HIV-infected individuals with normal or near-normal chest radiographs and normal arterial oxygen tensions at rest. A normal exercise test, with no desaturation, virtually excludes a diagnosis of *P. carinii* pneumonia [34].

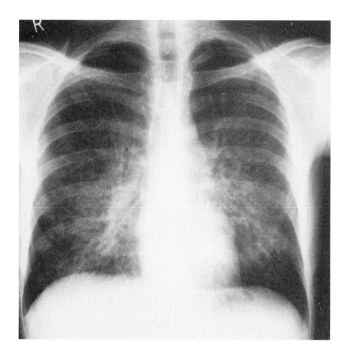

Fig. 4.2 Later presentation of *Pneumocystis carinii* pneumonia: chest radiograph showing more marked bilateral consolidation, which resembles the appearance of pulmonary oedema.

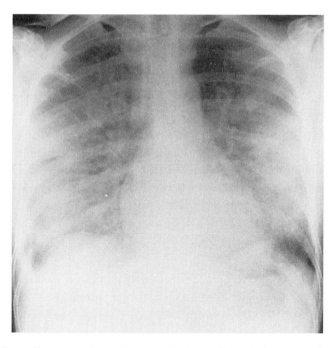

Fig. 4.3 Severe *Pneumocystis carinii* pneumonia: chest radiograph showing confluent alveolar shadowing, which spares the lung apices and costophrenic angles.

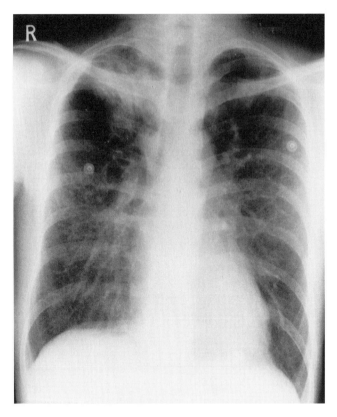

Fig. 4.4 *Pneumocystis carinii* pneumonia: chest radiograph showing right upper-lobe collapse and consolidation radiographically mimicking tuberculosis.

Pulmonary-function tests

The single-breath carbon monoxide transfer factor ($T_L$co) is a sensitive but non-specific measure of pulmonary abnormality in HIV-infected individuals. A value of $\leq 70\%$ of normal is frequently found in patients with *P. carinii* pneumonia, but also in other infections and in some HIV-infected individuals without respiratory disease [35]. The measurement of $T_L$co has a good negative predictive value, as a normal $T_L$co value excludes the presence of *P. carinii* pneumonia [35,36].

Lactate dehydrogenase enzyme

Serum lactate dehydrogenase (LDH) enzyme levels are raised in the majority of patients with *P. carinii* pneumonia and also in bacterial pneumonia and pulmonary Kaposi's sarcoma [37]. Widespread use of prophylaxis, especially with nebulized pentamidine (see below), has led to concerns that if relapse of *P. carinii* pneumonia occurs it may be clinically

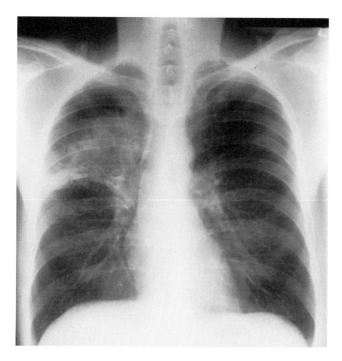

Fig. 4.5 *Pneumocystis carinii* pneumonia: chest radiograph showing lobar consolidation of the right upper lobe.

and radiographically atypical. In this situation, a raised LDH enzyme level may be diagnostically useful [38].

Nuclear medicine techniques

Diffuse or focal intrapulmonary accumulation of gallium-67-citrate occurs in inflammatory conditions, including *P. carinii* pneumonia and bacterial and mycobacterial infection. No accumulation of gallium-67-citrate occurs in Kaposi's sarcoma [39]. In an HIV-infected patient with an abnormal chest radiograph, imaging of the lungs with this radiotracer may help distinguish *P. carinii* and other infections from pulmonary Kaposi's sarcoma.

The rate of clearance of an inhaled aerosol technetium-diethylenetri-amine penta-acetate (DTPA) from alveoli to capillary is a measure of alveolar 'leakiness'. The rate of clearance is markedly increased in HIV-positive patients with *P. carinii* pneumonia, which is in contrast to those with pulmonary Kaposi's sarcoma and bacterial and mycobacterial infection [3]. Thus this test has a good specificity for diagnosis of *P. carinii* pneumonia; its clinical usefulness is restricted as it is not routinely available in the majority of hospitals.

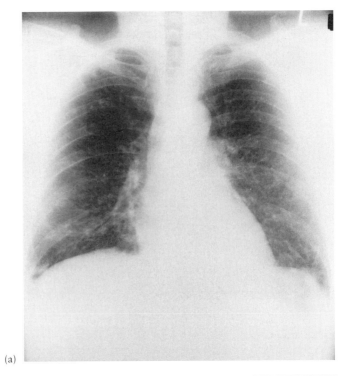

(a)

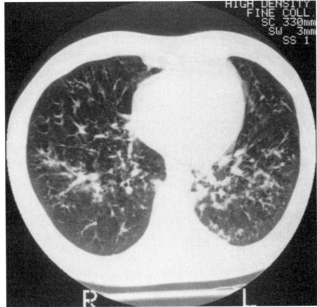

(b)

Fig. 4.6 *Pneumocystis carinii* pneumonia. (a) Chest radiograph showing a diffuse nodular appearance due to a granulomatous inflammatory response to *P. carinii*. (b) Same patient as (a). CT scan through lower lobes (lung window) showing diffuse bilateral intrapulmonary nodules

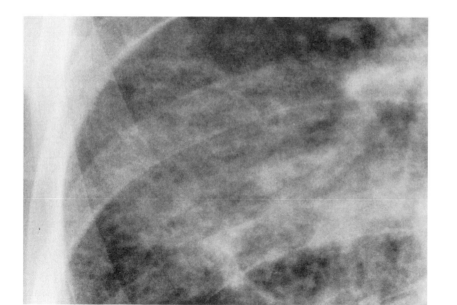

Fig. 4.7 *Pneumocystis carinii* pneumonia: chest radiograph; coned view of right upper lobe showing cystic air spaces.

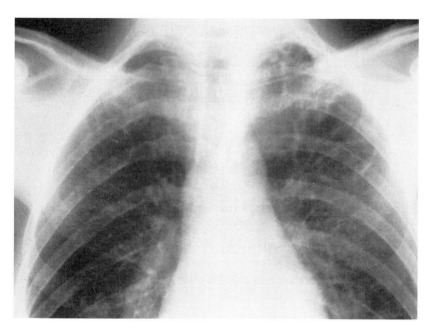

Fig. 4.8 *Pneumocystis carinii* pneumonia: chest radiograph showing multiple pneumatocoeles in both upper lobes.

4.5.3 Invasive tests

Sputum induction, fibre-optic bronchoscopy with bronchoalveolar lavage (with or without transbronchial biopsy) and open-lung biopsy enable a specific diagnosis to be made.

Hypertonic saline-induced sputum

As HIV-infected patients with suspected *P. carinii* pneumonia usually have a non-productive cough, sputum expectoration may be provoked by the patient inhaling an aerosol of hypertonic 2.7% (3 N) saline, generated by a high-output ultrasonic nebulizer, such as the UltraNeb 99m (Devillbliss) nebulizer [40]. For best results, the technique requires careful patient preparation, including careful cleaning of the mouth, so that oral debris does not contaminate the specimen, and the procedure should ideally be supervised by an experienced nurse or physiotherapist [40]. In prospective studies in which sputum induction has been compared with fibre-optic bronchoscopy, the yield from sputum induction for *P. carinii* (and other pathology) is lower than that from bronchoscopy [40]. In addition, some patients find the procedure of sputum induction unpleasant, and dyspnoea, cough, retching and unpredictable hypoxaemia [41] may develop during inhalation of saline and persist for up to 20 minutes afterwards. It is recommended that the patient's arterial oxygen saturation be monitored during the procedure, using a transcutaneous oximeter [41].

Bronchoscopy

Many centres do not routinely perform transbronchial biopsy, as fibre-optic bronchoscopy with bronchoalveolar lavage has a high diagnostic yield for *P. carinii*. Transbronchial biopsy adds little, if any, diagnostic information [42] and is associated with complications, including pneumothorax, in 20% of cases (which occurs whether or not fluoroscopic screening is used), and haemorrhage, which may be fatal.

In an HIV-positive patient with suspected *P. carinii* pneumonia, treatment should not be deferred until results of bronchoscopy are known. The diagnostic yield from bronchoalveolar lavage remains high, as cysts of *P. carinii* persist in the lung for many days after antimicrobial therapy is commenced.

Open-lung biopsy

This technique is occasionally performed in HIV-positive patients with diffuse pneumonia and negative results from two or more fibre-optic bronchoscopies and also in those patients who deteriorate despite treatment for bronchoscopically confirmed *P. carinii* pneumonia, in whom a second pathology is suspected [43]. In this group of patients, the procedure has a surprisingly low morbidity and a high diagnostic yield [43].

4.5.4 Molecular diagnostic techniques

Although still largely a research tool, the technique of DNA amplification using *P. carinii* oligonucleotide primers has been shown in prospective clinical studies to be superior to conventional silver staining of bronchoalveolar lavage [26] and induced sputum [44] for the diagnosis of *P. carinii* pneumonia. A single pilot study has shown that *P. carinii* DNA can be detected by molecular biological techniques in samples of saliva in up to 80% of patients with bronchoscopically confirmed *P. carinii* pneumonia [45].

4.6 Prognosis

Several clinical and laboratory features have prognostic significance in an HIV-infected patient with *P. carinii* (Table 4.2) [46]. A severity score based on serum LDH levels, the $D(A–a)O_2$ and the percentage of

Table 4.2 Prognostic factors predictive of a poor outcome in HIV patients with *Pneumocystis carinii* pneumonia. Modified from [46].

On admission
No previous knowledge of HIV status
Recurrent *P. carinii* pneumonia (second, third or fourth episode)
Prolonged history of dry cough/dyspnoea (>4 weeks)
Tachypnoea(>30 breaths/min)
Poor oxygenation
  $Pa,O_2 < 7.0\,kPa$
  Alveolar–arterial oxygen gradient $\geq 4.0\,kPa$
Marked chest radiographic abnormalities (diffuse bilateral interstitial infiltrates with or
  without alveolar consolidation)
Peripheral blood leucocytosis ($>10.8 \times 10^9$ cells/l)
Low serum albumin (<35 g/l)
Raised serum lactate dehydrogenase enzyme levels (>300 U/l)

Following admission
Bacterial copathogen in induced sputum or bronchoalveolar lavage fluid
Neutrophilia (>5%) in bronchoalveolar lavage fluid
Marked interstitial oedema in transbronchial biopsy specimens
Serum lactate dehydrogenase enzyme levels that remain elevated despite specific anti-
  P. carinii therapy

Table 4.3 Grading of severity of *Pneumocystis carinii* pneumonia. Modified from [3] and [76].

	Mild	Moderate	Severe
Symptoms and signs	Dyspnoea on exertion, with or without cough and sweats	Dyspnoea on minimal exertion and occasionally at rest. Cough and fever	Dyspnoea and tachypnoea at rest. Persistent fever and cough
Arterial oxygen tension (Pa,o_2) (at rest)	>11.0 kPa	8.0–11.0 kPa	<8.0 kPa
Arterial oxygen saturation (Sa,o_2)	>96%	91–96%	<91%
Chest radiograph	Normal or minor perihilar shadowing	Diffuse interstitial shadowing	Extensive interstitial shadowing with or without diffuse alveolar shadowing

neutrophils in bronchoalveolar fluid has a high prognostic significance — with the highest scores indicating the poorest outcome [47].

4.7 Treatment

Before instituting treatment, it is important to make an assessment of the severity of the pneumonia, using the history, examination findings, results of arterial blood-gas estimations and chest radiograph in order to stratify patients into those having mild, moderate or severe disease. Table 4.3 [3]. In severe disease, some drugs are known to be ineffective and others are of unproved benefit. Those with moderate and severe disease should receive adjunctive steroids (see below) [48].

Co-trimoxazole, dapsone and primaquine should not be used in patients with glucose-6-phosphate dehydrogenase deficiency, as this increases the risk of haemolysis. When patients are receiving high-dose co-trimoxazole, ganciclovir and zidovudine should be stopped because of the potential for severe marrow toxicity.

4.7.1 Co-trimoxazole

Co-trimoxazole — 100 mg/kg/day of sulphamethoxazole and 20 mg/kg/day trimethoprin — given in two to four divided doses either orally or intravenously for 21 days is the drug of first choice to treat *P. carinii* pneumonia of any severity (Table 4.4) [49,50]. For intravenous use, the drug is diluted 1:25 in 0.9% saline or 5% dextrose in water and is infused over

Table 4.4 Treatment of *Pneumocystis carinii* pneumonia. From [76].

	Severity of *P. carinii* pneumonia		
	Mild	Moderate	Severe
First line	Co-trimoxazole	Co-trimoxazole	Co-trimoxazole
Second line	i.v. pentamidine or Clindamycin and primaquine or Dapsone and trimethoprim	i.v. pentamidine or Dapsone and trimethoprim	i.v. pentamidine
Third line	Atovaquone	Clindamycin and primaquine or Tremetrexate or Atovaquone	Clindamycin and primaquine or Tremetrexate
Fourth line	Trimetrexate	Eflornithine	Eflornithine
Fifth line	Nebulized pentamidine* Eflornithine		
Adjunctive steroids	Unproved benefit	Benefit	Benefit

* If used, combine with i.v. pentamidine for the first 3–5 days of therapy.
For doses and route of administration see text. Co-trimoxazole is the best treatment for
P. carinii pneumonia of all severity; if co-trimoxazole used, stop zidovudine. Avoid co-
trimoxazole, dapsone and primaquine in patients with glucose-6-phosphate dehydrogenase
deficiency.

$1\frac{1}{2}$–2 hours. Used orally, two 'double-strength' (1960 mg) tablets are
given three or four times daily. Up to 80% of patients will respond to
therapy [49,50].

Adverse reactions to co-trimoxazole, which usually become evident at
between 6 and 14 days of treatment, are common. Neutropenia and
anaemia occur in up to 40% of patients, rash in approximately 25%,
fever in greater than 20% and abnormalities of liver function in approximately 10% [49,50]. Folic or folinic acid does not prevent or attenuate
co-trimoxazole-induced haematological toxicity and it may be associated
with increased therapeutic failure [51]. This may be due to folinic acid
antagonizing the action of trimethoprim and sulphamethoxazole on the
folic acid metabolism of *P. carinii*. If the dose of co-trimoxazole is reduced
to 75% of the dose given above, there is an improved toxicity profile and
efficacy is maintained [49].

There is no clear explanation for the high frequency of adverse reactions to co-trimoxazole in HIV-infected individuals [52]. HIV-induced

changes in acetylator status-dependent metabolism of co-trimoxazole to toxic metabolites, such as hydroxylamines, glutathione deficiency, alterations in immunoglobulin E (IgE) synthesis and immunopathogenic effects of HIV and herpesviruses, such as cytomegalovirus (CMV) or Epstein–Barr virus (EBV), have all been suggested as possible explanations [52]. The optimal strategy for a patient who becomes intolerant of co-trimoxazole remains to be elucidated. Many physicians 'treat through' minor rash, often with addition of antihistamines and a short course of oral steroids (typically prednisolone 30 mg once daily reducing to zero, for 5–7 days). Desensitization has been successful in some individuals who develop adverse reactions to co-trimoxazole [53,54].

4.7.2 Pentamidine

Intravenous (i.v.) pentamidine (4 mg/kg) as a single daily infusion to 250 ml of 5% dextrose in water over 1–2 hours for 21 days is second-choice therapy for *P. carinii* pneumonia, whatever the severity. Pentamidine is not given by intramuscular (i.m.) injection because of the risk of sterile abscesses. In patients with renal impairment, reduced doses of pentamidine are given; when the glomerular filtration rate falls to between 10 and 50 ml/min, the drug is given every 36 hours and, if less than 10 ml/min, it is given every 48 hours [48]. Compared with high-dose co-trimoxazole, pentamidine is of almost equivalent efficacy but has greater toxicity [49,50]. Over half of patients given pentamidine develop nephrotoxicity (usually an isolated elevation of serum creatinine), approximately 50% develop leucopenia and up to a quarter experience hypotension or nausea and vomiting [49]. Hypoglycaemia occurs in approximately 20% of patients. Toxicity is improved, but efficacy is not compromised, if the dose is reduced to 3 mg/kg/day [49]. Coadministration of i.v. pentamidine and high-dose co-trimoxazole is associated with a much higher rate of toxicity than occurs with either drug used alone and confers no therapeutic advantage [55].

4.7.3 Other therapy

If co-trimoxazole or pentamidine is not tolerated by the patient or if treatment fails, several alternative therapies are available (Table 4.4).

4.7.4 Dapsone with trimethoprim

In patients with mild and moderately severe *P. carinii* pneumonia, the combination of oral dapsone (100 mg/day) and trimethoprim (20 mg/kg/day) is as effective as oral co-trimoxazole (dose as above) and is better tolerated [56]. Rash, nausea and vomiting, and asymptomatic methaemoglobinaemia (due to dapsone) are the major side-effects with this combination. Up to half of patients develop mild hyperkalaemia (<6.1 mmol/l). The drug has not been shown to be of benefit in severe disease.

4.7.5 Clindamycin with primaquine

The combination of clindamycin, a broad-spectrum antibiotic, and the antimalarial drug primaquine was originally used to 'salvage' patients with mild and moderate-severity disease who were failing to respond to co-trimoxazole or pentamidine [57]. In doses of clindamycin 300–450 mg four times a day (q.d.s.) and primaquine 15 mg once a day (o.d.) given orally, the combination is as effective as oral dapsone/trimethoprim and co-trimoxazole for initial treatment of mild and moderate-severity *P. carinii* pneumonia [58]. In severe disease, clindamycin is usually given i.v. (450–600 mg q.d.s.). Rash occurs in almost two-thirds of patients and approximately 25% develop diarrhoea [58]. If diarrhoea occurs, the stool should be analysed for the presence of *Clostridium difficile* toxin.

4.7.6 Atovaquone

Oral atovaquone in a dose of 750 mg three times daily is less effective than either high-dose co-trimoxazole [59] or i.v. pentamidine [60] for mild and moderate-severity *P. carinii* pneumonia, but is better tolerated than either of these drugs. There are no data to support its use in patients with severe disease. Common adverse reactions include rash, nausea and vomiting and constipation. Absorption of atovaquone tablets from the gastrointestinal tract is highly variable [59]; taking the tablets with food increases their absorption. The formulation as a suspension offers increased bioavailability of atovaquone but may be associated with a higher frequency of adverse reactions consequent upon increased absorption of drug.

4.7.7 Trimetrexate

Trimetrexate, a methotrexate analogue, used at a dose of 45 mg/m^2 given i.v. (with folinic acid 20 mg/m^2 q.d.s. by mouth to protect human cells from trimetrexate-induced toxicity) for 21 days is less effective than co-trimoxazole when used as initial treatment of moderate and severe *P. carinii* pneumonia; the two regimens have similar rates of toxicity [61]. when used to 'salvage' patients who have failed to respond to co-trimoxazole or i.v. pentamidine, approximately two-thirds of patients will respond to trimetrexate [62].

4.7.8 Eflornithine

Intravenous eflornithine (in a dose of 400 mg/kg/day in divided doses) has been used as 'salvage' therapy in patients who have failed to respond to treatment with i.v. co-trimoxazole or pentamidine. In this situation, it is >60% effective. The main side-effects include neutropenia and phlebitis, both of which occur in approximately half of patients [63].

4.7.9 Nebulized pentamidine

This form of therapy is less effective than i.v. pentamidine, and it is now only rarely used to treat mild and moderate-severity *P. carinii* pneumonia [64]. It should not be used to treat severe disease. Patients given nebulized pentamidine in a dose of 600 mg/day for 21 days respond very slowly. It may take 10–14 days for reduction in fever and dyspnoea and improvements in radiographic appearances and blood gases to occur [64,65]. Following treatment of *P. carinii* pneumonia with nebulized pentamidine, there is a greater rate of relapse when compared with patients given parenteral pentamidine or co-trimoxazole. As very little, if any, drug is systemically absorbed, development of extrapulmonary pneumocystosis may not be suppressed [4]. Some centres advocate combining nebulized pentamidine with i.v. pentamidine (doses as above) for the first 3–5 days of therapy to ensure rapid accumulation of drug within the lungs [66].

4.7.10 Corticosteroids

Adjunctive therapy with corticosteroids for patients with moderate and severe *P. carinii* pneumonia has been shown to reduce the risk of respiratory failure (by up to half) [67] and the risk of death (by up to one-third) [68]. It is thought that corticosteroids act by reducing the body's intrapulmonary inflammatory response to *P. carinii*. It is recommended that glucocorticoids are given to HIV-infected patients with proved or suspected *P. carinii* pneumonia who have an arterial partial pressure of oxygen (Pa,o_2) of ≤ 9.3 kPa or a $D(A–a)o_2$ of ≥ 4.7 kPa (both measured while breathing room air) [69]. Oral or i.v. corticosteroids should be started at the same time as or within 72 hours of specific anti-*Pneumocystis* therapy. In some patients, it will be necessary to begin treatment on a presumptive basis, pending confirmation of the diagnosis as soon as possible. Several regimens of corticosteroids have been used; the most commonly used is oral prednisolone 40 mg given twice daily for 5 days, thereafter 40 mg given once daily for days 6 to 10 and then 20 mg once daily for 10 further days [48]. Intravenous methylprednisolone may be given at 75% of these doses; alternatively, higher doses may be given for a shorter period of time. A regimen widely used in the UK is methylprednisolone 1 g once daily for 3 days, then 0.5 g on days 4 to 6, followed by oral prednisolone initially 40 mg once daily and thereafter reducing to zero over 10 days. There is no evidence that adjunctive corticosteroids are of benefit in patients with mild *P. carinii* pneumonia, although it would be difficult to demonstrate benefit, as the expected outcome in mild disease is good.

4.7.11 General management

Patients with mild *P. carinii* pneumonia may be treated with oral co-trimoxazole as out-patients under close medical supervision. Clearly, patients should be able to cope at home and be willing and able to attend the out-patient department for regular review. If oral co-trimoxazole is not tolerated despite clinical recovery, the drug may be given i.v., or treatment may be changed to oral clindamycin with primaquine, dapsone with trimethoprim or atovaquone (Table 4.4).

All patients with moderate and severe *P. carinii* pneumonia should always initially be treated in hospital with i.v. co-trimoxazole or pentamidine and adjunctive steroids. If within 7–10 days the patient has not responded to either regimen or has deteriorated before this time, he/she should be switched to the other drug, where possible allowing ≥48 hours' overlap with therapy to allow intrapulmonary accumulation of the new drug. If there is still no evidence of response, i.v. clindamycin with oral primaquine, i.v. trimetrexate with folinic acid or i.v. eflornithine should be used. Patients with moderate and severe *P. carinii* pneumonia at presentation who respond to i.v. co-trimoxazole and adjunctive steroids and show a good response by 7–10 days of i.v. therapy can be switched to oral co-trimoxazole to complete the remaining 11–14 days of therapy.

4.7.12 The deteriorating patient

Deterioration in a patient with *P. carinii* pneumonia may be due to a severe progressive *P. carinii* pneumonia, to side-effects of treatment, such as anaemia, to other diseases, such as pulmonary Kaposi's sarcoma or bacterial pneumonia mimicking *P. carinii* pneumonia, to coinfections or to other complications of treatment (which may be iatrogenic), such as pneumothorax or left ventricular failure secondary to fluid overload [46,70]. Before therapy is changed, it is important to consider these possible alternative explanations for the patient's deterioration. Consideration should be given to treating any copathogens present in sputum or bronchoalveolar lavage fluid, to performing fibre-optic bronchoscopy if treatment has been on an empirical basis or repeating the investigation if the patient has already been bronchoscoped or to proceeding to open-lung biopsy in order to confirm that the diagnosis is correct [43,46,70].

4.7.13 Intensive care

Pulmonary oedema and fluid overload may complicate severe *P. carinii* pneumonia. Myocardial ischaemia, shown by electrocardiogram (ECG) abnormalities, occurs in many severely ill, hypoxaemic patients with *P. carinii* pneumonia. This may lead to impaired left ventricular compliance and an increase in left atrial pressure, with development of pulmonary oedema [43]. The large volumes of fluid required to give i.v. co-trimoxazole may produce fluid overload and left ventricular failure: the drug can be administered diluted in 5% dextrose in water at a ratio of 10:1 [70].

All patients with *P. carinii* pneumonia who are hypoxaemic should receive supplementary oxygen via a tight-fitting Venturi-principle face-mask, with the aim of maintaining the $Pa,o_2 \geq 8.0\,kPa$ (or the arterial oxygen saturation $\geq 91\%$) [43]. Once an inspired oxygen concentration of 60% is needed to maintain a $Pa,o_2 \geq 8.0\,kPa$ by non-invasive ventilatory support with a nasal or face-mask, continuous positive airway pressure (CPAP) should be considered [71]. CPAP probably acts as a pneumatic splint, holding open narrow, poorly compliant airways and so improving oxygenation. CPAP is particularly useful when a patient deteriorates following bronchoscopy; CPAP will frequently tide the patient over this self-limiting deterioration, once a pneumothorax has been excluded as the cause of the deterioration. CPAP is well tolerated by patients, who often report a significant reduction in dyspnoea. Rare complications of the technique include pneumothorax, mediastinal emphysema, gastric aspiration and mask-pressure necrosis [71].

If adequate oxygenation is not maintained by CPAP ventilation or the patient becomes tired or the arterial partial pressure of carbon dioxide (Pa,co_2) rises, consideration should be given to transferring the patient to the intensive care unit for intubation and mechanical ventilation. Most centres would offer mechanical ventilation for a first episode of *P. carinii* pneumonia and for rapid and severe postbronchoscopy deterioration [70]. In patients with severe *P. carinii* pneumonia and respiratory failure, the interval between the start of specific anti-*P. carinii* therapy and the need for mechanical ventilation and also the duration of HIV seropositivity are factors which discriminate between survivors and non-survivors. Mortality rates of approximately 50% are seen in patients who receive less than 5 days of co-trimoxazole and adjunctive corticosteroids and 95% in those who receive more than 5 days of therapy before ventilation is commenced. Survivors tend to have a shorter HIV history [70,72]. Use of adjunctive corticosteroids may have influenced the natural history of *P. carinii*-associated respiratory failure by selecting out a subgroup of patients with severe *P. carinii* pneumonia in whom treatment has failed [72,73]. Before deciding to institute ventilation, it is important to carefully consider the patient's previous HIV history, current quality of life and likely prognosis, not only from the episode of pneumonia but also in the long term from HIV disease itself, and to take into account the wishes of their partner or next of kin [43,70]. Once a patient has been mechanically ventilated, it is important to set clear goals and objectives so that the patient will not remain mechanically ventilated with an ever-decreasing chance of recovery [70].

4.8 Prophylaxis

With the progressive immunosuppression induced by HIV, associated with falls in CD4 (T-helper-lymphocyte count), individuals are at increased risk of developing *P. carinii* pneumonia [74]. Primary prophylaxis is given, to prevent a first episode of *P. carinii* pneumonia, to patients who have CD4 counts $<0.20 \times 10^9$ cells/l, a CD4-to-total lymphocyte count ratio <1.5 or HIV-related constitutional symptoms, such as fever or oral *Candida*, regardless of the CD4 lymphocyte count, and to those with other AIDS-defining illnesses such as Kaposi's sarcoma. Secondary prophylaxis is given in order to prevent a recurrence [48,75]. Once started, prophylaxis is lifelong and so regimens used should ideally be easily administered, in order to optimize compliance, cheap and effective, have low toxicity and not interact adversely with antiretroviral therapy [76].

4.8.1 Co-trimoxazole

Oral co-trimoxazole 960 mg once daily or three times a week is the first-choice regimen for both primary and secondary prophylaxis (Table 4.5) [48,75]. Trimethoprim is not an effective drug when used alone [77]. Co-trimoxazole may also protect against bacterial infections and reactivation of cerebral toxoplasmosis and does not react adversely with zidovudine at these doses. Rash, which occurs in about 20% of individuals, nausea, headache and bone-marrow suppression (usually neutropenia and thrombocytopenia) are the commonest adverse reactions. It is worth attempting desensitization in a patient who has developed an adverse reaction to co-trimoxazole before considering a change to an alternative agent for prophylaxis [53,54].

The efficacy and toxicity of oral co-trimoxazole as primary prophylaxis given at doses of 480 mg and 960 mg once daily have been compared with nebulized pentamidine 300 mg per month administered by a Respir-

Table 4.5 Prophylaxis of *Pneumocystis carinii* pneumonia. From [76].

	Drug	Dose	Route	Comment
First line	Co-trimoxazole	960 mg o.d.	Oral	480 mg o.d. or 960 mg 3 times a week may be equally effective. May protect against bacterial infection and reactivation of cerebral toxoplasmosis
Second line	Pentamidine	300 mg once a month	Jet nebulizer	Consider increasing dose to fortnightly if CD4 count $<0.05 \times 10^9$ cells/l
Third line	Dapsone with or without pyrimethamine	100 mg o.d.	Oral	Pyrimethamine may protect against reactivation of cerebral toxoplasmosis
Fourth line	Pentamidine	300 mg once every 2–4 weeks	i.v. or i.m.	May cause severe side-effects
Fifth line	Sulfadoxine and pyrimethamine	1 g and 50 mg both once a week	Oral Oral	Less effective than other regimens
Anecdotal	Dapsone with trimethoprim	100 mg o.d. 20 mg/kg o.d.	Oral Oral	
	Atovaquone	750 mg t.d.s.	Oral	
	Clindamycin with primaquine	300–450 mg t.d.s.–q.d.s. 1.5 mg o.d.	Oral Oral	

t.d.s., three times a day.

gard II jet nebulizer in HIV-infected individuals with CD4 lymphocyte counts $<0.20 \times 10^9$ cells/l [78]. During follow-up (mean $=9$ months), none of those receiving either dose of co-trimoxazole but 11% of those receiving pentamidine developed *P. carinii* pneumonia. In the first 3 months, the incidence of toxic events was 21, 26 and 3% for low- and high-dose co-trimoxazole and pentamidine, respectively. Adverse reactions to co-trimoxazole occurred sooner in those who received 960 mg compared with those who received 480 mg.

Co-trimoxazole at dose of 960 mg given three times a week has been prospectively compared with monthly inhaled pentamidine 300 mg and dapsone 100 mg once daily with pyrimethamine 25 mg once a week [79]. During follow-up, the yearly attack rate for *P. carinii* pneumonia in co-trimoxazole-treated patients was 3% but adverse reactions were commoner in those who received co-trimoxazole and dapsone with pyrimethamine compared with those who received inhaled pentamidine. Compliance with intermittent therapy is a potential problem for some patients, as missing any one of the doses may result in inadequate prophylaxis and breakthrough infection may occur.

Co-trimoxazole 960 mg once daily, dapsone 100 mg once daily and nebulized pentamidine 300 mg per month have been compared as primary prophylaxis in HIV-infected patients with CD4 counts $<0.20 \times 10^9$ cells/l who were receiving zidovudine. The cumulative risk of *P. carinii* pneumonia over 36 months was 18, 17 and 21% in those receiving co-trimoxazole, dapsone and pentamidine, respectively [80]. Co-trimoxazole 960 mg once daily was compared with nebulized pentamidine 300 mg monthly given by a Respigard II nebulizer for secondary prophylaxis in AIDS patients who were also taking zidovudine [81]. The risk of recurrent *P. carinii* pneumonia was more than three times greater in the pentamidine-treated group. Previous adverse drug reactions occurring during treatment of *P. carinii* pneumonia with high-dose co-trimoxazole did not predict subsequent toxicity when the drug was used for secondary prophylaxis [81].

4.8.2 Nebulized pentamidine

Nebulized pentamidine is the second choice for primary and secondary prophylaxis [75] (Table 4.5). Nebulized pentamidine given by a Respirgard II nebulizer 300 mg per month has been shown to be superior to either 30 mg or 150 mg given once a fortnight [82]. However, nebulized pentamidine is less effective than oral co-trimoxazole for both primary and secondary prophylaxis [78,81].

The most common adverse reactions to pentamidine are cough and bronchospasm [82]; hypersalivation, a bitter metallic taste and nausea also occur. A bronchodilator, such as salbutamol 200 µg, via a metered-dose inhaler, is routinely given before administering the pentamidine [66]. The nebulized pentamidine should deposit in the alveoli and not in the upper airways and oropharynx. Conventional nebulizers produce an heterogeneous aerosol, containing some large particles which deposit in the upper respiratory tract, and so they are inappropriate for pentamidine aerosol delivery [66]. The Respirgard II jet nebulizer contains several internal 'baffles', which prevent the passage of larger droplets into the aerosol; with this delivery system, the frequency of adverse reactions is markedly reduced [65,66]. Nebulized pentamidine prophylaxis is approximately eight times more expensive than treatment with co-trimoxazole [48]. The process of nebulization and any associated coughing may increase the risk of nosocomial transmission of respiratory disease, such as tuberculosis, to other patients or healthcare workers [66]. Adverse reactions, including cough, bronchoconstriction, circumoral paraesthesia and metallic taste, due to environmental contamination have been reported among healthcare workers supervising the process of pentamidine nebulization [3,48,66]. It is recommended that nebulization of pentamidine in hospital wards or out-patient departments should be carried out in a separate room, with its own extraction and ventilation system. Once the nebulizer is loaded with drug and connected to the piped air supply or compressor, healthcare workers should leave the room and not return until nebulization is complete [66]. Nebulized pentamidine prophylaxis may also alter the clinical presentation of *P. carinii* pneumonia. An increased proportion of patients have atypical radiographs, with upper-zone abnormalities [3,83]. Nebulized pentamidine is unlikely to prevent extrapulmonary pneumocystosis, as very little drug is absorbed systemically [4].

In profoundly immunosuppressed patients with CD4 lymphocyte counts $<0.05 \times 10^9$ cells/l who are intolerant of co-trimoxazole, nebulized pentamidine is often given more frequently, for example 300 mg once a fortnight, although the relapse rate with this regimen may not be any lower [84]. Anecdotally, some centres are combining nebulized pentamidine, given every fortnight, with oral medication, such as dapsone 100 mg per day, for patients who have had multiple episodes of *P. carinii* pneumonia (M.A. Johnson, personal communication).

4.8.3 Dapsone

Dapsone 50 mg or 100 mg daily is effective primary and secondary prophylaxis [85]. Dapsone may be combined with pyrimethamine, but this adds little to the effect of dapsone against *P. carinii* [86]. In a randomized trial, dapsone 50 mg per day with pyrimethamine 50 mg per week was as effective as nebulized pentamidine 300 mg per month for primary prophylaxis. By 18 months of follow-up, 5.5% of patients receiving either regimen had developed *P. carinii* pneumonia. Although nebulized pentamidine was better tolerated than dapsone with pyrimethamine, the combination appeared to protect against reactivation of cerebral toxoplasmosis [87]. In another study, dapsone 100 mg given three times weekly with pyrimethamine 25 mg given once per week was less effective prophylaxis than co-trimoxazole 960 mg three times weekly [88].

4.8.4 Parenteral pentamidine

I.v. [89] or i.m. [90] pentamidine at a dose of 4 mg/kg every 2–4 weeks has been used in patients intolerant of other therapy and in those who have recurrent *P. carinii* pneumonia while taking other regimens of prophylaxis. With this method of prophylaxis, there is often severe local (muscle abscess or phlebitis) or systemic (hypotension, dysrhythmias, hypoglycaemia) toxicity [89,90].

4.8.5 Other drugs

The combination of sulfadoxine 1 g with pyrimethamine 50 mg, both given once a week, appears to be the least effective [91]. There is only anecdotal evidence for the efficacy of dapsone with trimethoprim, clindamycin with primaquine and atovaquone as primary or secondary prophylaxis.

References

1 Gottlieb M.S., Schanker K., Pan P. *Pneumocystis* pneumonia — Los Angeles. *Morbidity, Mortality Weekly Report* 1981; **30**: 250–252.

2 Foley N.M., Griffiths M.H., Miller R.F. Histologically atypical *P. carinii* pneumonia. *Thorax* 1993; **48**: 996–1001.

3 Miller R.F., Mitchell D.M. *Pneumocystis carinii* pneumonia. *Thorax* 1992; **47**: 303–314.

4 Coker R.J., Clark D., Claydon E.L. *et al.* Disseminated *Pneumocystis carinii* infection in AIDS. *Journal of Clinical Pathology* 1991; **44**: 820–823.

5 Stringer J.R. The identity of *Pneumocystis carinii:* not a single protozoan, but a diverse group of exotic fungi. *Infectious Agents and Disease* 1993; **2**: 109–117.

6 Pixley F.J., Wakefield A.E., Banerji S., Hopkin J.M. Mitochondrial gene sequences show fungal homology for *Pneumocystis carinii. Molecular Microbiology* 1991; **5**: 1347–1351.

7 Van de Peer Y., Hendrick L., Goris A. *et al.* Evolution of basidiomycetous yeasts as deduced from small ribosomal sub-unit RNA sequences. *Systematic and Applied Microbiology* 1992; **15**: 250–258.

8 Edlind T.D., Bartlett M.S., Weinberg G.A., Prah G.N., Smith J.W. The β tubulin gene from rat and human isolates of *Pneumocystis carinii. Molecular Microbiology* 1992; **6**: 3365–3373.

9 Banerji S., Wakefield A.E., Allen A.G., Maskell D.J., Peters S.E., Hopkin J.M. The cloning and characterisation of the *arom* gene in *Pneumocystis carinii. Journal of General Microbiology* 1993; **139**: 2901.

10 Wakefield A.E., Fritscher C., Malin A., Gwanzura L., Hughes W.T., Miller R.F. Analysis of genetic diversity in human-derived *Pneumocystis carinii* isolated from four geographical locations. *Journal of Clinical Microbiology* 1994; **32**: 2959–2961.

11 Bauer N.L., Paulsrud J.R., Bartlett M.S., Smith J.W., Wilde C.E. *Pneumocystis carinii* organisms from rats, ferrets and mice are antigenically different. *Infection and Immunity* 1993; **61**: 1315–1319.

12 Kovacs J.A., Halpern J.L., Suran J.C., Moss P., Parillo J.E., Masur H. Identification of antigens and antibodies specific for *Pneumocystis carinii. Journal of Immunology* 1988; **140**: 2023–2031.

13 Hong S.-T., Steele P.E., Cushion M.T., Walzer P.D., Stringer S.L., Stringer J.R. *Pneumocystis carinii* karyotypes. *Journal of Clinical Microbiology* 1990; **28**: 1785–1795.

14 Sinclair K., Wakefield A.E., Banerji S., Hopkin J.M., *Pneumocystis carinii* organisms

derived from rat and human hosts are genetically distinct. *Molecular and Biochemical Parasitology* 1991; **45**: 183–184.

15 Stringer J.R., Stringer S.L., Zhang J., Baughman R., Smulian A.G., Cushion M.T. Molecular genetic distinction of *Pneumocystis* from rats and humans. *Journal of Eukaryotic Microbiology* 1993; **40**: 733–741.

16 Banerji S., Lugli E.B., Miller R.F., Wakefield A.E., Analysis of genetic diversity at the *arom* locus in isolates of *Pneumocystis carinii*. *Journal of Eukaryotic Microbiology* 1995; **42**: 676–679.

17 Cushion M.T., Zhang J., Kaselis M., Giuntoli D., Stringer S.L., Stringer J.R. Evidence for two genetic variants of *Pneumocystis carinii* co-infecting laboratory rats. *Journal of Clinical Microbiology* 1993; **31**: 1217–1223.

18 Lee C.H., Bartlett M.S., Durkin M.M. *et al.* Nucleotide sequence variation in *Pneumocystis carinii* strains that infect humans. *Journal of Clinical Microbiology* 1993; **31**: 754–757.

19 Lu J.-J., Bartlett M.S., Shaw M.M. *et al.* Typing of *Pneumocystis carinii* strains that infect humans based on nucleotide sequence variations of internal transcribed spacers of the rRNA gene. *Journal of Clinical Microbiology* 1994; **32**: 2904–2912.

20 Keely S.P., Stringer J.R., Banghman R.P., Lenke M.J., Waltzer P.D., Smulian A.C. Genetic variations among *Pneumocystis carinii hominis* isolates in recurrent pneumocystosis. *Journal of Infectious Diseases* 1995; **172**: 595–598.

21 Wakefield A.E., Stewart T.J., Moxon E.R., Marsh K., Hopkin J.M. Infection with *Pneumocystis carinii* is prevalent in healthy Gambian children. *Transactions of the Royal Society of Tropical Medicine and Hygiene* 1990; **84**: 800–802.

22 Peglow S.L., Smulian A.G., Linke M.J. *et al.* Serological responses to *Pneumocystis carinii* in health and disease. *Journal of Infectious Diseases* 1990; **161**: 296–306.

23 Millard P.R., Heryet A.R. Observations favouring *Pneumocystis carinii* pneumonia as a primary infection: a monoclonal antibody study on paraffin sections. *Journal of Pathology* 1988; **154**: 365–370.

24 Peters S.E., Wakefield A.E., Sinclair K., Millard P.J., Hopkin J.M. A search for latent *Pneumocystis carinii* infection in post-mortem lungs by DNA amplification. *Journal of Pathology* 1991; **166**: 195–198.

25 Matusiewicz S.P., Ferguson R.J., Greening A.P., Cromptom G.K., Burns S.M. *Pneumocystis carinii* in bronchoalveolar lavage fluid and bronchial washings. *British Medical Journal* 1994; **308**: 1206–1207.

26 Wakefield A.E., Pixley F.J., Banerjis, Miller R.F., Moxon E.R., Hopkin J.M. Detection of *Pneumocystis carinii* with DNA amplification. *Lancet* 1990; **336**: 451–453.

27 Wakefield A.E. Detection of DNA sequences identical to *Pneumocystis carinii* in samples of ambient air. *Journal of Eukaryotic Microbiology* 1994; **41**: 116S.

28 Bartlett M.S., Lee C.H., Lu J.-J. *et al. Pneumocystis carinii* detection in air. *Journal of Eukaryotic Microbiology* 1994; **41**: 75S.

29 Miller R.F., Grant A.D., Foley N.M. Seasonal variation in presentation of *Pneumocystis carinii* pneumonia. *Lancet* 1992; **339**: 747–748.

30 Hoover D.R., Saah A.J., Bacellar H. *et al.* Clinical manifestations of AIDS in the era of *Pneumocystis* prophylaxis. *New England Journal of Medicine* 1993; **329**: 1922–1926.

31 Malin A., Miller R.F. Diagnosis and investigation of *Pneumocystis carinii* pneumonia in the acquired immunodeficiency syndrome. *Reviews in Medical Microbiology* 1992; **3**: 80–87.

32 Miller R.F., Millar A.B., Weller I.V.D., Semple S.J.G. Empirical treatment without bronchoscopy for *Pneumocystis carinii* pneumonia in the acquired immunodeficiency syndrome. *Thorax* 1989; **44**: 559–564.

33 Tu J.V., Biem H.J., Detsky A.S. Bronchoscopy versus empirical therapy in HIV infected patients with presumptive *Pneumocystis carinii* pneumonia: a decision analysis. *American Review of Respiratory Disease* 1993; **148**: 370–377.

34 Chouaid C., Maillard D., Housset F., Febvre M., Zaoui D., Lebean B. Cost effectiveness

of non-invasive oxygen saturation measurements during exercise for the diagnosis *Pneumocystis carinii* pneumonia. *American Review of Respiratory Disease* 1993; **147**: 1360–1363.

35 Mitchell D.M., Fleming J., Pinching A.J. *et al*. Pulmonary function in human immunodeficiency virus infection. *American Review of Respiratory Disease* 1992; **146**: 745–751.

36 Mitchell D.M., Fleming J., Harris J.R.W., Shaw R.J. Serial pulmonary function tests in the diagnosis of *P. carinii* pneumonia. *European Respiratory Journal* 1993; **6**: 823–827.

37 Zaman M.K., White G.A. Serum lactate dehydrogenase levels and *Pneumocystis carinii* pneumonia: diagnostic and prognostic significance. *American Review of Respiratory Disease* 1988; **137**: 796–800.

38 Meeker D.P., Matysck G.A., Stelmach K., Rehm S. Diagnostic utility of lactate dehydrogenase levels in patients receiving aerosolized pentamidine. *Chest* 1993; **104**: 386–388.

39 Buscombe J.R., Oyen W.J.G., Corstens F.H.M., Ell P.J., Miller R.F. Localization of infection in HIV antibody positive patients with fever: comparison of the efficacy of [67]gallium citrate and radiolabelled human IgG (HIG). *Clinical Nuclear Medicine* 1995; **20**: 334–339.

40 Miller R.F., Kocjan G., Buckland J., Holton J., Malin A., Semple S.J.G. Sputum induction for the diagnosis of respiratory disease in HIV positive patients. *Journal of Infection* 1991; **23**: 5–16.

41 Miller R.F., Buckland J., Semple S.J.G. Arterial desaturation in HIV positive patients undergoing sputum induction. *Thorax* 1991; **46**: 449–451.

42 Griffiths M.H., Kocjan G., Miller R.F., Godfrey-Faussett P. Diagnosis of pulmonary disease in human immunodeficiency virus infection: role of transbronchial biopsy and bronchoalveolar lavage. *Thorax* 1991; **44**: 554–558.

43 Miller R.F., Pugsley W.B., Griffiths M.H. Open lung biopsy for investigation of acute respiratory episodes in patients with HIV infection and AIDS. *Genitourinary Medicine* 1995; **71**: 280–285.

44 Wakefield A.E., Guiver L., Miller R.F., Hopkin J.M. DNA amplification on induced sputum samples for diagnosis of *Pneumocystis carinii* pneumonia. *Lancet* 1991; **337**: 1378–1379.

45 Wakefield A.E., Miller R.F., Guiver L., Hopkin J.M. Oropharyngeal samples for detection of *Pneumocystis carinii* by DNA amplification. *Quarterly Journal of Medicine* 1993; **86**: 401–406.

46 Jeffrey A.A., Bullen C., Miller R.F. Intensive care management of *Pneumocystis carinii* pneumonia. *Care of the Critically Ill* 1993; **9**: 258–260.

47 Speich R., Opravil M., Weber R., Hess T., Lenthy R., Russi W. Prospective evaluation of a prognostic score for *Pneumocystis carinii* pneumonia in HIV infected patients. *Chest* 1992; **102**: 1045–1048.

48 Miller R.F. Prevention and treatment of *Pneumocystis carinii* pneumonia in patients infected with HIV. *Drug and Therapeutics Bulletin* 1994; **32**: 12–15.

49 Sattler F.R., Cowan R., Nielson D., Ruskin J. Trimethoprim–sulfamethoxazole compared with pentamidine for treatment of *Pneumocystis carinii* pneumonia in the acquired immunodeficiency syndrome. *Annals of Internal Medicine* 1988; **109**: 280–287.

50 Klein N.C., Duncanson F.P., Lenox T.H. *et al*. Trimethoprim–sulphamethoxazole versus pentamidine for *Pneumocystis carinii* pneumonia in AIDS patients: results of a large prospective randomized treatment trial. *AIDS* 1992; **6**: 301–305.

51 Safrin S., Lee B.L., Sande M.A. Adjunctive folinic acid with trimethoprim–sulphamethoxazole for *Pneumocystis carinii* pneumonia in AIDS patients is associated with an increased risk of therapeutic failure and death. *Clinical Infectious Diseases* 1994; **170**: 912–917.

52 Koopmans P.P., van der Ven A.J.A.M., Vree T.B., van der Meer J.W.M. Pathogenesis of hypersensitivity reactions to drugs in patients with HIV infection: allergic or toxic? *AIDS* 1995; **9**: 217–222.

53 Jung A.C., Paauw D.S. Management of adverse reactions to trimethoprim–sulfamethoxazole in human immunodeficiency virus-infected patients. *Archives of Internal Medicine* 1994; **154**: 2402–2406.

54 Bachmeyer C., Salmon D., Guerin C. *et al.* Trimethoprim–sulphamethoxazole densitization in HIV-infected patients: an open study. *AIDS* 1995; **9**: 299–300.

55 Haverkos H.W. Assessment of therapy for *Pneumocystis carinii* pneumonia. *American Journal of Medicine* 1994; **76**: 501–508.

56 Medina I., Mills J., Leoung G. *et al.* Oral therapy for *Pneumocystis carinii* pneumonia in the acquired immunodeficiency syndrome: a controlled trial of trimethoprim–sulfamethozazole versus trimethoprim–dapsone. *New England Journal of Medicine* 1990; **323**: 776–782.

57 Toma F., Fournier S., Poisson M., Morisset R., Phaneuf D., Viega C. Clindamycin with primaquine for *Pneumocystis carinii* pneumonia. *Lancet* 1989; **i**: 1046–1048.

58 Black J.R., Feinberg J., Murphy R.L. Clindamycin and primaquine therapy for mild-to-moderate episodes of *Pneumocystis carinii* in patients with AIDS: AIDS clinical trial group 044. *Clinical Infectious Diseases* 1994; **18**: 9095–9013.

59 Hughes W., Leoung G., Kramer F. *et al.* Comparison of atovaquone (566C80) with trimethoprim–sulfamethoxazole to treat *Pneumocystis carinii* pneumonia in patients with AIDS. *New England Journal of Medicine* 1993; **328**: 1521–1527.

60 Dohn M.N., Weinberg W.G., Torres R.A. *et al.* Oral atovaquone compared with intravenous pentamidine for *Pneumocystis carinii* pneumonia in patients with AIDS. *Annals of Internal Medicine* 1994; **121**: 174–180.

61 Sattler F.R., Frame P., Davis R. *et al.* Trimetrexate with leucovorin versus trimethoprim–sulfamethoxazole for moderate to severe episodes for *Pneumocystis carinii* pneumonia in patients with AIDS. *Journal of Infectious Diseases* 1994; **170**: 166–172.

62 Allegra C.J., Chabner B.A., Tuazon C.U. *et al.* Trimetrexate for the treatment of *Pneumocystis carinii* pneumonia in patients with the acquired immunodeficiency syndrome. *New England Journal of Medicine* 1987; **317**: 978–985.

63 Smith D., Davies S., Nelson M., Youle M., Gleeson J., Gazzard B. *Pneumocystis carinii* pneumonia treated with eflornithine in AIDS patients resistant to conventional therapy. *AIDS* 1990; **4**: 1019–1021.

64 Conte J.C., Chernof D., Feigal D.W., Jr., Joseph P., McDonald C., Golden J.A. Intravenous or inhaled pentamidine for treating *Pneumocystis carinii* pneumonia in AIDS. *Annals of Internal Medicine* 1990; **113**: 203–209.

65 Miller R.F., Godfrey-Faussett P., Semple S.J.G. Nebulised pentamidine as treatment for *Pneumocystis carinii* pneumonia in the acquired immunodeficiency syndrome. *Thorax* 1989; **44**: 565–569.

66 Miller R.F., O'Doherty M.J. Nebulisers for patients with HIV infection and AIDS: British Thoracic Society standards of care. *Thorax* 1997 (in press).

67 Bozette S.A., Sattler F.R., Chiu J. *et al.* A controlled trial of early adjunctive treatment with corticosteroids for *Pneumocystis carinii* in the acquired immunodeficiency syndrome. *New England Journal of Medicine* 1990; **323**: 1451–1457.

68 Gagnon S., Boota A.M., Fischl M.A., Baier H., Kirksey O.W., La Voie L. Corticosteroids as adjunctive therapy for severe *Pneumocystis carinii* pneumonia in the acquired immunodeficiency syndrome. *New England Journal of Medicine* 1990; **323**: 1444–1450.

69 National Institutes of Health—University of California Expert Panel for Corticosteroids as Adjunctive Therapy for Pneumocystis Pneumonia. Consensus statement on the use of corticosteroids as adjunctive therapy for *Pneumocystis carinii* in the acquired immunodeficiency syndrome. *New England Journal of Medicine* 1990; **323**: 1500–1504.

70 Miller R.F., Mitchell D.M. Management of respiratory failure in patients with the acquired immune deficiency syndrome and *Pneumocystis carinii* pneumonia. *Thorax* 1990; **45**: 140–144.

71 Miller R.F., Semple S.J.G. Continuous positive airway pressure ventilation for respiratory failure associated with *Pneumocystis carinii* pneumonia. *Respiratory Medicine* 1991; **85**: 135–138.

72 Staikowsky F., Lafon B., Guidet B., Denis M., Mayaud C., Offenstadt G. Mechanical ventilation for *Pneumocystis carinii* pneumonia in patients with the acquired syndrome. *Chest* 1993; **104**: 756–762.

73 Miller R.F., Mitchell D.M. *Pneumocystis carinii* pneumonia. *Thorax* 1995; **50**: 191–200.

74 Phair J.P., Munoz A., Detels R. *et al.* The risk of *Pneumocystis carinii* pneumonia among men infected with human immunodeficiency virus type 1. *New England Journal of Medicine* 1990; **322**: 161–165.

75 US Public Health Service Task Force on Antipnuemocystis Prophylaxis in Patients Infected with Human Immunodeficiency Virus Infection. Recommendations for prophylaxis against *Pneumocystis carinii* pneumonia for persons infected with human immunodeficiency virus. *Journal of AIDS* 1993; **6**: 161–165.

76 Miller R.F., LeNoury J., Corbett E.L., Felton J.M., De Cock K.M. *Pneumocystis carinii* infection: current treatment and prevention. *Journal of Antimicrobial Therapy* 1996; **37** (Suppl. B): 33–53.

77 Waltzer P.D., Foy J., Steele P., White M. Treatment of experimental pneumocystosis: development of a new system for classifying anti microbial drugs. *Antimicrobial Agents and Chemotherapy* 1992; **36**: 1934–1950.

78 Schneider M.N.E., Hoepelman A.I.M., Efftinck-Schattenkerk J.K.M. *et al.* A controlled trial of an aerolized pentamidine or trimethoprim–sulfamethoxazole as primary prophylaxis against *Pneumocystis carinii* pneumonia in patients with human immunodeficiency virus infection. *New England Journal of Medicine* 1992; **327**: 1836–1841.

79 Mallolas J., Zamora L., Gatell J.M. *et al.* Primary prophylaxis for *Pneumocystis carinii* pneumonia: a randomized trial comparing co-trimoxazole, aerolized pentamidine and dapsone plus pyrimethamine. *AIDS* 1993; **7**: 59–64.

80 Bozette S.A., Finkelstein D.M., Spector S.A., Fame P., Powderly W.G., He W. A randomized trial of three anti *Pneumocystis* agents in patients with advanced human immunodeficiency virus infection. *New England Journal of Medicine* 1995; **332**: 693–699.

81 Hardy W.D., Feinberg J., Finkelstein D.M. *et al.* A controlled trial of trimethoprim–sulfamethoxazole or aerosolized pentamidine for secondary prophylaxis against *Pneumocystis carinii* pneumonia in patients with the aquired immunodeficiency syndrome. *New England Journal of Medicine* 1992; **327**: 1842–1848.

82 Leoung G.S., Feigal D.W., Montgomery A.B. *et al.* Aerosolised pentamidine for prophylaxis against *Pneumocystis carinii* pneumonia—the San Francisco Community Prophylaxis Trial. *New England Journal of Medicine* 1990; **323**: 769–775.

83 Fahy J.V., Chin D.P., Schnapp L.M. *et al.* Effect of aerosolized pentamidine prophylaxis on the clinical severity of *Pneumocystis carinii* pneumonia. *American Review of Respiratory Disease* 1992; **146**: 844–848.

84 Golden J.A., Katz M.H., Chernoff D.N., Duncan S.M., Conte J.E., Jr. A randomised trial of once-monthly or twice-monthly high dose aerosolized pentamidine prophylaxis. *Chest* 1993; **104**: 743–750.

85 Kemper C.A., Tucker R.M., Lang O.S. *et al.* Low-dose dapsone prophylaxis of *Pneumocystis carinii* pneumonia in AIDS and AIDS related complex. *AIDS* 1990; **4**: 1145–1148.

86 Falloon J., Lavelle J., Ogata-Arakaki D. Pharmacokinetics and safety of weekly dapsone and dapsone plus pyrimethamine for prevention of *Pneumocystis* pneumonia. *Antimicrobial Agents and Chemotherapy* 1994; **38**: 1580–1587.

87 Girard P.M., Landman R., Gaudebout C., Olivares R., Saimot A.G., Jelazko P. Dapsone–pyrimethamine compared with aerosolised pentamidine as primary prophylaxis against *Pneumocystis carinii* pneumonia and toxoplasmosis in HIV infection. *New England Journal of Medicine* 1993; **328**: 1514–1520.

88 Coker R.J., Nieman R., McBride M., Mitchell D.M., Harris J.R.W., Weber J.N. Co-

trimoxazole versus dapsone–pyrimethamine for prevention of *Pneumocystis carinii* pneumonia. *Lancet* 1992; **340**: 1099.

89 Ena J., Amador C., Pasqua F. *et al.* Once-a-month administration of intravenous pentamidine to patients infected with human immunodeficiency virus: a prophylaxis for *Pneumocystis carinii*. *Clinical Infectious Diseases* 1994; **18**: 901–904.

90 Cheung T.W., Matta R., Neibart E. Intramuscular pentamidine for the prevention of *Pneumocystis carinii* in patients infected with human immunodeficiency virus. *Clinical Infectious Diseases* 1993; **16**: 22–25.

91 Gottlieb M.S., Knight S., Mitsuyasu R., Weisman J., Roth M., Young L.S. Prophylaxis of *Pneumocystis carinii* infection in AIDS with pyrimethamine–sulfadoxine. *Lancet* 1984; **2**: 398–399.

5 Pulmonary Kaposi's sarcoma

A.L. POZNIAK

5.0 Introduction

Kaposi's sarcoma (KS) was one of the first harbingers of the AIDS epidemic and yet its aetiology is unclear. For example, it is not known whether different clinical forms of KS are all manifestations of the same disease. Is KS a true clonal malignancy? Are the clinical forms of the disease hyperproliferative states induced by an excess of cytokines and growth factors?

KS often involves the lung. Most studies of pulmonary KS have been observational, describing features in small numbers of patients. Consequently, a number of different views about diagnosis and treatment have arisen. To differentiate the important from the irrelevant, the cause and effect from the chance and coincidence, is not an easy task. With this aim in mind, this chapter will discuss fact and theory of this enigmatic disease.

5.1 Epidemiology of Kaposi's sarcoma

The incidence of KS as an index diagnosis for AIDS has decreased from 61% in the early 1980s to 14% [1,2], although it is still the most prevalent neoplasm in HIV-infected persons [3–5]. KS occurs unequally in the different groups at risk of HIV infection. The highest incidence is found in those groups where sexual intercourse is the mode of transmission for HIV, the lowest incidence being in those who are infected by blood products. Twenty per cent of homosexuals, 6% of heterosexuals, but only 3% of intravenous drug users (IVDUs) and 1% of haemophiliacs develop KS [6,7]. This phenomenon remains unexplained.

The occurrence of KS in young male homosexuals was first reported in 1981 [8,9]. Since then the Centers for Disease Control (CDC) have reported over 24 000 cases of HIV-related (epidemic) KS. Epidemic KS is the most common neoplastic manifestation of AIDS in the USA and Europe [2,8] and was the AIDS-defining manifestation in 15% of patients reported to CDC in 1990 [7]. It is uncommon in women, accounting for only 2.1% of AIDS diagnoses [10], and is even rarer in children [11].

5.2 Aetiology

Although the epidemiology of this disease has suggested that an infectious agent, such as cytomegalovirus (CMV) [12] or HIV itself [13], might play a causative role, there is evidence that a newly discovered KS-associated herpesvirus (KSHV) may be vital in its pathogenesis. In December of 1994, Chang *et al.* reported the discovery of a unique herpes-like deoxyribonucleic acid (DNA) sequence in KS lesions [14]. It is found in both classical and African forms of KS. Subsequent studies have shown that KSHV is present in more than 90% of AIDS-related KS tissue but is found less frequently in uninvolved skin. DNA sequences of the virus are detected more frequently in the peripheral blood of patients with KS than in other HIV-infected patients [15,16].

This viral sequence is not specific for KS and has been detected in sperm samples from adults without HIV, in body-cavity lymphomas and Castleman's disease and in various skin lesions from transplant patients. It is likely that when this virus is fully characterized it will be called human herpesvirus 8 (HHV-8). It is possible that this virus is able to replicate well in immunodeficient patients and KS lesions without itself playing a causal role. In spite of this doubt, KSHV (HHV-8) is the most attractive candidate to date for the infectious agent of KS and seems to fit the epidemiological evidence. This evidence thus far suggests that KS is caused by such an infectious agent, which is then transmitted sexually, rather than by any blood-borne route.

5.3 History and natural history

Dr Moriz Kaposi (pronounced KOP-osh-eee) [17], a Hungarian dermatologist/dermatopathologist, described idiopathic multiple pigmented sarcoma in 1872 [18]. This classical form usually involved one or more limbs and associated lymph nodes and ran a long indolent course; 20% of patients died of visceral involvement, especially of the lung and gut [19]. This was the only form described in the literature until the 1950s, when an endemic form of KS was recognized in Africa as a lymphadenopathic disease, usually affecting children. It accounted for up to 10% of all tumours in some regions [20]. With the era of iatrogenic immunosuppression, another form of KS was reported in renal transplant patients and for the first time a link with immune suppression was observed. Fascinatingly, in these transplant patients the disease, even if it involved the lung, could regress on stopping immunosuppressant therapy [21,22]. Finally, in the last 15 years, infection with HIV has led to the emergence of a generalized aggressive or 'epidemic' form of KS. Unlike transplant patients, the relationship between the risk of developing KS and the degree of immune suppression in HIV patients is not as straightforward. Patients can present with KS as the sole manifestation of AIDS when their immune system is relatively well preserved. Most patients, however, present with KS as a subsequent AIDS diagnosis when severely immune suppressed [23]. Occasionally, KS will even regress in patients with untreated HIV infection [24].

5.4 Pathogenesis

KS is probably of lymphatic endothelial origin. It has been postulated that it may well not be a true cancer—that is, due to a monoclonal proliferation of cells—but is polyclonal in origin and arises due to an overexpression of oncogene products thought to have angiogenic activity. Mouse experiments suggest that the HIV *tat* gene may induce cells to produce angiogenic factors and that these cellular products, such as basic fibroblast growth factor and interleukin 1β (IL-1β) messenger ribonucleic acid (mRNA), cause a positive feedback on the tumour and promote increased growth [25,26]. This process may explain why KS appears to arise at multiple and differing primary sites contemporaneously, rather than spreading contiguously or by metastasis [27].

5.5 Pulmonary involvement

The lung is rich in lymphatics and blood-vessels. This and other factors, such as lack of natural killer-cell activity in pulmonary lymphocytes, crucial to tumour lysis [28], and local changes in pulmonary immune status may explain the predilection of KS for the lung.

Pulmonary KS may occur either as a primary, usually multicentric tumour or, more usually, as part of systemic involvement. It has been described in patients without known immunodeficiency [29–31] and in patients with iatrogenic immune deficiency [32]. Compared with the low risk of visceral involvement in the classical forms, visceral KS occurs in up to 50% of patients with HIV-associated KS and can involve almost every organ [33]. Pulmonary and gut involvement together can be found in 27% of cases, but because of diagnostic difficulties this is probably an underestimate.

So how common is lung involvement? The data are variable. Two autopsy studies had very different results and found that 3.7% and 48% [26] of Kaposi patients have lung involvement. Likewise the overall incidence of pulmonary involvement diagnosed in life in patients with KS varies from study to study, from 3.4 to 35% being reported [34,35]. In three studies of hospitalized patients with mucocutaneous or lymphatic KS, the incidences of pulmonary involvement were 6 [31], 18 [33] and 32% [26]. When the selection criteria were narrowed down to patients with known KS and respiratory symptoms and/or abnormal chest radiographs, the reported incidence varied from 21 to 49% [36–40].

The true incidence of pulmonary involvement may be dependent on duration and rate of progression of disease. However, it should be noted that lung involvement can be completely asymptomatic and thus unsuspected and can even present as the sole manifestation of KS [41,42].

5.5.1 Clinical features (Table 5.1)

By the time patients develop pulmonary KS, they are usually severely immunosuppressed. Between 35 and 79% of patients have previously developed at least one opportunistic infection.

Table 5.1 Pulmonary Kaposi's sarcoma: clinical features.

	Miller *et al.* [64]	Mitchell *et al.* [106]	Pozniak *et al.* [56]	Other [43–47]
Number of patients	20	19	47	5–50
Cough (%)	100	100	89	83–100
Breathless (%)	100	100	81	—
Chest pain (%)	0	11	34	17–47
Haemoptysis (%)	0	5	49	33
Symptoms (median weeks)	4	4	—	—
Smokers (%)	85	—	43	—
Palatal lesions (%)	95	—	77	—
Fever >38.5°C	—	—	—	30–53
CD4 count (median cells/µl)	—	—	—	77–170
Pa,o_2 (kPa)	—	—	8.0	8.0–10.2

Symptoms of pulmonary involvement mimic those of both opportunistic infection and tuberculosis. Even when coexisting infection is excluded, weight loss, fever, night sweats, prolonged cough, breathlessness and haemoptysis are common and often of long duration [36,43–45] (Table 5.1).

Cough and breathlessness occur in almost all patients [36,37,43]. Haemoptysis can be recurrent and life-threatening [41,46,47]. Wheezing, stridor and hoarseness are due to upper-airway or vocal-cord involvement [43,48,49].

A careful clinical examination is always required. KS lesions may be few in number or only occur in the mouth or around the anus. Occasionally, only lymph nodes are clinically involved. Chest examination may reveal some crackles but is usually unhelpful. The extent and rate of progression of any cutaneous disease do not always correlate with the extent of pulmonary disease [37]. The clinician should be aware that concomitant pulmonary infection can occur with pulmonary KS. Suggestive of this would be rapid onset of new symptoms, such as fever, productive cough or worsening breathlessness. Purulent phlegm production, lobar consolidation and rapid radiographic change or progression, such as cavitation or new widespread shadowing, also suggest a concomitant infection.

5.5.2 Pleural effusions

Extensive parenchymal disease is often associated with pleural disease, and pleural effusions are common, occurring in up to 30% of patients [3,43,50]. These may develop as a result of direct involvement of the pleura or lymphatic obstruction to mediastinal or hilar nodes (Fig. 5.1).

Effusions presenting as pleurisy are more likely to be due to KS than to a coexisting opportunistic infection, especially if cutaneous KS is present [36,37]. They usually consist of a mononuclear exudate but, when doubt exists about the diagnosis, pleural fluid cytology is unhelpful [43,50].

Because of the patchy nature of the disease and the parietal pleura being spared, closed pleural biopsy is not useful diagnostically [50,51]. Up to 80% of effusions are bilateral [46] and most are bloodstained [46,51], but they can be straw-coloured or chylous [50,52]. Unfortunately, effusions can cause respiratory compromise [46] and are often unresponsive to systemic or local treatment [37,50,51]. They are probably best treated with drainage and pleural sclerosis if symptomatic, but the development of an effusion in KS is regarded as a factor for poor prognosis [50,53].

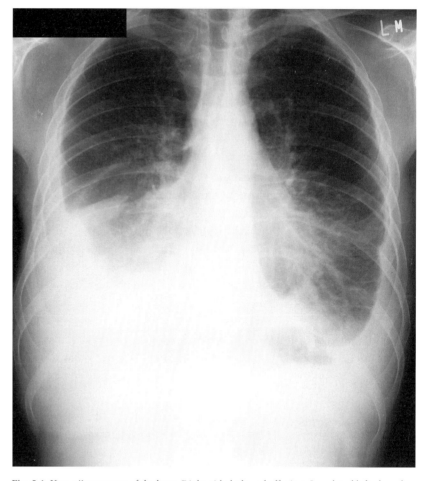

Fig. 5.1 Kaposi's sarcoma of the lung. Right-sided pleural effusion. Loculated left pleural effusion.

5.6 Radiology

Radiological features of pulmonary KS have been well documented [36,37,43,54,55] (Table 5.2). The chest radiograph can be normal [36,46,54] in spite of involvement. Localized disease, represented as focal opacities [55], masses [56] and cavities [57], have been described, but most patients have widespread infiltrates (Fig. 5.2). These can be alveolar, interstitial, mixed alveolar–interstitial or, most commonly, nodular. Mediastinal- and hilar-node involvement with KS has been described in 26–63% [46,55,58] of patients, either alone or in association with opportunistic fungal or mycobacterial infection.

In patients with cutaneous KS, certain radiological changes suggest lung involvement. Parenchymal nodular and reticular opacities had a 100% positive predictive value for lung involvement in AIDS patients

Table 5.2 Pulmonary Kaposi's sarcoma: chest radiographic changes.

	Miller *et al.* [64]	Mitchell *et al.* [106]	Pozniak *et al.* [56]	Other [36,37,43,46,54–58]
Number of patients	20	19	47	5–50
Normal (%)	35	25	7	5–20
Bilateral interstitial shadowing (%)	45	48	53	—
Lobar consolidation (%)	5	11	21	—
Pleural effusion (%)	20	11	15	7–50
Hilar enlargement (%)	15	5	4	8–46

Total percentages are greater than 100% as some patients had more than one feature present.

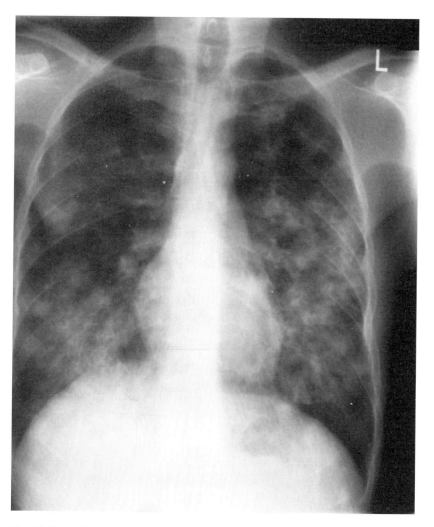

Fig. 5.2 Kaposi's sarcoma of the lung. Bilateral nodular infiltrates.

with and without autopsy-proved pulmonary KS [46]. Mediastinal and hilar nodes had a predictive value of 92% and pleural effusions 89%. An important radiological differential diagnosis is *Pneumocystis carinii* pneumonia (PCP). Pulmonary involvement with KS tends to progress over many months, but the pattern and tempo of progression are distinctly different from that of PCP, which tends to progress over days and weeks. The typical ground-glass perihilar radiological appearance of PCP contrasts with the usually lower-zone nodular opacities, occasionally associated with lymphatic lines, seen in KS. Localized pulmonary involvement can be masked by the presence of concurrent disease [46] and can, for example, be the cause of 'persistent' radiological changes after an acute pneumonic event.

There is some correlation between the type of radiographic changes and pulmonary histology [55]. In patients with predominantly nodular lesions on chest X-ray, histological examination of the lung also shows a predominance of nodules, and those with a predominantly interstitial pattern on X-ray have a thickened interstitium, characterized by invasive angiomatous proliferation of slit-like vessels with atypical endothelial cells.

5.6.1 Computer-assisted tomography

Computer-assisted tomography (CAT) scanning has been used as a diagnostic tool in KS of the lung [59,60]. In 22/24 patients with chest radiograph findings of non-specific, bilateral perihilar infiltrates, corresponding CAT scans documented abnormal hilar densities extending into the adjacent pulmonary parenchyma along distinct perivascular and peribronchial paths (Fig. 5.3). This CAT appearance was felt to be characteristic of pulmonary KS. Discrete, poorly marginated nodules were seen in 10 patients and were randomly distributed throughout the lung. Mediastinal adenopathy was unusual. In spite of the improved definition of pulmonary change, the amount of additional information gained from CAT scans in the diagnosis of pulmonary KS probably does not justify their routine use [61]. New techniques using helical CAT scanning have yet to be evaluated in this disease.

5.6.2 Magnetic resonance imaging

No role for magnetic resonance imaging (MRI) in pulmonary KS has yet been defined. A few groups have used it as a research tool. In one study, spin-echo (T_1) enhancement of gadolinium with a marked reduction of the second echo of the spin-echo (T_2) in the pathological areas was observed in patients with pulmonary KS but not in patients with PCP

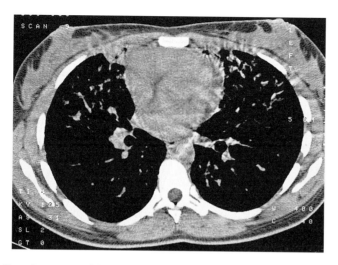

Fig. 5.3 Kaposi's sarcoma of the lung. Computed tomography (CT) scan showing confluent nodules with involvement along perivascular tracts.

[64]. Both the vascular and the fibrous components of KS would account for this finding. MRI would be most useful if it could be used to definitively diagnose pulmonary KS or as a means of monitoring progress and response to treatment.

5.7 Lung-function tests

Although spirometry may be normal in the early stages of lung involvement, the infiltrative nature of the disease can eventually result in a restrictive pattern of lung-function tests (Table 5.3). Occasionally, with extensive upper-airway involvement, airflow obstruction can occur [43,49]. A decreased forced expiratory volume in 1 second (FEV_1)/forced vital capacity (FVC) has limited diagnostic value in individual patients, as

Table 5.3 Pulmonary Kaposi's sarcoma: pulmonary-function tests.

	Miller *et al.* [64]	Mitchell *et al.* [106]	Pozniak *et al.* [56]
	(%)	(%)	(%)
FEV_1	61*	56*	1.81
FVC	70*	59*	63
PEF	59*	55*	—
$T_L$co	72*	45*	—

* For widespread disease only.
FEV_1, forced expiratory volume in 1 second; FVC, forced vital capacity; PEF, peak expiratory flow; $T_L$co, carbon monoxide transfer factor; %, per cent of predicted.

these changes can also occur in some patients with PCP. Arterial desaturation with exercise and a low diffusion capacity are also suggestive of lung involvement [43,63] but are not specific. Blood-gas analyses are unhelpful in the differential diagnosis of pulmonary KS but do help in monitoring response to treatment [64]. A normal carbon monoxide diffusing capacity (D_LCO) is more likely in patients with KS than in patients with PCP, but if alveolar haemorrhage has occurred the diffusing capacity may even be increased.

5.8 Isotope scanning

Although gallium-67-citrate scans do not localize KS [65], they do have a high sensitivity (but low specificity) for PCP. Therefore gallium scanning is helpful in patients with known pulmonary KS who have progression of symptoms or radiological progression, when a negative scan usually suggests that a second disease is not present [61]. Cutaneous Kaposi lesions take up thallium-201 [66] and might be useful in diagnosing lung involvement. Further evaluation is needed of this and other isotopes, such as technetium pertechnetate immunoglobulin G (IgG) and indium-111-labelled immunoglobulin. Their role in diagnosis and in attempting to differentiate tumour from infection needs to be defined.

5.9 Bronchoscopy

There are no non-invasive techniques which allow clinicians to diagnose pulmonary KS with certainty and so bronchoscopy remains the diagnostic gold standard. In most cases, bronchoscopy will exclude concomitant infection and demonstrate suggestive lesions which will suffice for diagnosis. At bronchoscopy, lesions may be seen in the nose, pharynx and larynx. Any tracheal and bronchial lesions are highly characteristic [35,43,67]. They resemble the skin lesions but are usually less violaceous and more erythematous [68]. Bronchi may be normal, but, if lesions are present, they have a variety of appearances, such as well-defined discrete macules, early or well-formed plaques, frank nodules or large masses. Diffuse erythema may be the only visible evidence of extensive involvement and may accompany the lesions described above.

5.9.1 Bronchial/transbronchial biopsy

It is not easy to make a tissue diagnosis of pulmonary KS from bronchial biopsies. Even when lesions are seen, a bronchial biopsy may show no abnormality. Two factors which cause difficulties in tissue diagnosis are that biopsies are easier to perform when lesions are found at orifices of segmental bronchi [68,69] and that early lesions of KS can histologically resemble inflammatory or granulation tissue [69,70]. Bleeding from biopsy sites is usually self-limiting, but can be significant [71], especially with biopsies of the upper respiratory tract. Obviously, bronchoscopy should only be performed when there is adequate provision for resuscitation, intubation, ventilation and surgical support.

When endobronchial disease is not obvious, should transbronchial biopsy be performed? Transbronchial biopsy may be useful in diagnosing pulmonary KS in many more patients than is generally appreciated [72] and may be useful in excluding coexisting disease. Five out of nine patients were diagnosed by this technique in one study [72] and other small studies have found it useful, with diagnostic yields of up to 50% or more, close to that obtained at open-lung biopsy [73]. Others, having found transbronchial biopsy unhelpful [36,48,70,74–76], argue that if a definitive diagnosis is needed it should be made at open-lung biopsy. The patchy nature of the disease [41] and the difficulties in interpreting early histological changes have led to these differing viewpoints.

5.9.2 Bronchoalveolar lavage

Since an associated infection has been reported in 17–27% of patients with pulmonary KS, bronchoalveolar lavage (BAL) is usually performed at bronchoscopy and is safe even in thrombocytopenia [70]. Finding bacterial organisms, such as *Staphylococcus aureus* and *Pseudomonas aeruginosa*, in the lavage may signify active infection rather than colonization and should be taken seriously, especially as patients may be on or starting chemotherapy. CMV was often found in the lungs of patients with pulmonary KS but its role in causing pulmonary disease in patients with HIV infection is controversial. The majority of patients with CMV found in BAL have either no clinical disease or another more serious opportunistic or neoplastic HIV-related condition [77].

Haemorrhagic lavage fluid is suggestive of pulmonary KS [69,78] but can also be found in pneumonia [79]. The examination of lavage specimens for haemosiderin-laden macrophages is neither sensitive nor specific for KS. The lavage cytology can be entirely normal, although lymphocytosis is often observed whether or not patients with AIDS have pulmonary KS. It is probably due to mild lymphoid infiltrates in bronchovascular connective tissue and interlobular septa [80]. Bronchial brushings are not usually helpful [43] and their routine use cannot be recommended.

5.10 Histology

The problems that some studies had with low diagnostic yields from bronchial, transbronchial and even open-lung biopsy are not only due to the patchy nature of KS but also due to the difficulty in interpreting the early histological changes of KS. These histological changes can be misdiagnosed as inflammation [81], organizing pneumonia, fibrosis [82] or granulation tissue [60]. The presence of abnormally shaped vessels, especially those with an irregular jagged outline, is said to be the best single criterion for early KS [81].

When KS involves the lung, it grows along lymphatic and bronchovascular tracts in interlobular septa and into the pleura [72]. The disease can be divided into an early stage, with an interstitial infiltrate in the alveolar wall, bronchovascular sheaths and interlobular septa, and a later stage, which evolves into nodular tumour masses that obliterate tissue and have a predilection for airways and vesels [83]. Death may be caused by hypoxia due to the envelopment of blood-vessels and filling of the lungs by tumour and haemorrhage [54]. Histologically there is a wide differential diagnosis, including capillary haemangiomatosis, haemangioendothelioma, angiosarcoma, pulmonary artery sarcoma and intravascular sclerosing bronchoalveolar tumour [84].

5.11 Staging

There is no uniformly accepted staging system for HIV-related KS. This causes problems for treatment decisions and for clinical-trial monitoring. Tumour progression and survival are probably related to the degree of immune deficiency rather than the tumour bulk, unless there is extensive visceral involvement. Patients with CD4 counts less than 300 cells/μl [85,86] and signs and symptoms of systemic infection have a worse prognosis [88]. Earlier staging systems used the site of the disease and visceral involvement for staging, but these had no relationship to prognosis [7,88], either in endemic disease or in HIV-related KS. A newer staging system from San Francisco divides patients up into limited and extensive disease on the basis of immunological function, clinical stability, patient tolerance of zidovudine and evaluation of tumour-associated complications [89]. This categorization decides treatment protocols and prognostic information and its use is still being assessed.

5.12 Treatment—chemotherapy

Treatment for pulmonary KS has usually involved combination chemotherapy. The best-documented regimens use bleomycin 10 international units (iu)/m^2 and vincristine 1.2 mg/m^2, often with adriamycin 10 or 20 mg/m^2. The exact role for antineoplastic agents remains undefined [90] and there is concern that their use may exacerbate immunosuppression and increase morbidity by drug side-effects. Although chemotherapy does not appear to significantly shorten or prolong survival in AIDS–KS [91], a satisfactory and rapid clinical response can be obtained with single-agent chemotherapy (with responses of 20–40%) using vinblastine, etoposide, doxorubicin, vincristine [90] and epirubicin. Response rates vary from 30% for vinblastine [92] to more than 80% for etoposide [93]. These differing responses may be due to the different entry criteria applied to trials and the different response criteria used. Combination chemotherapy with bleomycin, vincristine and doxorubicin may increase the response rates but also increases toxicity and the rate of opportunistic infections [94], and higher response rates do not necessarily mean longer survival. Liposomal preparations of daunorunicin and doxorubicin may decrease toxicity and limit neutropenia.

In the analysis of clinical studies which use various regimens from response to survival, the following conclusions may be drawn. Firstly, in pulmonary KS there appears to be a discrepancy between the effectiveness of chemotherapy on respiratory symptoms and that on radiographic changes. There is often a major improvement in respiratory symptoms, even with the first course of chemotherapy, and this can be associated with a large rise in arterial partial pressure of oxygen (Pa,o_2) [95]. Complete radiological responses are unusual but partial responses can occur in 50–90%. Secondly, beneficial effects persist for a mean period of 2–4 weeks but do not usually exceed 2 months. Thirdly, the average survival after the first course of chemotherapy is 5–6 months, although survival longer than 2 years has been reported. Prognostic factors for survival vary from study to study, but three series have indicated that haemoglobin values of $\leq 10\,g/dl$, leucopenia of ≤ 1500 cells/l, a CD4 count of ≤ 100 cells/µl and the presence of opportunistic infection before chemotherapy are all predictors of rapid progression to death [53,95]. Some other series have stated that bilateral effusions, a Karnofsky index of $\leq 70\%$, poor response on radiography and the absence of cutaneous lesions are associated with a short survival. Finally, although patients experience some side-effects of chemotherapy, leucopenia may have a detrimental effect on outcome, as up to 50% of patients develop bacterial infections, requiring longer breaks between courses of chemotherapy. This may indirectly lead to progression of pulmonary KS, with acute respiratory failure. Growth factors may help overcome this problem but in theory might make KS lesions proliferate because of their 'cytokine' effect.

5.12.1 Radiotherapy

Local radiotherapy to the lungs has been used to palliate the disease [96]. Doses of 5–35 Gy whole-lung irradiation have been reported to cause subjective and objective improvement in patients [37,44]. These patients often have severe disease, with survival being a mean of 12 weeks. Local palliative irradiation can be given for haemoptysis and upper-airway obstruction [97,98].

5.12.2 Other therapies

Other treatments using systemic interferon alpha therapy [99–101], alone or with zidovudine [102], or other antivirals may have clinical effects against KS as well as the benefit of anti-HIV effects. They tend not to be effective in patients with CD4 counts less than 150 cells/μl and so have a limited use. Most patients with lung involvement are severely immunosuppressed. Antiangiogenic therapy is another interesting area of research, as heparin and steroid do inhibit angiogenesis in some tumour models [103], but this type of treatment is still in the experimental stage.

Paclitaxel, a drug with an action similar to that of vincalkaloid [104], has substantial activity in KS. Four out of five patients with pulmonary disease had a good response in one study. As KS lesions are highly vascular, theoretically antiangiogenesis agents may be useful. Such agents include the fumagillin analogue TNP-470, tecogalan, platelet factor 4 and IL-4. All are being tested at present. Analogues of retinoic acid are found to be active against spindle cells, but variable results have been obtained with all-*trans*-retinoic acid. There are also anecdotal reports of KS resolving in patients receiving foscarnet, a drug with both antiherpesvirus and anti-HIV effects. Human chorionic gonadotrophin (HCG) may have an effect on reversing the angiogenic factor responsible for KS, especially fibroblast growth factor. HCG has been given to humans in large doses — between 150 and 700 000 iu intramuscularly three times a week. HCG is extremely expensive and, although it appeared to have an effect on patients' lesions, if less than 100 000 iu was given the tumour regrew [105].

5.13 Prognosis

There is no doubt that patients with pulmonary involvement have a worse prognosis compared with those who do not. Various small studies have found median survivals of 3.8–9 months [57,107], but many of these patients have been treated. The ranges for survival again vary and individual patients do less well. Two studies which have looked at untreated patients estimate that survival from onset of symptoms was 3.8 and 3.2 months.

5.14 Conclusions

KS remains an enigma and pulmonary involvement a diagnostic and therapeutic challenge. Bronchoscopy and BAL may be sufficient to diagnose pulmonary KS, even without histological confirmation. Transbronchial biopsy could be performed in those with a normal tracheobronchial tree at bronchoscopy. Open-lung biopsy should be reserved for those cases in whom a diagnosis has not been made. Once diagnosed, pulmonary KS may progress slowly over many months. At any point in a patient's illness, careful evaluation is needed in order to differentiate between progressive radiological change due to the KS and superimposed opportunistic infection. Isotope scanning may well prove useful in this situation. At present, treatment would best be planned as part of clinical trials, which should include the assessment of the role of radiotherapy and new compounds. In the developing world, symptomatic therapy may be the only option, especially when there are restraints on money, resources and staffing levels.

References

1 Beral V. The epidemiology of Kaposi's sarcoma. *Cancer Surveys* 1991; **10**: 5–22.
2 Martin R.W., Hood A.F., Farmer E.R. Kaposi's sarcoma. *Medicine* 1993; **72**: 245–261.
3 Rutherford G.W., Schwarcz S.K., Lemp G.F. *et al.* The epidemiology of AIDS-related Kaposi's sarcoma in San Francisco. *Journal of Infectious Diseases* 1989; **159**: 569–572.
4 Boylston A.W., Cook H.T., Francis N.D., Goldin R.D. Biopsy pathology of acquired immune deficiency syndrome (AIDS). *Journal of Clinical Pathology* 1987; **40**: 1–8.
5 Steis R.G., Longo D.L. Clinical, biologic, and therapeutic aspects of malignancies associated with the acquired immunodeficiency syndrome: Part I and Part II. *Annals of Allergy* 1988; **60**: 310–323.
6 Curran J.W., Morgan W.M., Hardy A.M., Jaffe H.W., Darron W.W., Dowdle W.R. The epidemiology of AIDS: current status and future prospects. *Science* 1985; **229**: 1352–1357.
7 Beral V., Peterman T.A., Berkelman R.L., Jaffe H.W. Kaposi's sarcoma among persons with AIDS: a sexually transmitted infection? *Lancet* 1990; **335**: 123–128.
8 Friedman-Kein A.E., Laubenstein L.J., Ribinstein P. *et al.* Disseminated Kaposi's sarcoma in homosexual men. *Annals of Internal Medicine* 1982; **120**: 693–700.
9 Hymes K.B., Cheung T., Greene J.B. *et al.* Kaposi's sarcoma in homosexual men — a report of eight cases. *Lancet* 1981; **ii**: 598–600.
10 Albrecht H., Helm E.B., Plettenberg A. *et al.* Kaposi's sarcoma in HIV infected women in Germany: more evidence for sexual transmission. A report of 10 cases and review of the literature. *Genitourinary Medicine* 1994; **70**: 394–398.
11 Athale U.H., Patil P.S., Chintu C., Elem B. Influence of HIV epidemic on the incidence of Kaposi's sarcoma in Zambian children. *Journal of Acquired Immune Deficiency Syndromes and Human Retrovirology* 1995; **8**: 96–100.
12 Giraldo G., Beth E. Involvement of CMV in AIDS and Kaposi's sarcoma. *Progress in Allergy* 1986; **37**: 319–331.

13 Nakamura S., Salahuddin S.Z., Bilberfeld P. *et al*. Kaposi's sarcoma cells: long-term culture with growth factor from retrovirus-infected CD4+ T cells. *Science* 1988; **242**: 426–430.

14 Chang Y., Cesarman E., Pessin M. *et al*. Identification of herpesvirus-like DNA sequences in AIDS-associated Kaposi's sarcoma. *Science* 1994; **266**: 1865–1869.

15 Huang Y.Q., Li J.J., Kaplan M.H. *et al*. Human herpes virus-like nucleic acid in various forms of Kaposi's sarcoma. *Lancet* 1995; **345**: 759–761.

16 Whitby D., Howard M.R., Tennant-Flowers M. *et al*. Detection of Kaposi's sarcoma-associated herpes virus in peripheral blood of HIV-infected individuals: a progression to Kaposi's sarcoma. *Lancet* 1995; **346**: 799–802.

17 Dirckx J. Kaposi. In: Gottlieb G.J., Ackerman A.B., eds. *Kaposi's Sarcoma: a Text and Atlas*. Philadelphia: Lea and Faber, 1988: pp. 25–26.

18 Kaposi M. Idiopathisches multiples Pigmentsarkom der Haut. *Archives of Dermatology and Syphilis* 1872; **4**: 265–277.

19 Cox F.H., Helwig E.G. Kaposi's sarcoma. *Cancer* 1959; **12**: 289–298.

20 Taylor J.F., Templeton A.C., Vogel C.L., Zeigler J.L., Kyalwazi S.K. Kaposi's sarcoma in Uganda: a clinicopathological study. *International Journal of Cancer* 1971; **8**: 122–135.

21 Harwood A.R., Osoba D., Hofstader S.K. *et al*. Kaposi's sarcoma in recipients of renal transplant. *American Journal of Medicine* 1979; **67**: 759–765.

22 Penn I. Kaposi's sarcoma in organ transplant recipients: report of 20 cases. *Transplantation* 1979; **27**: 8–11.

23 Krown S.E. AIDS-associated Kaposi's sarcoma: pathogenesis, clinical course and treatment. *AIDS* 1988; **2**: 71–80.

24 Real F.X., Krown S.E. Spontaneous regression of Kaposi's sarcoma in patients with AIDS. *New England Journal of Medicine* 1985; **313**: 1659.

25 Salahuddin S.Z., Nakamura S., Biberfeld P. *et al*. Angiogenic properties of Kaposi's sarcoma derived cells after long-term culture *in vitro*. *Science* 1988; **242**: 430–433.

26 Vogel J., Hinrichs S.H., Reynolds R.K., Luciw P.A., Jay G. The HIV-*tat* gene induces dermal lesions resembling Kaposi's sarcoma in transgenic mice. *Nature* 1988; **335**: 606–611.

27 Mitsuyasu R.T., Groopman J.E. Biology and therapy of epidemic Kaposi's sarcoma. *Seminars in Oncology* 1984; **11**: 53–59.

28 Bach M.C., Bagwell S.P., Fanning J.P. Primary pulmonary Kaposi's sarcoma in the acquired immunodeficiency syndrome: a cause of persistent pyrexia. *American Journal of Medicine* 1988; **85**: 274–275.

29 Dantzig P.I., Richardson D., Rayhanzadeh S., Mauro J., Shoss R. Thoracic involvement of non-African Kaposi's sarcoma. *Chest* 1974; **66**: 522–525.

30 Misra D.P., Sunderrajan E.V., Hurst D.J., Maltby J.D. Kaposi's sarcoma of the lung: radiography and pathology. *Thorax* 1982; **37**: 155–156.

31 Antman K.H., Nadler L., Mark E.J., Montela D.L., Kirkpatrick P., Halpern J. Primary Kaposi's sarcoma of the lung in an immunocompetent 32-year of heterosexual white man. *Cancer* 1984; **54**: 1696–1698.

32 Gunawardena K.A., al-Hasani M.K., Haleem A., al-Suleiman M., al-Kahder A.A. Pulmonary Kaposi's sarcoma in two recipients of renal transplants.*Thorax* 1988; **43**: 653–656.

33 Gill P.S. Recent advances in AIDS-related Kaposi's sarcoma. *Current Opinion in Infectious Diseases* 1990; **3**: 94–99.

34 Murray J.F., Felton C.P., Garay S.M. *et al*. Pulmonary complications of AIDS: report of a National Heart, Lung, and Blood Institute Workshop. *New England Journal of Medicine* 1984; **310**: 1682–1688.

35 Zibrak J.D., Silvestri R.C., Costello P. *et al*. Bronchoscopic and radiologic features of Kaposi's sarcoma involving the respiratory system. *Chest* 1986; **90**: 476–479.

36 Garay S.M., Belenko M., Fazzini E., Schinella R. Pulmonary manifestations of Kaposi's sarcoma. *Chest* 1987; **91**: 39–43.

37 Ognibene F.P., Steis R.G., Macher A.M. Kaposi's sarcoma causing pulmonary infiltrates and respiratory failure in the acquired immunodeficiency syndrome. *Annals of Internal Medicine* 1985; **102**: 471–475.

38 Tapper O.J., Corian M., Wolfe S., Berger T. Kaposi's sarcoma: epidemiology, pathogenesis, histology, clinical spectrum, staging criteria and therapy. *Journal of American Academy of Dermatology* 1993; **28**: 371–395.

39 Safai B. Pathophysiology and epidemiology of epidemic Kaposi's sarcoma. *Seminars in Oncology* 1987; **14** (Suppl.), 7.

40 Nash G., Fligiel S. Pathological features of the lung in the acquired immunodeficiency syndrome (AIDS): an autopsy study of seventeen homosexual males. *American Journal of Clinical Pathology* 1984; **81**: 6–12.

41 Agostini C., Poletti V., Zambello R. *et al.* Phenotypical and functional analysis of bronchoalveolar lavage lymphocytes in patients with HIV infection. *American Review of Respiratory Diseases* 1988; **138**: 1609–1615.

42 Nash G., Fligiel S. Kaposi's sarcoma presenting as pulmonary disease in the acquired immune deficiency syndrome: diagnosis by lung biopsy. *Human Pathology* 1984; **15**: 999–1001.

43 Meduri G.U., Stover D.E., Lee M., Myskowski P.L., Caravelli J.F., Zaman M.B. Pulmonary Kaposi's sarcoma in the acquired immune deficiency syndrome: clinical, radiographic, and pathologic manifestations. *American Journal of Medicine* 1986; **81**: 11–18.

44 Niedt G.W., Schinella R.A. AIDS: clinicopathological study of 56 autopsies. *Archives of Pathology and Laboratory Medicine* 1985; **109**: 727–734.

45 Kornfeld H., Axelrod J.L. Pulmonary presentation of Kaposi's sarcoma in a homosexual patient. *American Review of Respiratory Diseases* 1983; **127**: 248–249.

46 Davis S.D., Henschke C.I., Chamides B.K., Westcott J.L. Intrathoracic Kaposi's sarcoma in AIDS patients: radiographic–pathologic correlation. *Radiology* 1987; **163**: 495–500.

47 Ramaswamy G., Jagadha V., Tchertkoff V. Diffuse alveolar damage and interstitial fibrosis in AIDS patients without concurrent pulmonary infection. *Archives of Pathology and Laboratory Medicine* 1985; **109**: 408–412.

48 Ognibene F.P., Shelhamer J.H. Kaposi's sarcoma. *Clinical Chest Medicine* 1988; **9**: 459–465.

49 Greenberg J.E., Fischl M.A., Berger J.R. Upper airway obstruction secondary to AIDS related Kaposi's sarcoma. *Chest* 1985; **88**: 638–640.

50 O'Brien R.F., Cohn D.L. Serosanguinous pleural effusions in AIDS-associated Kaposi's sarcoma. *Chest* 1989; **96**: 460–466.

51 Cohn D.L., O'Brien R.F., Arnel M.F. Pleuropulmonary Kaposi's sarcoma in AIDS: clinical, radiographic and pathological manifestations. *American Review of Respiratory Diseases* 1985; **131**: A82.

52 Pandya K., Lal C., Tuchschmidt J., Boylen C.T., Sharma O.P. Bilateral chylothorax with pulmonary Kaposi's sarcoma. *Chest* 1988; **94**: 1316–1317.

53 Gill P.S., Akil B., Colletti P. *et al.* Pulmonary Kaposi's sarcoma: clinical findings and results of therapy. *American Journal of Medcine* 1989; **87**: 57–61.

54 Naidich D.P., Garay S.M., Leitman B.S., McCauley D.I. Radiographic manifestations of pulmonary disease in the acquired immunodeficiency syndrome (AIDS). *Seminars in Roentgenology* 1987; **22**: 14–30.

55 Sivit C.J., Schwartz A.M., Rockoff S.D. Kaposi's sarcoma of the lung in AIDS: radiologic–pathologic analysis. *American Journal of Radiology* 1987; **148**: 25–28.

56 Pozniak A.L., Latif A.S., Macleod D., Neill P., Ndemere B. Pulmonary Kaposi's sarcoma. *Thorax* 1992; **7**: 730–733.

57 Lai K.K. Pulmonary Kaposi's sarcoma presenting as diffuse reticular nodular infiltrates with cavitatory lesions. *Southern Medical Journal* 1990; **83**: 1096–1098.

58 McCauley D.I., Naidich D.P., Leitman B.S., Reede D.L., Laubenstein L. Radiographic

patterns of opportunistic lung infections and Kaposi's sarcoma in homosexual men. *American Journal of Radiology* 1982; **139**: 653–658.

59 Naidich D.P., Tarras M., Garay S.M., Birnbaum B., Rybak B.J., Schinella R. Kaposi's sarcoma: CT–radiographic correlation. *Chest* 1989; **96**: 723–728.

60 Kuhlman J.E., Fishman E.K., Hruban R.H., Knoles M., Zerhouni E.A., Siegelman S.S. Diseases of the chest in AIDS: CT diagnosis. *Radiographics* 1989; **9**: 827–857.

61 White D.A., Mattay R.A. Non-infectious pulmonary complications of infection with the human immunodeficiency virus. *American Review of Respiratory Diseases* 1989; **140**: 1763–1787.

62 Khalil A., Carett M., Cadranel J., Mayaud C., Akoun G., Bigot J. Magnetic resonance imaging findings in pulmonary Kaposi's sarcoma: a series of 10 cases. *European Respiratory Journal* 1994; **7**: 1285–1289.

63 Stover D.E., White D.A., Romano P.A., Gellene R.A., Robeson W.A. Spectrum of pulmonary diseases associated with the acquired immune deficiency syndrome. *American Journal of Medicine* 1995; **1985**: 429–437.

64 Miller R.F., Tomlinson M.C., Cottrill C.P., Donald J.J., Spittle M.F., Semple S.J.G. Bronchopulmonary Kaposi's sarcoma in patients with AIDS. *Thorax* 1992; **47**: 721–725.

65 Woolfenden J.M., Carrasquillo J.A., Larson S.M. *et al.* Acquired immunodeficiency syndrome: GA-67 citrate imaging. *Radiology* 1987; **167**: 383–387.

66 Lee V.W., Rosen M.P., Baum A., Cohen S.E., Cooley T.P., Liebman H.A. AIDS-related Kaposi's sarcoma: findings on thallium-201 scintigraphy. *American Journal of Radiology* 1988; **151**: 1233–1235.

67 MacLeod D.T., Neill P., Robertson V.F. *et al.* Pulmonary disease in patients affected with the human immunodeficiency virus in Zimbabwe, Central Africa. *Transactions of the Royal Society of Tropical Medicine and Hygiene* 1989; **83**: 694–697.

68 Hamm P.G., Judson M.A., Aranda C.P. Diagnosis of pulmonary Kaposi's sarcoma with fiberoptic bronchoscopy and endobronchial biopsy: a report of five cases. *Cancer* **59**: 807–810.

69 Fouret P.J., Touboul J.L., Mayaud C.M., Akoun G.M., Roland J. Pulmonary Kaposi's sarcoma in patients with acquired immune deficiency syndrome: a clinicopathological study. *Thorax* 1987; **42**: 262–287.

70 Stover D.E., White D.A., Romano P.A., Gellene R.A. Diagnosis of pulmonary disease in acquired immune deficiency syndrome (AIDS): role of bronchoscopy and bronchoalveolar lavage. *American Review of Respiratory Diseases* 1984; **130**: 659–662.

71 Pitchenik A.E., Fischl M.A., Saldana M.J. Kaposi's sarcoma in the tracheobronchial tree: clinical, bronchoscopic and pathologic features. *Chest* 1985; **87**: 122–124.

72 Purdy L.J., Colby T.V., Yousem S.A., Battifora H. Pulmonary Kaposi's sarcoma: premortem histologic diagnosis. *American Journal of Surgical Pathology* 1986; **10**: 301–311.

73 Hanson P.J., Harcourt-Webster J.N., Gazzard B.G., Collins J.V. Fiberoptic bronchoscopy in diagnosis of bronchopulmonary Kaposi's sarcoma. *Thorax* 1987; **42**: 269–271.

74 McKenna R.J., Campbell A., McMurtrey M.J., Mountain C.F. Diagnosis for interstitial lung disease in patients with acquired immune deficiency syndrome (AIDS): a prospective comparison of bronchial washing, alveolar lavage, transbronchial lung biopsy, and open lung biopsy. *Annals of Thoracic Surgery* 1986; **41**: 318–321.

75 Griffiths M.H., Kocjan G., Miller R.F., Godfrey-Faussett P. Diagnosis of pulmonary disease in human immunodeficiency virus infection: role of transbronchial biopsy and bronchoalveolar lavage. *Thorax* 1989; **44**: 554–558.

76 Pass H.I., Potter D., Shelhammer J. *et al.* Indications for and diagnostic efficacy of open-lung biopsy in the patient with acquired immunodeficiency syndrome (AIDS). *Annals of Thoracic Surgery* 1986; **41**: 307–312.

77 Millar A.B., Patou G., Miller R.F. *et al.* Cytomegalovirus in the lungs of patients with AIDS. *American Review of Respiratory Diseases* 1990; **141**: 1474–1477.

78 Touboul J.L., Mayaud C.M., Fouret P., Akoun G.M. Pulmonary lesions of Kaposi's sarcoma, intra-alveolar hemorrhage, and pleural effusion. *Annals of Internal Medicine* 1985; **103**: 808.

79 Drew W.L., Finley T.N., Golde D.W. Diagnostic lavage and occult pulmonary hemorrhage in thrombocytopoenic immunocompromised patients. *American Review of Respiratory Diseases* 1977; **116**: 215–221.

80 Fouret P.J., Touboul J.L., Picard F., Mayaud C., Roland J. Value of the cytological examination of the bronchoalveolar lavage fluid in patients with acquired immunodeficiency syndrome and related syndromes. *Annales de Pathologie* 1986; **6**: 45–52.

81 Blumenfeld W., Egbert B.M., Sagbiel W.R. Differential diagnosis of Kaposi's sarcoma. *Archives of Pathology and Laboratory Medicine* 1985; **109**: 123–127.

82 Suffredini A.F., Ognibene F.P., Lack E.E. *et al.* Nonspecific interstitial pneumonitis: a common cause of pulmonary disease in the acquired immunodeficiency syndrome. *Annals of Internal Medicine* 1987; **107**: 7–13.

83 Sidawi M.K. The lungs. In: Harawi S.J., O'Hara C.J., eds. *Pathology and Pathophysiology of AIDS and HIV-related Diseases*. London: Chapman and Hall Medical, 1989: 301–326.

84 Harawi S.J. Kaposi's sarcoma. In: Harawi, S.J., O'Hara C.J., eds. *Pathology and Pathophysiology of AIDS and HIV-related Diseases*. London: Chapman and Hall Medical, 1989; 83–133.

85 Taylor J., Afrasiabi R., Fahey J.L., Korns E., Weaver J., Mitsuysau R. Prognostically significant classification of immune changes in AIDS with Kaposi's sarcoma. *Blood* 1986; **67**: 666–671.

86 Chachoua A., Krigel R., Lafleur F. *et al.* Prognostic factors and staging classification of patients with epidemic Kaposi's sarcoma. *Journal of Clinical Oncology* 1989; **7**: 774–780.

87 Mitsuyasu R.T., Groopman J.E. Biology and therapy of Kaposi's sarcoma. *Seminars in Oncology* 1984; **11**: 53–59.

88 Krigel R.L., Laubenstein L.J., Muggia F.M. Kaposi's sarcoma: a new staging classification. *Cancer Treatment Review* 1983; **67**: 531–534.

89 Krown S.E., Metroka C., Wernz J.C. Kaposi's sarcoma in the acquired immunodeficiency syndrome: a proposal for uniform evaluation, response and staging criteria. *Journal of Clinical Oncology* 1989; **4**: 1201–1207.

90 Volberding P.A. The role of chemotherapy for epidemic Kaposi's sarcoma. *Seminars in Oncology* 1987; **2** (Suppl. 3): 23–26.

91 Volberding P.A., Cusick P.S., Feigal D.W. Effect of chemotherapy for HIV-associated Kaposi's sarcoma on long-term survival. *American Society of Clinical Oncology, San Francisco* 1989; **11**.

92 Volberding P.A., Abrahams D.I., Conant M.A., Kaslow K., Vranizan K., Zieglar J. Vinblastine therapy for Kaposi's sarcoma in the acquired immunodeficiency syndrome. *Annals of Internal Medicine* 1985; **103**: 335–338.

93 Laubenstein L.J., Krigel R.J., Odajnyk C.M. *et al.* Treatment of epidemic Kaposi's sarcoma with etoposide or a combination of doxorubicin, bleomycin and vinblastine. *Journal of Clinical Oncology* 1984; **2**: 1115–1120.

94 Gelmann E.P., Longo D., Lane H.C. *et al.* Combination chemotherapy of disseminated Kaposi's sarcoma in patients with the acquired immunodeficiency syndrome. *American Journal of Medicine* 1987; **82**: 456–462.

95 Cadranel J., Kammoun S., Chevret S. *et al.* Results of chemotherapy in 30 AIDS patients with symptomatic pulmonary Kaposi's sarcoma. *Thorax* 1994; **49**: 101–103.

96 Nobler M.P. Pulmonary irradiation for Kaposi's sarcoma in AIDS. *American Journal of Clinical Oncology* 1985; **8**: 441–444.

97 Nisce L.Z., Safai B. Radiation therapy of Kaposi's sarcoma in AIDS: Memorial Sloan-Kettering experience. *Frontiers in Radiation Therapy and Oncology* 1985; **19**: 133–137.

98 Murray J.F., Garay S.M., Hopewell P.C., Mills J., Snider G.L., Stover D.E. Pulmonary

complications of the acquired immunodeficiency syndrome: an update. *American Review of Respiratory Diseases* 1987; **135**: 504–509.

99 DeWit R., Boucher C.B., Veenhof K.N., Schatenkerk J., Bakker P., Danner S. Clinical and virological effects of high dose recombinant interferon-alpha in disseminated AIDS-related Kaposi's sarcoma. *Lancet* 1988; **ii**: 1214–1217.

100 Krigel R.L., Slywotzky C.M., Lonberg M. *et al.* Treatment of epidemic Kaposi's sarcoma with a combination of interferon-alpha 2β and etoposide. *Journal of Biological Response* 1988; **7**: 359–364.

101 Lane H.G., Feinberg J., Davey V. *et al.* Anti-retroviral effects of interferon-alpha in AIDS-associated Kaposi's sarcoma. *Lancet* 1988; **ii**: 1218–1222.

102 Kovacs J.A., Deyton L., Davey R. *et al.* Combined zidovudine and interferon alpha therapy in patients with Kaposi's sarcoma and the acquired immunodeficiency syndrome. *Annals of Internal Medicine* 1989; **111**: 280–287.

103 Folkman J., Langer R., Linhardt R.J., Haudenschild C., Taylor S. Angiogenesis, inhibition and tumour regression caused by heparin or a heparin fragment in the presence of cortisone. *Science* 1983; **221**: 719–725.

104 Saville M.W., Lietzau J., Pluda J.M. *et al.* Treatment of HIV-associated Kaposi's sarcoma with paclitaxel. *Lancet* 1995; **346**: 26–28.

105 Harris P.J. Treatment of Kaposi's sarcoma and other manifestations of AIDS with human chorionic gonadotrophin [letter]. *Lancet* 1995; **346**: 118–119.

106 Mitchell D.M., McCarty M., Fleming J., Moss F.M. Bronchopulmonary Kaposi's sarcoma in patients with AIDS. *Thorax* 1992; **47**: 726–729.

6 Hodgkin's lymphoma, non-Hodgkin's lymphoma and carcinoma of the bronchus

S.J.G. SEMPLE

6.0 Introduction

It is now well known and established that HIV infection is associated with a marked increase in the incidence of Kaposi's sarcoma and non-Hodgkin's lymphoma (NHL), both of which are included in the case definition of AIDS [1–3]. In a cohort study of 1756 newly diagnosed malignancies in HIV-infected persons, 99% occurred in males, 83% were Kaposi's sarcomas, 13% were NHLs and 1% were Hodgkin's disease [2]. In this cohort study, some other malignancies, not traditionally thought to be HIV-associated, occurred more frequently than expected; these were Hodgkin's disease, cancers of the rectum, anus and nasal cavity and rare non-melanoma skin cancers [2]. The temporal increase, since the start of the AIDS epidemic, of NHL (and possibly of Hodgkin's disease) has been substantial and continues to be so [2,4]. Cohort studies linking HIV infection and malignancy have predominantly been in homosexual or bisexual men and the incidence of NHL in these men has been found to be four times greater than in other groups at risk of acquiring AIDS [5]. In Italy, where HIV infection is predominantly due to intravenous drug use, at least 15% of AIDS cases are associated with tumours, of which Kaposi's sarcoma and high-grade malignancy are the most common [6]. The association between malignancy and HIV may be a general feature of immune deficiency, which has been shown to be related to the development of neoplasia in conditions other than AIDS [7,8].

CHAPTER 6
*Hodgkin's
lymphoma,
non-Hodgkin's
lymphoma and
carcinoma of the
bronchus*

Improved antiretroviral treatment and the introduction of prophylaxis have prolonged survival and hence provided an increased opportunity for the development of NHL. In a retrospective analysis of the development of NHL in a cohort of HIV-infected patients treated with zidovudine between 1985 and 1987, the estimated probability of developing lymphoma by 30 months of survival was 28.6% (confidence interval 13.7–50.3%) and by 36 months 46% (confidence interval 19.6–75.5%). In this series, those patients who did develop lymphoma were profoundly immunosuppressed, with CD4 counts of less than 50 cells/mm^3 [9]. The patients in this study were not on the combination antiretroviral therapy now available (in the mid-1990s) and there is no mention of prophylaxis for *Pneumocystis carinii* pneumonia (PCP). However, these estimates, in spite of wide confidence limits, suggest that prolonged survival and severe immunosuppression are important predisposing factors in the development of NHL. These factors are unlikely to be the sole explanation for the increased incidence of NHL in HIV-infected people, because in North America there has been a substantial increase in the incidence of NHL in patients who are not infected with HIV.

6.1 Non-Hodgkin's lymphoma

6.1.1 Early reports of non-Hodgkin's lymphoma in HIV-infected people

In the original description of the association between NHL and persistent generalized lymphadenopathy (PGL) in homosexual men at risk of AIDS, not all patients had an AIDS diagnosis at their presentation with NHL; thus, of 90 homosexual men, 15 had no prodromal illness or symptoms and 33 patients had PGL [10]. Two other studies of patients at risk of AIDS report similar results. In one series, of 84 patients with NHL, 27 patients were diagnosed as having AIDS on presentation, 15 patients had PGL and 10 patients had the AIDS-related complex (ARC); the remainder had none of these three complications of HIV infection [11]. In another series, of 89 patients with NHL, 15 patients had ARC and 20 patients were classified as 'at risk of AIDS'. In this series, in a further 15 patients the diagnosis of AIDS was made on the basis of the simultaneous finding of NHL and a positive serological test for HIV infection [12]. These three series cover a period of time starting in 1981, when serological testing for HIV infection was not available, so some patients were only classified as 'at risk of AIDS'; hence infection was presumed and not always proved. However, after 1985 all patients with NHL were HIV antibody-tested and were found to be positive, so the earlier assumption that those 'at risk of AIDS' were truly HIV-infected was reasonable [11,12].

CHAPTER 6
*Hodgkin's
lymphoma,
non-Hodgkin's
lymphoma and
carcinoma of the
bronchus*

6.1.2 Non-Hodgkin's lymphoma and the Epstein–Barr virus

Genomic sequences of HIV are not present in clones of B cells derived from patients with NHL or PGL [13–15]. Studies of AIDS-related lymphoproliferative disorders at a cellular and molecular level have shown that the majority of NHL is B-cell-specific and that multiple B-cell clonal expansion is a feature of NHL and PGL, being common in the former and less so in the latter [13]. The second cellular feature is the finding of translocations or rearrangements of the oncogene, c-*myc*, which has been found in NHL but not in PGL [13,15]. Only a single rearranged c-*myc* gene has been detected in NHL, suggesting that only one clone of the B-cell expansion carries the rearranged gene [13]. Specific chromosomal translocations of the c-*myc* locus are also a feature of Burkitt's lymphoma and this leads on to the possible role of the Epstein–Barr virus (EBV) in the development of NHL.

EBV may immortalize B cells *in vitro*, but not transform them, and this effect may also be associated with c-*myc* activation. It is, however, the combined action of EBV and c-*myc* which is likely to be responsible for malignant transformation, as shown by the ability of these cells to form tumours *in vivo* in immunodeficient mice [16].

With the information from these studies, a hypothesis for the generation of lymphoma in AIDS has been formulated. In summary, this is that EBV infection leads to the expansion of B-cell clones (as in PGL), which is not suppressed in patients with HIV infection because of lack of immune surveillance. This facilitates an increased occurrence of c-*myc* rearrangements and hence malignant transformation [13–15,17]. In favour of this hypothesis is the high level of EBV titres found in AIDS patients with lymphoma compared with those without HIV infection [5] and the identification of EBV deoxyribonucleic acid (DNA) in tumour cells of AIDS-related lymphoma [18]. However, it is unlikely that this hypothesis can be extended to all NHLs [17], because EBV can only be demonstrated by *in situ* hybridization in approximately 50% of cases [18] and EBV genomic sequences have been found in only five out of 15 biopsies from lymphoma in patients with AIDS [11].

6.1.3 Histology and phenotype of non-Hodgkin's lymphoma in HIV infection

The histological and phenotypic origin of the NHLs which are used for the case definition of AIDS is high-grade B-cell lymphoma, which may be variously reported as large-cell lymphoma (immunoblastic lymphoma, large-cell non-cleaved lymphoma) and small-cell non-cleaved lymphoma (either Burkitt's or non-Burkitt's). Not included are T-cell lymphoma, and

CHAPTER 6
*Hodgkin's
lymphoma,
non-Hodgkin's
lymphoma and
carcinoma of the
bronchus*

Table 6.1 The histological description of 100 cases of B-cell lymphoma [19].

Diffuse, large cell (cleaved and non-cleaved)	40%
Large-cell immunoblastic (plasmacytoid and polymorphous)	31%
Small non-cleaved cell (Burkitt's and Burkitt's-like)	24%
Diffuse, small cleaved cell	4%
Small lymphocytic	1%

those described as lymphocytic, lymphoblastic, small cleaved or plasma-cytoid lymphocytic [3].

NHLs are almost exclusively of the B-cell phenotype. In a large series of 100 cases reported from New York [19], all were B-cell lymphomas. The histology of the NHLs as described is shown in Table 6.1. The last two histological types, comprising five patients, were low-grade lymphomas and would therefore not be classed as AIDS-defining conditions. Over 60% of the extranodal NHLs were of the two most aggressive types, namely large-cell immunoblastic and Burkitt's, and these accounted for the majority of NHLs involving the brain and gastrointestinal (GI) tract [19]. NHL has been found to occur following development of lymphadenopathy, which initially on biopsy was found to be non-neoplastic and had the histological features of HIV infection [19,20].

6.1.4 Clinical presentation of non-Hodgkin's lymphoma in HIV infection

The special clinical characteristics of NHL in patients with HIV infection are that the initial presentation is late in the disease (stage III–IV), the course is 'aggressively' downhill and the involvement is extranodal in the majority of patients [10–12,20]. These extranodal sites include the central nervous system (CNS), GI tract, including the rectum, bone marrow and myocardium. When the presentation is nodal, the initial feature may be a rapid enlargement of a lymph node or group of nodes. Occasionally, patients may present with HIV 'constitutional' symptoms — namely weight loss, fatigue and fever [21]. The mode of presentation and course of the illness are related to the histological findings. Stage IV disease at presentation is more common in patients with high-grade as opposed to low-grade lymphoma, and this may be associated with a higher frequency of bone-marrow involvement in the former group [12]. On the basis of the incidence of HIV infection in patients with NHL, it has been suggested that, overall, low-grade B-cell lymphoma in homosexual men may be a fortuitous occurrence and may not be related to HIV infection [22].

Overall, survival has been found to be short, the median survival being 10.5 months in one series [23] and 4.3 in another [11], the cause of death usually being an opportunistic infection [23]. Poor prognostic indicators at presentation are a low CD4 lymphocyte count, a previous AIDS-defining illness, a poor Karnofsky performance score and the presence of extranodal disease [11]. In those with good prognostic indicators, satisfactory improvement or complete remissions may be achieved with chemotherapy [11,24,25]. In those patients with poor indicators (especially CD4 counts under 100 cells/m^3), chemotherapy may cause significant morbidity, with little improvement in survival, while 'aggressive' chemotherapy may increase immunosuppression and shorten survival [11,25].

These early disappointing results in the treatment of NHL in HIV-infected persons have led to a modification in therapeutic approach. In patients who are profoundly immunosuppressed, with low CD4 counts and poor prognostic indicators, chemotherapeutic agents are used in low doses (e.g. less than 1 g/m^2 of cyclophosphamide), together with granulocyte colony-stimulating factor to ameliorate neutropenia [4,11]. The use of intensive regimens of chemotherapy is reserved for those patients with good prognostic factors, where satisfactory complete response rates can be achieved, as well as longer periods of survival (for review see [4]).

6.1.5 Pulmonary complications of patients with non-Hodgkin's lymphoma and HIV infection

Opportunistic and non-opportunistic infection of the lung is common before, during and following treatment of patients with NHL, and indeed it is often the cause of death. The frequency of extranodal disease in patients with NHL and the number of patients with lung disease can be approximately estimated from several reports in the literature (Table 6.2). In these studies, lung involvement in all patients with NHL has varied from 2.0 to 17%. Extranodal involvement, including all sites, was high, varying from 61 to 98%. When lung involvement is expressed as a percentage of patients with extranodal disease (with or without associated nodal involvement), the frequency varies from 2 to 25%. These data suggest that the lung is not a common site for extranodal disease in patients with NHL. The precise nature of the pulmonary involvement is often not quoted but in some reports details are available. Out of 84 patients with NHL, five had lung involvement and two patients had upper-lobe nodules as the sole site of their disease [11]. In a report of three patients with NHL and lung involvement, one patient had PCP among

CHAPTER 6
*Hodgkin's
lymphoma,
non-Hodgkin's
lymphoma and
carcinoma of the
bronchus*

Table 6.2 Extranodal disease and lung involvement in patients with NHL at risk of AIDS.

No. of patients with NHL [reference]	No. of patients with extranodal involvement (%)	No. of patients with NHL and pulmonary involvement (%)	Patients with lung involvement by NHL expressed as a percentage of patients with extranodal disease
100 [19]	61 (61.0)	1 (1.0)	1.6
84 [9]	62 (73.8)	5 (6.0)	8.1
90 [10]	88 (97.8)	8 (8.9)	9.1
43 [23]	28 (65.1)	7* (16.3)	25.0
31 [24]	26 (83.9)	4 (12.9)	15.4
24 [5]	23 (95.8)	4 (16.7)	17.4

* These seven patients had pulmonary involvement but a further two patients were reported as having pleural effusions without details of the cause.

many other non-respiratory complications, one had bilateral pleural effusions without mediastinal lymphadenopathy and a third had superior vena-caval obstruction associated with an anterior mediastinal mass [20]. There are two reports of NHL presenting as isolated primary pulmonary lymphoma; one was in the left lower lobe and the other in the left hilar region [4,26]. The lymphoma in the left lower lobe was removed at thoracotomy and there was no relapse 8 months after resection; no chemotherapy was given. The tumour was a high-grade malignant lymphoma of the large-cell immunoblastic type [26].

In a group of 20 patients with AIDS-related lymphoma, five presented with lesions in the thorax, four localized to the chest. The abnormalities seen were: (i) in one patient a large anteroposterior mass (10 cm diameter) in the mediastinum which invaded the sternum; (ii) a pleuropulmonary mass in another patient which invaded the chest wall; and (iii) in three patients pulmonary nodules were seen without mediastinal or pleural involvement. Computed tomography (CT) scanning was useful in identifying the best site for biopsy and in revealing pulmonary nodules or mediastinal lymphadenopathy which were not evident on the plain chest radiograph [27].

In the reports of lung involvement by NHL described so far, it is not always clear whether the lung is one of several extranodal sites and is a manifestation of diffuse widespread disease or whether the lung is the primary extranodal site of presentation and contains the main bulk of disease. The latter presentation is compatible with the current operational definition of an extranodal lymphoma [28]. This distinction between lung involvement as part of widespread disease and lung involvement as the primary extranodal site has been made in a comprehensive review of the radiographic manifestations of AIDS-related lymphoma in the thorax.

Table 6.3 Radiographic findings in the thorax of 20 patients with AIDS-related lymphoma.

CHAPTER 6
*Hodgkin's
lymphoma,
non-Hodgkin's
lymphoma and
carcinoma of the
bronchus*

Normal	Mediastinal lymph nodes	Pleural effusions		Multiple nodules	Single nodules	Parenchymal changes
		Single	Bilateral			
5	5	5	2	2	9	5

Subsequent CT scanning revealed in the five normal chest radiographs three patients with small mediastinal lymph nodes and two patients with peripheral masses, 2–5 cm in diameter. The number of patients with pleural effusions was increased from seven to nine.

This was a retrospective study of 116 consecutive cases of AIDS-related lymphoma [29]. Abnormalities were seen on the chest X-ray or CT scan in 52 of these patients, but in 32 the abnormalities were due to the complications of AIDS rather than NHL (e.g. mycobacterial infection, PCP, Kaposi's sarcoma and bacterial or viral infection). In 20 patients, the abnormal chest radiology was due to NHL, nine of whom had direct histological or cytological confirmation of lymphoma in the chest. The remaining patients had biopsy evidence of lymphoma at a distant site and the radiological changes in the chest were attributed to lymphoma, no other causes being found on the chest radiograph or CT scan to account for the findings. In 15 patients the thorax was the principal site of disease, on the basis of symptoms, radiology and clinical examination. Dyspnoea, cough, haemoptysis and chest pain were the principal symptoms. The most frequent findings on imaging were pleural or intrapulmonary masses, frequently peripheral and sometimes with cavitation; in one case, this cavitation simulated mycetoma formation. The presence of effusions, pulmonary nodules and lymphadenopathy were the findings most suggestive of AIDS-related lymphoma. In two patients mediastinal involvement was a direct extension of an extrathoracic mass, while in another two patients lymphoma involvement of the pericardium led to pericardial effusions. Table 6.3 summarizes the radiographic findings in this review [29].

CT scanning provided useful additional information to the chest radiograph, particularly in the assessment of mediastinal lymph-node involvement, as well as in the identification of small parenchymal nodules. CT scanning was also helpful in determining the best approach for percutaneous biopsy of the lesion, thereby avoiding open-lung biopsy.

6.1.6 T-cell lymphoma

Occasionally, in patients with NHL the phenotypic origin of the cells has been T rather than B. In a series of 105 patients with lymphoid neoplasia

CHAPTER 6
*Hodgkin's
lymphoma,
non-Hodgkin's
lymphoma and
carcinoma of the
bronchus*

associated with disease due to HIV, three patients were shown to have lymphocytes belonging to the suppressor–cytotoxic T-cell subset giving rise to chronic lymphocytic leukaemia [12]. One of the patients developed multiple opportunistic infection and died from PCP. The other two patients showed no progression of their lymphoid disease following presentation. T-cell chronic lymphocytic leukaemia usually pursues an aggressive fulminant downhill course, but a small subgroup have been identified with a chronic indolent disease [30] and these two patients could be a manifestation of this subgroup. However, this subgroup has special morphological and phenotypic features which were not found in these two patients and therefore they may represent a previously unrecognized form of chronic T-cell leukaemia [12]. In another series, of 84 patients with AIDS-associated NHL, two patients had T-cell lymphoma and in a further three patients the cell type was less clear but may have been T-cell [11]. Five of the 84 patients had involvement of the lung but the report does not specify whether any of these patients belonged to the T-cell subgroup.

Infection with the human T-cell lymphotrophic virus I (HTLV-I) is associated with adult T-cell leukaemia/lymphoma and the two reports of T-cell lymphoma in patients with HIV infection quoted above [11,12] do not state if the patients were tested for evidence of HTLV-I infection. There is, however, a report of a patient with a combined HTLV-I and HTLV-III (HIV) infection with T_8 'proliferative' disease [31]. The patient had a T_8 lymphocytosis with a low T_4/T_8 ratio, which is not characteristic of HTLV-I infection. The patient suffered a long debilitating illness more like AIDS than T-cell leukaemia, with frequent chest infections, including a left lower pneumonia and a pleural effusion. There is further discussion in Chapter 9 (section 9.6) of HTLV-I infection and lymphoproliferative disorders of the lung.

Peripheral T-cell lymphoma has also been recorded in patients with AIDS. Two such patients have been reported, both with lymphoma within the lung. One patient developed a lymphoma of the left lung, proved on open biopsy. Antibodies to HTLV-I were not detected and the patient responded poorly to chemotherapy and died shortly after presentation; the cause of death was not specified [32]. The second patient developed a lymphoma of the right middle lobe, which was removed at thoracotomy. The patient died of his AIDS with no clinical evidence of recurrence of the lymphoma [33].

In view of the small number of T-cell leukaemia/lymphomas reported in patients with HIV infection, it is not possible to determine if they are associated with AIDS. It is possible, however, that the features and course of the illness may be affected by infection with HIV.

6.2 Hodgkin's lymphoma

CHAPTER 6
*Hodgkin's
lymphoma,
non-Hodgkin's
lymphoma and
carcinoma of the
bronchus*

In a large registry-linkage study in San Francisco, Hodgkin's lymphoma (HL) occurred more often than expected in members of an AIDS cohort [2]. The early reports of HL in patients with HIV infection certainly raised the possibility of this association but the numbers were too small to give statistical certainty [12,23,34–39]. At present, HL is not an AIDS-defining condition.

Two recent studies of the association of HL with HIV infection are based on substantial numbers of patients (46 and 114, respectively), compared with the earlier reports [40,41]. However, 85% of the patients were intravenous drug users (IVDUs) and evidence was provided in both series that the occurrence of HL in IVDUs is higher than in homosexuals [40,41]. In spite of this difference in incidence, the clinical picture and response to treatment of patients in these two series in IVDUs is very similar to those of earlier reports, which were based on findings in male homosexuals or bisexuals [12,23,34–39].

The presentation of HL in HIV-infected persons differs in many respects from that found in patients free of HIV. In a comparison of HL between two groups of patients (HIV-infected versus non-HIV-infected), it was found at presentation that HIV-infected persons were younger (29 vs. 38 years) and that there was a prevalence of males (90% vs. 56%), a higher percentage of stage IV disease (52% vs. 15%) and the presence of B symptoms (77% vs. 35%) and extranodal disease (63% vs. 29%). Mediastinal involvement was significantly less common in patients who were HIV-infected than in those who were not (23% vs. 58%). There was a predominance of mixed-cellularity and lymphocyte-depletion histological subtypes in HIV-infected persons, whereas in those not infected with HIV lymphocyte predominance together with nodular sclerosis was the more common subtype. The association with EBV was also compared between the two groups, the association being detected in 14 out of 18 patients infected with HIV (78%) and 12 out of 44 (38%) of HIV-unassociated HL. Evidence of monoclonal expansion of EBV-infected cells was found in eight out of 10 HIV-associated HL but only 12 of 44 lymphomas which were not HIV-related [41].

The clinicopathological features of Hodgkin's disease associated with HIV infection are shown in Table 6.4; the data are obtained from two recent studies [40,41].

Treatment has consisted of various chemotherapeutic regimens, often combined with radiotherapy. In one series the median survival was 15 months (range = 1–44 months), with 44% achieving a complete response and 37% a partial response [40], while in another series the correspond-

CHAPTER 6
*Hodgkin's
lymphoma,
non-Hodgkin's
lymphoma and
carcinoma of the
bronchus*

Table 6.4 Clinicopathological features of Hodgkin's disease associated with HIV infection.

	Series 1 [40] n = 44 (%)	Series 2 [41] n = 114 (%)
Risk group		
IVDUs	84.8	85.6
Homosexual	8.7	8.1
AIDS in past or on presentation	6.5	16.7
Histopathology		
Mixed cellularity	41.3	44.9
Lymphoid depletion	21.7	21.5
Nodular sclerosis	21.7	30.0
Lymphocyte predominance	4.3	3.7
Advanced stages (III/IV)	89.1	80.6
B symptoms	82.6	72.2
Extranodal involvement	50.0	63.0
Bone-marrow involvement	41.3	39.0
CD4 lymphocytes <250 cells/mm^3	43.7	—
Response to chemotherapy		
Complete response	44.0	58.0
Partial response	37.0	27.0

ing figures were 13 months, 58% and 27% [41]. Poor prognostic factors were CD4 count <200 cells/mm^3, diagnosis of AIDS at onset, presence of B symptoms and no response to chemotherapy. The poor prognosis and survival of HIV-infected persons with HL is in part due to the unfavourable stage of disease together with the presence of B symptoms at presentation, and in part due to the progression of disease due to HIV unrelated to the concomitant lymphoma.

Lung involvement (apart from opportunistic infection) does not appear to be a common feature of HL in HIV-infected persons. There is a report of one patient with a large mediastinal mass [35] and of another with lower-lobe infiltrates of the lung without hilar or mediastinal lymphadenopathy [37].

6.3 Mediastinal and hilar lymphadenopathy

In a study of 30 homosexual men with PGL, posterior–anterior and lateral chest radiographs showed no evidence of mediastinal or hilar lymphadenopathy and the lung fields were normal. Peripheral lymph-node biopsy was carried out on the patients and in all instances non-specific reactive hyperplasia with a predominantly follicular pattern was seen [42]. In general, the patients were well and free of pulmonary disease.

This group of patients was compared in the same study with 45 patients with AIDS [42]. In nine of those patients thoracic adenopathy was seen on the chest radiograph and in four of these patients the lungs were abnormal, showing a combination of a local or diffuse ground-glass pattern, patchy consolidation and small pleural effusions. All nine patients were ill with a variety of symptoms, including fever, malaise, weight loss, diarrhoea and vomiting. Five had respiratory symptoms, including cough and dyspnoea. After investigation the diagnoses were: PCP in four, *Mycobacterium tuberculosis* in one, *Mycobacterium avium intracellulare* in one, *Cryptococcus neoformans* in two, cytomegalovirus in four and tracheobronchial candidiasis in four. Two patients had Hodgkin's disease, one diagnosed by lymph-node biopsy at mediastinoscopy and one by axillary-node biopsy. In the ninth patient no cause for the lymphadenopathy was found, even after open-lung biopsy. In those patients who responded to specific therapy, there was some reversibility of the lymphadenopathy [42].

In summary, it would appear that, in homosexuals, mediastinal and/or hilar lymphadenopathy is not a complication of PGL. In patients with AIDS mediastinal lymphadenopathy when it occurs is likely to have an infective or neoplastic cause, requiring appropriate investigation and treatment.

6.4 Lung cancer

Early in the AIDS epidemic, there were reports of small-cell carcinoma of the lung in single patients who had AIDS or ARC [43,44]. This raised the possibility that infection with HIV rendered patients more susceptible to carcinoma of the lung, in line with the known increase in malignancy in the immunosuppressed. Since these initial reports, there have been studies on larger groups of patients to determine if there is an increased rate of lung cancer in persons who are infected with HIV. This has been done by comparing the incidence of lung cancer in the years before the start, or soon after the start, of the AIDS epidemic with the incidence when that epidemic was firmly established. In this section on lung cancer, this comparison is assessed together with a description of the clinical presentation of carcinoma of the lung in HIV-infected persons as reported in the literature.

The average age of HIV-infected persons is young compared with that of the majority of patients with lung cancer, which is in the range of 50–70 years of age. Lung cancer is uncommon in individuals under the age of 40 and it is relevant to determine if the presentation of this cancer is different in this age group independent of infection with HIV. In a review of a cancer registry in a hospital in North America (1971–89), there were 50

CHAPTER 6
*Hodgkin's
lymphoma,
non-Hodgkin's
lymphoma and
carcinoma of the
bronchus*

(3%) out of 1678 patients with lung cancer under the age of 42 (range 24–40). A smoking history was available in 37 patients, of whom 35 were heavy smokers (>20 packs per year). Four patients were IVDUs but only one out of the four was HIV-seropositive. Twenty-seven (54%) had adenocarcinoma, which was significantly higher than that found in all age groups (28%). The majority of the patients (78%) had advanced unresectable disease at presentation (stage III/IV). The length of survival was available for 49 of the 50 patients, of whom 47 died during the study. The overall median survival was 26 weeks; in those with small-cell carcinoma it was 24 weeks and in those with non-small-cell carcinoma it was 30 weeks [45].

In a retrospective analysis, a comparison was made between 1335 patients with lung cancer registered between the years 1977 and 1986, and 19 patients who were HIV-seropositive and were diagnosed as having lung cancer between the years 1986 and 1991 [46]. Of the 19 patients, four were IVDUs. The following differences between the two groups of patients were statistically significant.
• All 19 HIV-infected patients were men, whereas the male preponderance in the larger 'control' group was 69%.
• The median age of the seropositive patients was 48 compared with 61 in the HIV-indeterminate group.
• The median survival was 3 months in 16 of the HIV-infected patients and 10 months in 32 HIV-indeterminate control patients matched for the stage of their cancer, age, sex and race.
• Histological features and smoking history were not significantly different between the two groups.
• There were no 1-year survivors in the HIV-seropositive group.

There is a report on the chest radiographs and CT scans of 30 HIV-seropositive patients with proved bronchial carcinoma [47]. Fourteen of the patients had AIDS at the time of diagnosis, all but one were men and most (27) had a history of smoking, on average 57 pack-years. The radiological findings were as follows.
• Eighteen tumours were peripheral, and 17 occurred in the upper lobes. Three were initially mistaken for inflammatory disease
• Eleven tumours were central (hilar or mediastinal) and showed consolidation in the distribution of the affected airways
• Lymphadenopathy was present in 63% of the patients and pleural effusions or masses seen in 33%
• A history of tuberculosis or PCP was present in 83% of the patients with peripheral tumours and 27% of the patients with central lesions.

In a review of the tumour registry at the San Francisco Hospital for lung cancer between 1985 and 1993, 13 patients were found to be HIV-seropositive [48]. All were heavy smokers, 12 were male and the mean age was 41.1 years (range 33–52 years). Six patients were IVDUs, five were homo/bisexual and two were both homosexual and IVDUs. In 10 patients there was no index diagnosis of AIDS on clinical evaluation alone at the time lung cancer was diagnosed. However, five patients had a CD4 count of under 200 cells/mm^3 and, if this is also used as an AIDS-defining criterion, eight out of 13 patients had AIDS. The initial findings on the chest radiograph was a solitary nodule or mass in five, a nodule or mass with hilar or mediastinal adenopathy in five, lobulated pleural disease in one and diffuse small parenchymal nodules in one further patient. CT scanning often revealed more widespread disease than was evident on the plain chest radiograph and nine of the patients had advanced disease (stage III or IV). Only two patients survived more than a year and both had squamous-cell carcinomas which were not poorly differentiated. At this hospital, where an estimated 30% of medical patients are HIV-positive, there has been no change in the incidence of lung cancer in young patients between the pre-AIDS era (1976–79) and the years 1987–90. Further support for no change in the incidence of lung cancer comes from a study of a cohort of 1101 patients with haemophilia followed for up to 12 years. Sixty-three of the subjects were HIV-seropositive [49]. There was no evidence of an increased incidence of cancers in those who were HIV-infected apart from NHL and Kaposi's sarcoma.

In conclusion, there is no evidence at present that the incidence of lung cancer is increased in HIV-infected persons, but the number of patients reviewed is small. A large prospective study with a long-term follow-up will be needed to establish whether the incidence is increased or not. Patients are affected at a significantly younger age than expected but this may be due to the young average age of HIV-infected persons. It does, however, raise the possibility that HIV infection may bring forward in time the development of cancer which would otherwise occur at a later time. A surprisingly high number of IVDUs have been identified in the series reported here, both in those uninfected and those infected with HIV. This has led to speculation that a transmissible agent may be involved in pathogenesis. However, IVDUs are usually heavy smokers and this is more likely to be one of the precipitating causes of lung cancer in the young and is therefore not directly related to HIV infection.

Lung cancer presented at an advanced stage of disease in HIV-infected patients, with a correspondingly poor outcome, but this was also a feature of presentation and outcome in the young age group who were not so infected. There is one report of three patients who were seropositive for HIV infection who developed carcinoma of the bronchus at a later age, namely at ages 50, 51 and 60 [50]. The presentation and outcome were similar to those seen in patients in the younger age group.

CHAPTER 6
*Hodgkin's
lymphoma,
non-Hodgkin's
lymphoma and
carcinoma of the
bronchus*

CHAPTER 6
*Hodgkin's
lymphoma,
non-Hodgkin's
lymphoma and
carcinoma of the
bronchus*

References

1 Biggar R.J., Horm J., Goedert J.J., Melbye M. Cancer in a group of acquired immunodeficiency syndrome (AIDS) through 1984. *American Journal of Epidemiology* 1987; **126**: 578–581.

2 Reynolds P., Saunders L.D., Layefsky M.E., Lemp G.F. The spectrum of acquired immunodeficiency syndrome (AIDS)-associated malignancies in San Francisco, 1980–1987. *American Journal of Epidemiology* 1993; **137**: 19–30.

3 Centers for Disease Control. Revision of the CDC surveillance case definition for acquired immunodeficiency syndrome. *Morbidity and Mortality Weekly Report* 1987; **36** (Suppl. 1S): 3S–13S.

4 Denton A.S., Brook M.G., Miller R.F., Spittle M. AIDS-related lymphoma: an emerging epidemic. *British Journal of Hospital Medicine* 1996; **55**: 282–288.

5 Beckhardt R.N., Farady N., May M., Torres R.A., Strauchen J.A. Increased incidence of malignant lymphoma in AIDS. *The Mount Sinai Journal of Medicine* 1988; **55**: 383–389.

6 Montfardini S., Vaccher E., Lazzarin H. *et al.* Characterization of AIDS-associated tumours in Italy: report of 435 cases of an IVDA-based series. *Cancer Detection and Prevention* 1990; **14**: 391–393.

7 Gatti R.A., Good R.A. Occurrence of malignancy in immunodeficiency diseases. *Cancer* 1971; **28**: 89–98.

8 Penn I. Lymphomas complicating organ transplantation. *Transplantation Proceedings* 1983; **15** (Suppl. 1): 2790–2797.

9 Pluda J.M., Yarchoan R., Jaffe E.S. *et al.* Development of non-Hodgkin's lymphoma in a cohort of patients with severe human immunodeficiency virus (HIV) infection of long-term antiretroviral therapy. *Annals of Internal Medicine* 1990; **113**: 276–282.

10 Zeigler J.L., Beckstead J.A., Volberding P.A. *et al.* Non-Hodgkin's lymphoma in 90 homosexual men: relation to generalized lymphadenopathy and the acquired immunodeficiency syndrome. *New England Journal of Medicine* 1984; **311**: 565–570.

11 Kaplan L.D., Abrams D.I., Feigal E. *et al.* AIDS-associated non-Hodgkin's lymphoma in San Francisco. *Journal of the American Medical Association* 1989; **261**: 719–724.

12 Knowles D.M., Chamulak G.A., Subar M. *et al.* Lymphoid neoplasia associated with the acquired immunodeficiency syndrome (AIDS). *Annals of Internal Medicine* 1988; **108**: 744–753.

13 Pelicci P., Knowles D.M., Arlin Z.A. *et al.* Multiple monoclonal B cell expansions and c-*myc* oncogene rearrangements in acquired immune deficiency syndrome-related lymphoproliferative disorders. *Journal of Experimental Medicine* 1986; **164**: 2049–2076.

14 Groopman J.E., Sullivan J.L., Mulder C. *et al.* Pathogenesis of B cell lymphoma in a patient with AIDS. *Blood* 1986; **67**: 612–615.

15 Rechavi G., Ben-Bassat I., Berkowicz M. *et al.* Molecular analysis of Burkitt's leukaemia in two haemophilic brothers with AIDS. *Blood* 1987; **70**: 1713–1717.

16 Lombardi L., Newcomb E.W., Dalla-Favera R. Pathogenesis of Burkitt lymphoma: expression of an activated c-*myc* oncogene causes the tumorigenic conversion of EBV-infected human B lymphoblasts. *Cell* 1987; **49**: 161–170.

17 Knowles D.M. Biologic aspects of AIDS-associated non-Hodgkin's lymphoma. *Current Opinion in Oncology* 1993; **5**: 845–851.

18 Hamilton-Dutoit S.J., Pallesen G., Karkov J., Skinhøj P., Franzmann M.B., Pedersen C. Identification of EBV-DNA in tumour cells of AIDS-related lymphomas by *in-situ* hybridisation. *Lancet* 1989; i: 554–555.

19 Ioachim H.L., Dorsett B., Cronin W., Maya M., Wahl S. Acquired immunodeficiency syndrome-associated lymphomas: clinical, pathologic and viral characteristics of 111 cases. *Human Pathology* 1991; **22**: 659–673.

20 Levine A.M., Meyer P.R., Begandy M.K. *et al.* Development of B-cell lymphoma in homosexual men. *Annals of Internal Medicine* 1984; **100**: 7–13.

21 Northfelt D.W., Kaplan L.D. Clinical manifestations and treatment of HIV related non-Hodgkin lymphoma. *Cancer Survey* 1991; **10**: 121–133.

22 Levine A.M., Gill P.S., Meyer P.R. *et al.* Retrovirus and malignant lymphoma in homosexual men. *Journal of the American Medical Association* 1985; **254**: 1921–1925.

23 Lowenthal D.A., Straus D.J., Campbell S.W., Gold J.W.M., Clarkson B.D., Kozimer B. AIDS-related lymphoid neoplasia. *Cancer* 1988; **61**: 2325–2337.

24 Bermudez M.A., Grant K.M., Rodvien R., Mendes F. Non-Hodgkin's lymphoma in a population with or at risk for acquired immunodeficiency syndrome: indications for intensive chemotherapy. *American Journal of Medicine* 1989; **86**: 71–76.

25 Gill P.S., Levine A.M., Krailo M. *et al.* AIDS-related malignant lymphoma: results of prospective treatment trials. *Journal of Clinical Oncology* 1987; **5**: 1322–1328.

26 Poelzleitner D., Huebsch P., Mayerhofer S., Chott A., Zielinski C. Primary pulmonary lymphoma in a patient with the acquired immune deficiency syndrome. *Thorax* 1989; **44**: 438–439.

27 Zompatori M., Canini R., Gavelli G. *et al.* Linfomi toracici nell'AIDS. *La Radiologia Medica* 1991; **82**: 270–274.

28 Isaacson P.G., Norton A.J. *Extranodal Lymphomas*. Churchill Livingstone, London 1994.

29 Blunt D.M., Padley S.P.G. Radiographic manifestations of AIDS-related lymphoma in the thorax. *Clinical Radiology* 1995; **50**: 607–612.

30 Williams W.J., Beutler E., Erslev A.J., Lichtman M.A. (eds). In: *Hematology*, 4th edn. McGraw-Hill, 1990: 1002–1003.

31 Harper M.E., Kaplan M.H., Marselle L.M. *et al.* Concomitant infection with HTLV-I and HTLV-III in a patient with T8 lymphoproliferative disease. *New England Journal of Medicine* 1986; **315**: 1073–1078.

32 Sternlieb J., Mintzer D., Kwa D., Gluckman S. Peripheral T-cell lymphoma in a patient with the acquired immunodeficiency syndrome. *American Journal of Medicine* 1988; **85**: 445.

33 Nasr S.A., Brynes R.K., Garrison C.P., Chan W.C. Peripheral T-cell lymphoma in a patient with acquired immune deficiency syndrome. *Cancer* 1988; **61**: 947–951.

34 Unger P.D., Strauchen J.A. Hodgkin's disease in AIDS complex patients. *Cancer* 1986; **58**: 821–825.

35 Baer D.M., Anderson E.T., Wilkinson L.S. Acquired immune deficiency syndrome in homosexual men with Hodgkin's disease. *American Journal of Medicine* 1986; **80**: 738–740.

36 Schoeppel S.L., Hoppe R.T., Dorfman R.F. *et al.* Hodgkin's disease in homosexual men with generalised lymph-adenopathy. *Annals of Internal Medicine* 1985; **102**: 68–70.

37 Scheib R.G., Siegel R.S. Atypical Hodgkin's disease and the acquired immunodeficiency syndrome. *Annals of Internal Medicine* 1985; **102**: 554.

38 Prior E., Goldberg A.F., Conjalka M.S., Chapman W.E., Tay S., Ames E.D. Hodgkin's disease in homosexual men: an AIDS-related phenomenon? *American Journal of Medicine* 1986; **81**: 1085–1088.

39 Robert N.J., Schneiderman H. Hodgkin's disease and the acquired immunodeficiency syndrome. *Annals of Internal Medicine* 1984; **101**: 142–143.

40 Rubio R. Hodgkin's disease associated with human immunodeficiency virus infection. *Cancer* 1994; **73**: 2400–2407.

41 Tirelli U., Errante D., Dolcetti R. *et al.* Hodgkin's disease and human immunodeficiency virus infection: clinicopathologic and virologic features of 114 patients from the Italian Cooperative Group on AIDS and tumours. *Journal of Clinical Oncology* 1995; **13**: 1758–1767.

42 Stern R.G., Gamsu G., Golden J.A., Hirji M., Webb W.R., Abrams D.I. Intrathoracic adenopathy: differential feature of AIDS and diffuse lymphadenopathy syndrome. *American Journal of Roentgenology* 1984; **142**: 689–692.

43 Nusbaum N.J. Metastatic small cell carcinoma of the lung in a patient with AIDS. *New England Journal of Medicine* 1985; **312**: 1706.

CHAPTER 6
*Hodgkin's
lymphoma,
non-Hodgkin's
lymphoma and
carcinoma of the
bronchus*

44 Weitberg A.B., Mayer K., Miller M.E., Mikolich D.J. Dysplastic carcinoid tumour and AIDS related complex. *New England Journal of Medicine* 1986; **314**: 1455.

45 Rocha M.P., Fraire A.E., Guntupalli K.K., Greenberg S.D. Lung cancer in the young. *Cancer Detection and Prevention* 1994; **18**: 349–355.

46 Sridhar K.S., Flores M.R., Raub W.A., Saldana M. Lung cancer in patients with human immunodeficiency virus infection compared with historic control subjects. *Chest* 1992; **102**: 1704–1708.

47 Fishman J.E., Schwartz D.S., Sais G.J., Flores M.R., Sridhar K.S. Bronchogenic carcinoma in HIV-positive patients: findings on chest radiographs and CT scans. *American Journal of Roentgenology* 1995; **164**: 57–61.

48 Gruden J.F., Webb W.R., Yao D.C., Klein J.S., Sandhu J.S. Bronchogenic carcinoma in 13 patients infected with the human immunodeficiency virus: clinical and radiographic findings. *Journal of Thoracic Imaging* 1995; **10**: 99–105.

49 Rabkin C.S., Hilgartner M.W., Hedberg K.W. *et al.* Incidence of lymphomas and other cancers in HIV-infected and HIV-uninfected patients with haemophilia. *Journal of the American Medical Association* 1992; **267**: 1090–1094.

50 Aaron S.D., Warmer E., Edelson J.D. Bronchogenic carcinoma in patients seropositive for human immunodeficiency virus. *Chest* 1994; **106**: 640–642.

7 Pulmonary complications of drug use

R.P. BRETTLE

7.0 Introduction

Recreational drug use has a number of complications, which include the excessive or withdrawal effects of the drugs as well as a number of diverse medical conditions (Table 7.1). The pulmonary problems associated with drug use vary from asymptomatic abnormalities of pulmonary-function tests to infections and immunological problems, such as polyarteritis nodosa. The advent of HIV has not only widened the pulmonary spectrum of disease in drug users but also increased the frequency of existing conditions.

7.1 Non-infectious pulmonary-related complications of drug use

7.1.1 Frequency

The frequency of respiratory problems associated with drug use varies between 1.5% for females and 8.5% for males (Table 7.2). A survey of 200 consecutive admissions over a 5-month period in 1973 to a specialized medical in-patient unit of a New York hospital devoted to drug addiction revealed that pulmonary disease accounted for 8.5% of the male and 1.45% of the female admissions [1]. The respiratory problems noted were pulmonary fibrosis (obstructive or restrictive), carcinoma of the lung, chronic bronchitis, pleural effusion, pulmonary

Table 7.1 Medical (non-infection) problems of drug use.

Problem	Medical complications
Drug effects	
Excess opiate	Narcosis, coma, small pupils, respiratory depression, aspiration pneumonia and rhabdomyolysis secondary to pressure
Opiate withdrawal	Mild 'URTI' (sweating, coryza, lacrimation), pupillary dilatation, insomnia, nausea, vomiting, diarrhoea, lethargy, muscle weakness, myalgia, muscle twitching, tachycardia and hypertension
Excess cocaine	Apprehension, dizziness, syncope, blurred vision, dysphoric states, paranoia, confusion and aggressive behaviour
	Seizures, coma, hyperthermia, respiratory depression, apnoea, sudden death, spontaneous rhabdomyolysis
Excess amphetamine	Headaches, anorexia, nausea, tremors, dilated pupils, tachycardia and hypertension
Stimulant withdrawal	Sleepiness, lethargy, increased appetite, food bingeing, depression or even suicide
Trauma	
Frequent injecting	Track marks and skin scars
	Lack of veins and thrombophlebitis
	Deep venous thrombosis
	Persistent peripheral oedema, venous stasis and ulcers secondary to chronic venous obstruction
Misplaced injections	Arterial damage and insufficiency with secondary tissue damage, muscle compartment syndrome and traumatic rhabdomyolysis
	False aneurysms and pulmonary emboli
	Traumatic neuropathy
Pulmonary	
Inhaled cocaine and excessive use of Valsalva	Spontaneous pneumomediastinum
	Spontaneous pneumopericardium
Excess sedatives or stimulants	Respiratory depression, coma and pneumonia
Opiate withdrawals	Mild 'URTI'
Stimulant use, e.g. cocaine	Tachypnoea
Opiates or cocaine	Pulmonary oedema
Hepatitis B	Polyarteritis nodosa
Foreign-body emboli (particles injected intravenously), e.g. talc granulomas	Pulmonary hypertension
	Abnormal pulmonary function, e.g. reduced $D_L\text{CO}$
	Restrictive defect due to interstitial lung disease

Continued

Table 7.1 *Continued.*

Problem	Medical complications
Smoking of tobacco, heroin, marijuana	Abnormal pulmonary function e.g. reduced $D_L$co
	COAD
'Snorting' stimulants	Chronic rhinitis, rhinorrhoea, anosmia, atrophy of the mucosal membranes, ulceration and perforation of the nasal septum
'Snorting' opiates	Recurrent sinusitis
Cardiology	
Cocaine	Cardiac arrhythmias, such as sinus tachycardia, ventricular tachycardia and fibrillation, as well as asystole
	Myocardial infarction
	Severe hypertension
Adulterants of illicit drugs, e.g. quinine	Cardiac arrhythmias and death
Immunology	
IDU	Enlarged lymph nodes
	Elevated serum IgM
	False-positive syphilis serology
Endocrinology	
Opiate use	Increased prolactin levels and gynaecomastia
	Amenorrhoea (may be secondary to weight loss)
Cannabis	Oligospermia, impotence and gynaecomastia
Neurology	
Stimulants	Psychosis
	Depression
	Cerebral infarcts and haemorrhages (cerebrovascular accidents)
Depressants, such as benzodiazepines or barbiturates	Brain damage

$D_L$co, carbon monoxide diffusing capacity; IDU, intravenous drug use; URTI, upper respiratory tract infection; COAD, chronic obstructive airways disease; IgM, immunoglobulin M.

Table 7.2 Pulmonary complications of IDU—frequency.

White [1]	8.5% males
	1.5% females
Helpern and Rho [2]	6.7%

emboli and bronchial asthma. Heavy cigarette smoking was regarded as a probable cause of many of the problems, although the injection of inert material was also thought to be a contributing cause of the pulmonary fibrosis [1].

A post-mortem study of deaths among narcotic drug users in New York from 1950 to 1961 found that 49% of the deaths were a consequence of drug excess, 19% a consequence of various infections and 6.7% because of respiratory problems (other than pulmonary oedema and drug overdose). A few of the lungs studied contained microscopic granulomas of the foreign-body type, which were thought to have occurred because of a reaction to injected foreign particulate matter which adulterates 'street heroin'. Particles of cotton fibres used to filter drugs before injection were also seen within these granulomas [2].

7.1.2 Drug effects

Before the advent of HIV infection, drug use itself had a relatively low mortality, with alternating periods of abstinence and drug use, together with natural recovery. Probably the commonest complication of opiate use is an excessive dose, with subsequent narcosis or coma and respiratory failure. It has been estimated that opiate overdoses kill around 1% of drug users each year [3–7]. The clinical features of excessive doses of opiates include coma of varying severity, small pupils and depressed respiration. This state may or may not be associated with a respiratory infection. There is an absence of focal neurology, poor peripheral circulation and possibly a fever, while investigations may reveal reduced oxygen tension and possibly hypercapnia. Management consists of supportive care and, where necessary, the use of antagonists, such as naloxone. While immediate improvement in respiratory function follows the intravenous or intramuscular injection of naloxone, caution is required, since mixed overdoses with benzodiazepines are common. Consequently, if respiratory function is still a problem, it is worth considering the benzodiazepine antagonist flumazenil. Early withdrawal from opiates simulates a mild upper respiratory-tract infection with sweating, coryza and even a fever. In a known drug user, sweating, involuntary sniffing and pupillary dilatation are helpful physical signs.

The excessive use of stimulants such as cocaine produces apprehension, dizziness, syncope, blurred vision, dysphoric states, paranoia, confusion and aggressive behaviour [8]. Seizures, coma, hyperthermia, respiratory depression, apnoea and sudden death have also been reported [8]. Cardiovascular problems can occur after apparently small doses, notably cardiac arrhythmias, such as sinus tachycadia, ventricular tachycardia and fibrillation, as well as asystole. Myocardial infarction, even in teenagers, severe hypertension and cerebrovascular accidents have all been noted [8].

Lung damage, in the form of spontaneous pneumomediastinum and pneumopericardium, as well as pulmonary oedema, has been associated with inhaling or smoking free-base cocaine. This method of drug use is associated with deep, forced and prolonged inspiratory efforts, together with a Valsalva's manoeuvre, which produces a sudden rise in intra-alveolar pressure and subsequent alveolar rupture. Inhaling or smoking cocaine has also been associated with a decreased diffusing capacity for carbon monoxide [8].

The commonest abnormality of pulmonary function in injecting drug users is a reduction of the carbon monoxide transfer factor, which occurred as the sole abnormality in 38% of one series. In 42%, the reduction was less than 75% of the predicted value. Obstructive lung disease (asthma or chronic bronchitis) was observed in 6% and a restrictive defect due to interstitial lung disease in 7%. Radiological evidence of pulmonary hypertension was not observed in any patient. The authors concluded that alterations of pulmonary function due to foreign-body emboli were common but that significant respiratory symptoms were unusual. Unfortunately, follow-up was not attempted and whether there are long-term pulmonary problems of intravenous drug use (IDU) has yet to be determined [9].

Regular smoking of marijuana (three to four cigarettes per day) is associated with the same frequency of symptoms of acute and chronic bronchitis as well as the same type and extent of epithelial damage in the central airways as the regular smoking of 20 tobacco cigarettes per day. The different methods of smoking marijuana compared with tobacco cigarettes results in a greater quantity of smoke particulates and noxious gases being delivered to and deposited in the lungs during the smoking of marijuana and this probably explains the greater propensity for lung damage associated with marijuana. In one study, smoking marijuana was associated with a fivefold increment in the blood carboxy-haemoglobin, a threefold increase in the amount of tar inhaled and a one-third increase in the amount of inhaled tar retained in the respiratory tract [10].

7.1.3 Sinusitis

The use of the nasal mucosa, also known as snorting, to absorb drugs is associated with a number of medical problems. The frequency of these upper-airway problems is unknown among snorters but they are probably fairly common. The use of amphetamine or cocaine has been associated with chronic rhinitis, rhinorrhoea, anosmia, atrophy of the mucosal membranes, ulceration and perforation of the septum, presumably as a consequence of intense vasoconstriction and necrosis of tissue [8]. Snorting as a cause of upper-airway symptoms is well worth considering in injecting drug users with limited access to injecting equipment but not drugs, e.g. inmates of prisons.

7.1.4 Pulmonary oedema

Heroin-related pulmonary oedema is a rare complication of heroin use if one considers the fact that most users inject three to four times each day [11,12]. It was reported in association with morphine by Osler as early as 1880, which was 18 years before heroin was first manufactured [13]. The majority of reports, however, have incriminated recreational injections of heroin, which may result in sudden unexpected death, often with the needle and syringe still *in situ* [6,14,15]. In one series, this problem accounted for 48% of all deaths in narcotic drug users in New York [6]. Estimates of one death per 150 000 injections have been made, which is less than for penicillin [15].

Since it was originally associated with sudden death in those injecting recreational opiates, a number of theories were suggested, including bacterial or endotoxin contamination [12]. However, it has also been described with sterile medical injections of opiates, as well as with orally administered opiates. Two cases of methadone-associated pulmonary oedema were reported in 1972 in individuals without previous drug use and unassociated with IDU [16].

It would therefore appear to be some form of idiosyncratic reaction, possibly as a result of activation of histamine-releasing cells [16,17]. Investigations have revealed that the pulmonary wedge pressure is normal and the resulting oedema fluid is rich in protein, supporting the hypothesis that it occurs because of altered capillary permeability and should therefore be considered as a form of adult respiratory distress syndrome (ARDS) [16,17].

7.1.5 Polyarteritis nodosa

In 1970, 14 injecting drug users were described with a necrotizing angiitis indistinguishable from polyarteritis nodosa. At that time, it was thought to be an idiosyncratic reaction to the use of amphetamines [18]. However, it is possible that this is in fact an example of polyartertis nodosa complicating chronic hepatitis B surface-antigen carriage, which was also described in 1970 [19–21]. Pneumonitis and pulmonary oedema are possible pulmonary presentations of polyarteritis nodosa.

7.1.6 Pulmonary hypertension

Post-mortem studies have revealed foreign-body emboli, thrombosis and granulomas in pulmonary arterioles [6,22,23]. In 1950, a pattern suggestive of pulmonary fibrosis was noted on the chest radiograph of a middle-aged, white, male, morphine addict, who eventually died of congestive right-heart failure [23]. The post-mortem demonstrated numerous foreign-body emboli in and around the pulmonary arterioles. Many of the pulmonary arterioles contained thrombi in various states of organization and canalization. The right ventricle was hypertrophied and dilated.

A number of particular foreign bodies have been associated with these granulomas including cotton fibre and talc. The majority of granulomas are apparently asymptomatic or subclinical (but see below) in life, but there have been reports of pulmonary hypertension in drug users. In 1964 Wendt *et al.* reported pulmonary hypertension secondary to arteritis and thrombosis of small pulmonary arteries, arterioles and capillaries [24]. These changes were associated with granulomatous reactions secondary to crystals induced by the injection of various drugs. While this report may also be an example of polyarteritis nodosa secondary to hepatitis B, the clinical features were not typical and subsequently similar pathological features were found after injecting rabbits with drugs containing talc [25]. It thus appears that tablets containing talc are able to induce this reaction when injected intravenously.

Evidence that granulomas may have some clinical effect comes from a case report of a 32-year-old drug user who presented with a 1-day history of low-grade fever, dyspnoea and dizziness. The chest radiograph showed diffuse, bilateral, miliary infiltrates. It appeared that these symptoms recurred each time he injected intravenously a mixture of drugs containing talc. Investigations failed to reveal any pathogens but a transbronchial biopsy revealed talc granuloma [26].

7.2 Injecting drug-use-related infections

7.2.1 Frequency

Drug-use-related infections are usually associated with IDU, although the use of animal excreta in the cultivation of marijuana and the subsequent outbreaks of *Salmonella* gastroenteritis is a notable exception [27]. IDU-related infections occur because of the use of either non-sterile equipment (needles, syringes, spoons, cups, etc.) or non-sterile solutions, both of which allow microorganisms direct access to subcutaneous tissues, muscle or blood and result in either local or systemic infections. Two particular practices associated with the sharing of injection equipment or associated paraphernalia seem to favour the spread of blood-borne microorganisms, notably hepatitis B and C as well as HIV. The first of these practices is washing the drug out of the syringe into the bloodstream by repeatedly drawing back and injecting the user's own blood (booting or flushing), which results in heavy blood contamination, which can be passed on to the next user. This practice may have originated with use of medicine droppers as syringes. The second practice is washing the equipment in a communal container of water, which rapidly becomes contaminated with blood.

The frequency of IDU-related infections varies with location and the type of study. Prior to the advent of HIV, a post-mortem study of narcotic drug users in New York, in which 49% of the deaths were a result of drug excess, noted that 19% of the deaths were a consequence of various infections [2]. The infection-related deaths were mainly bacterial sepsis, such as endocarditis (34.5%) and tetanus (44%), as well as viral hepatitis (10%). In comparison, the 1973 series of drug-related admissions to a New York hospital noted that 58% were related to infection [1]. While in that series acute viral hepatitis (30.5%) was the single largest reason for admission, the other infections, which accounted for 27.5% of the admissions, were endocarditis (3.5%), bacteraemia without a source (11%), chest infections (29%) and skin infections (43.5%). In Basel, Switzerland, between 1980 and 1986, 0.78% of all admissions to a university hospital involved narcotic drug users and of these 31% were infection-related; 24% were due to lower respiratory-tract infections, 20.3% were a consequence of viral hepatitis, 6% were soft-tissue infections and 3.2% were secondary to bacteraemia, including endocarditis [28].

In Edinburgh during 1983–84, the prevalence of opiate-related IDU was 0.6% for those between the ages of 15 and 35 and there was an estimated population of 2000 injecting drug users [5]. Twenty-three injecting drug users attended the accident and emergency department because of infection during a 4-month period, an incidence of clinical IDU infection requiring medical attention of around 3.5% (20% of which was viral hepatitis and less than 1% a consequence of serious infection) [5,29]. During 1984, there were 100 IDU-related admissions to Lothian hospitals for soft-tissue infections, hepatitis, endocarditis and pneumonia out of a population of 2000 drug users, an incidence of 5% for IDU infections that required admission [5,30]. Of these infections, 81% were bacterial and 15% were serious (pneumonia or endocarditis). Thus, the incidence of clinical IDU infection is probably somewhere between 3.5 and 5%, around 20% of these infections being viral. The incidence of serious drug-related infections is between 0.35 and 0.75%.

In summary, IDU-related medical problems account for between 0.1

and 1% of hospital medical problems and 20–60% of admissions are related to infections, i.e. 0.1–0.6% of all hospital admissions. Combined with the fact that 10–15% of IDU-related infections are serious systemic infections, we can conclude that at the most 0.1% of hospital admissions are related to serious IDU-related infections. Depending upon the year and geographical area, the commonest infection may well be viral hepatitis. However, once a population has been saturated by hepatitis, the next most likely reason to be admitted to hospital is for a respiratory-tract infection, which usually accounts for a third of the admissions.

7.2.2 Specific infections

The commonest organisms found in IDU-associated endocarditis are coagulase-positive staphylococci (up to 50%), enterococci and/or Gram-negative bacilli and *Candida* [3,31]. In the case of bacterial pneumonia, the predominant organism isolated tends to be pneumoccoci in between 30 and 50% of cases, followed by *Haemophilus influenzae* (2–10%), *Staphylococcus aureus* (2–5%) or *Klebsiella* [3,28,31].

Candida infection is a rare but well-recognized complication of intravenous heroin use, and disseminated candidiasis has been reported among intravenous heroin users worldwide in small epidemics [32–35]. This syndrome, caused by *Candida albicans*, is characterized by cutaneous, ocular, osteoarticular and pleuropulmonary involvement, alone or in combination [35]. At least 160 cases have been described in the literature, many of which have indicated the epidemic nature of this condition, the largest occurring in association with Iranian or brown heroin [35–37].

In disseminated candidiasis, all patients describe sudden-onset fever, shivers, myalgia, headaches and profuse sweating shortly after the intravenous injection of heroin. The fever usually lasts between 1 and 3 days and is followed by cutaneous signs in more than 90% of cases [34]. These are numerous painful nodules, 0.5–1 cm in diameter, occasionally surrounded by some erythema and usually located in the scalp and hairy parts of the body. Untreated, they gradually resolve within 4 weeks, generally leaving an area of alopecia. Sometimes, the nodule can discharge thick yellow pus. Painful pustules are also present in some patients; they are 2–3 mm in diameter on an inflamed base, from which the *Candida* can be easily identified. These can be found disseminated over the body and may appear like streptococcal or staphylococcal folliculitis. Patients often have high titres of anti-*C. albicans* antibodies, but *C. albicans* is readily isolated from the skin lesions [33].

Pleuropulmonary involvement was recorded in 8% of cases in one study, but *C. albicans* was always isolated in conjunction with other pathogens, such as *Staphylococcus* or other saprophytes, for instance *Torulopsis glabrata* [35].

7.3 The effect of HIV on injecting drug-use problems

7.3.1 Non-infective problems

There have been reports of pulmonary hypertension associated with HIV and, although some patients have been drug users, it has also been noted among non-drug-using homosexuals. Six patients with AIDS — four homosexuals and three drug users — developed moderate or severe pulmonary hypertension, associated with right-ventricular hypertrophy and cardiac failure [38]. The authors estimated an incidence of pulmonary hypertension of 0.5%. The patients presented with dyspnoea on exertion, hypoxaemia, restrictive lung disease, reduced transfer factor for carbon monoxide and pulmonary hypertension. The most distinguishing feature was right-ventricular hypertrophy in the electrocardiogram. The diagnosis was often obscured by the fact that the features developed during an episode of an opportunistic infection, although the symptoms and signs did not settle with treatment. Histology revealed that in two patients, in addition to *Pneumocystis carinii* pneumonia (PCP), medial hypertophy of the small pulmonary arteries and arterioles, endarteritis obliterans, intimal fibrosis of the pulmonary veins and lymphohistiocytic infiltration of the interstitium, associated with interstitial fibrosis, thickened alveolar septa and honeycombing, were present.

In a prospective evaluation of 74 patients with HIV and cardiopulmonary complaints, six patients (8%) had pulmonary hypertension, with elevated right-ventricular systolic pressures, as demonstrated by Doppler echocardiography [39]. This amounted to an incidence of 0.5% in a cohort of 1200 HIV-infected patients. In the latter series, the problem occurred in both early and late HIV and did not seem related to the level of immune deficiency. Five of the six patients were drug users but postmortem in two did not reveal evidence of foreign-body embolization, suggesting that it is distinct from the problem reported previously in drug users. In addition, there were no signs of inflammatory vessel changes and the pathology, like the others in the literature, consists of plexiform lesions typical of primary pulmonary hypertension.

In Edinburgh, 173 HIV patients underwent echocardiography and seven (4%) had isolated right-ventricular dilatation. Follow-up scans revealed that four of the patients reverted to normal after treatment of their chest infections, although the abnormality persisted in three (1.7%) patients. One had definitive pulmonary hypertension, demonstrated by

Doppler echocardiography, suggesting an incidence of pulmonary hypertension of at least 0.6% [40].

Emphysema-like pulmonary disease in association with HIV has been reported [41]. Four patients presented with dyspnoea (none were drug users), none had prior lung infections and chest X-rays did not show infiltrates. They were all late-stage in that the mean CD4 count was 100 cells/mm^3. No organisms were detected by bronchoalveolar lavage and the pulmonary-function tests suggested emphysema, with air trapping, hyperinflation and markedly reduced diffusion capacity. Only minimal airflow obstruction was present. Three of the patients had high-resolution computed tomographic scans of the chest, which revealed emphysema-like bullous changes [41].

7.3.2 Infection problems

There is surprisingly little variation with regard to the presentation of AIDS between patients with different risk activities. In drug users, Kaposi's sarcoma (KS), cytomegalovirus and chronic cryptosporidiosis are all significantly less common than for all other risk activities notified with AIDS, while PCP, tuberculosis, oesophageal candidiasis and extrapulmonary cryptococcosis are more common, probably partly because of the paucity of KS [42].

However, among drug users, data collected on AIDS cases greatly under-represents serious IDU-related HIV disease. In New York, there was a rapid increase in both AIDS and non-AIDS narcotic-related deaths between 1978 and 1986, such that, for every AIDS-related death in a drug user, there was one other as a consequence of conditions such as tuberculosis, endocarditis and bacterial pneumonia [43]. Similar data have been reported from Europe [44,45]. There had, however, been no increase in the non-infective causes of death [43].

IDU-related infections are very likely to become more common, since susceptibility to bacterial infections is increased by HIV infection [46–58]. For instance, in New York the rate of tuberculosis was 4% among HIV-positive compared with 0% in HIV-negative drug users [48]. The 36% increase in reported cases of tuberculosis between 1984 and 1986 in the USA has been largely ascribed to infection among HIV-positive drug users [49].

IDU-related HIV patients also have a higher incidence of bacterial infections, such as pneumonia — 12%, with a mortality of 2.2%, compared with 3%, with a mortality of 0%, in HIV-negative drug users [52]. The annual incidence of pneumonia was 9.7% for HIV-seropositive drug users, compared with under 2% for a population of mainly homosexual males with AIDS [53,54]. The rising mortality from pneumonia in young adults in New York City is primarily a consequence of IDU-related HIV, and other cities in the USA are showing similar trends [55,56].

The morbidity and mortality of bacterial endocarditis in HIV-seropositive individuals are greater than for seronegative individuals; the mortality was 24%, compared with 4%. The poorer outcome was related to more frequent embolization, a greater diversity of organisms, more prolonged fever, persistent bacteraemia and greater immunological dysfunction. It was not related to recognized opportunistic infections [57,58]. The combined effect of progressive immunodeficiency and attempts at harm reduction has had an influence on the predominant medical problems of drug users. A survey of methadone-maintenance patients from the Bronx, New York, in 1986–87 revealed that infection now accounted for 62% of the admissions, but infection that might be related to injecting, such as endocarditis or skin cellulitis, accounted for only 17% of admissions [59].

Estimates of the effect of HIV on IDU admissions are also available from Edinburgh, where the epidemic of IDU started around 1980 and peaked in 1983–84 [60–62]. The earliest known drug user infected with HIV as a consequence of drug use in Spain and Italy seroconverted in January 1983 [63]. The annual rate of admissions for pneumonia in Edinburgh during 1986 for individuals aged 15–44 was 0.6/1000, while the admission rate for pneumonia in drug users aged 15–44 rose from 1.4/1000 in 1983–85 (i.e. as HIV was spreading through the drug community) to 12/1000 by 1985–89, an eightfold increase, by, at the most, 5 years after infection with HIV [64].

The commonest single identifiable reason for an HIV admission in Edinburgh is because of a respiratory-tract infection (29% of the admissions) [64]. Unlike other UK centres, only 27% of these respiratory admissions were for PCP, while 54% were for a bacterial chest infection [64]. Despite the fact that 51.5% of the patients were regarded as being asymptomatic (Centers for Disease Control stage II, asymptomatic infection, and stage III, persistent generalized lymphadenopathy) as far as their HIV was concerned, the respiratory-tract infections were serious; 50% had radiological pneumonia, 43% were hypoxic, 28% were hypercapnic and the average length of stay was 10 days, reflecting the complicating factor of susceptibility to infection and drug use. Interestingly *H. influenzae* rather than *Streptococcus* pneumonia was the commonest organism isolated from these bacterial chest infections.

The reasons for the increased susceptibility to bacterial infections among HIV patients are not entirely clear. Although unsterile IDU exposes an individual to episodes of bacterial infection, the susceptibility is not specific for drug users, since bacteraemia is also increased in HIV-positive individuals in Africa [51]. In San Francisco, where IDU-related

HIV is unusual, the increase of pneumococcal bacteraemia in all HIV individuals has been shown to be 100 times that of the general population
[56]. In drug users and in Africa, it might be argued that limited access to
medical services is an additional contributory factor. However, antibody
production is impaired in HIV-infected patients, and low levels of immunoglobulin G (IgG_2) have been associated with bacterial infection
[65,66]. Additional susceptibility factors for drug users may be that
opiates themselves depress the cough reflex, as well as the immune system
[67–70].

7.4 Management of injecting drug-use-related pulmonary problems

There are no major differences in the management of HIV pulmonary
conditions complicated by drug use. The differences are essentially those
of differentiating drug-related conditions from HIV-related problems, as
well as coping with the problem of opiate excess in the presence of pulmonary conditions. The last section is dedicated to a method of investigat-
ing HIV-infected drug users with respiratory problems.

Unfortunately, many of the symptoms of HIV are mimicked by the
problems of drug use. For instance, shortness of breath and a persistent
cough are common early symptoms of PCP but can also occur with endocarditis, excessive smoking, recurrent bronchitis, obstructive airways
disease and pulmonary hypertension. An awareness of the fact that physical complaints may be drug-related or HIV-related is essential, and Table
7.3 details some drug-related versus HIV-related problems.

When opiated patients are admitted with respiratory problems, there
is the dilemma of how to manage the opiate dose. For those patients with
mild respiratory depression, a discussion over a temporary reduction in
oral drugs or splitting the daily dose into three or four doses may suffice.
In those with more severe respiratory depression, rapid improvement in
pulmonary function is required. However, if the opiate withdrawal is
excessive, as with intravenous bolus injections of naloxone, the patient
may become disruptive. Our preferred solution is to use naloxone infusions to achieve an acceptable improvement in respiratory rate (and therefore oxygenation) without too great an increase in physical arousal.
Essentially, the aim is to improve oxygenation rather than induce withdrawal from opiates. This improved oxygenation can be assessed by respiratory rate, oxygen desaturation or arterial blood gases.

7.4.1 Strategy for respiratory syndrome in injecting drug-use-related HIV

Patients with cough or breathlessness, with or without fever/weight loss

Table 7.3 Comparison of drug-, IDU- and HIV-related problems.

Symptom complex	Drug-related problems	HIV-related problems
Pulmonary		
Recurrent sinusitis	'Snorting' of drugs	Susceptibility to recurrent bacterial infection
Reduced transfer factor for carbon monoxide	Talc granuloma secondary to emboli, cocaine	PCP
Respiratory syndrome (cough, dyspnoea, etc.)	Chronic bronchitis secondary to tobacco and marijuana	Increased susceptibility to bacterial infections
	Emphysema (tobacco)	HIV-related emphysema
	Inhalation or aspiration pneumonia	PCP, TB, other OIs, bacterial pneumonia, KS, etc.
	Acute bronchitis	
	Endocarditis	
	'Heroin asthma' or pulmonary oedema	
	Polyarteritis nodosa-related pneumonitis	
Pulmonary hypertension (dyspnoea, hypoxaemia, restrictive lung disease)	Talc granuloma secondary to emboli	HIV-related pulmonary hypertension
Constitutional symptoms		
Fever	Endocarditis, septicaemia, etc.	CDC stage IVA, PCP and OIs such as MAI
	'Bad fix' or endotoxaemia	
Night sweats	Opiate withdrawals	CDC stage III, IVA, or early OI
Weight loss	Heavy addiction, poor diet and use of stimulants such as cocaine or amphetamines	CDC stage IVA, TB or other OI
Cardiology		
Heart murmurs	Endocarditis	
Cardiomyopathy	Alcohol	HIV
Pulmonary hypertension	Talc granulomas	HIV-related pulmonary hypertension

PCP, *Pneumocystis carinii* pneumonia; TB, tuberculosis; OIs, opportunistic infections; KS, Kaposi's sarcoma; CDC, Centers for Disease Control; MAI, *Mycobacterium avium intracellulare*.

of recent onset, are treated with broad-spectrum antibiotics while awaiting sputum-culture results. The antibiotics considered should have reasonable activity against *H. influenzae* and may have to be given intravenously. Examples are cefuroxime or amoxycillin–clavulanic acid

(Augmentin). In order to reduce the risk of masking PCP, we initially avoid co-trimoxazole. Nebulized bronchodilators are added if there is any evidence of obstructive airways disease.

Patients known to be receiving opiates and/or benzodiazepines and with a partial pressure of oxygen (Po_2) <10 kPa are closely monitored and advised to voluntarily reduce their intake and spread out their daily dose while in hospital. The reasons for this reduction are carefully explained in order to achieve the cooperation of the patient. Patients need to be reassured that doses will be restored once they are improving and that the reduction is not a form of punishment but a means of keeping them alive. Explanations that opiates reduce the cough reflex, reduce the effectiveness of neutrophils and reduce the respiratory drive and therefore oxygenation, which is important for cell killing, need to be carefully gone over.

If this fails to improve oxygenation or the situation worsens ($Po_2 <$ 8 kPa, respiratory rate falls, desaturation sets in or loss of consciousness occurs), some reversal of the opiated state is required in order to assess the contribution of the drugs to the respiratory failure. As noted previously, total and immediate withdrawal from opiates is difficult, if not impossible (i.e. with bolus injections), for the patient, despite the presence of life-threatening respiratory failure. It results in accompanying restlessness and agitation, which, if continued, usually results in interrupted venous access and self-discharge. The dramatic reversal of opiates with intravenous naloxone is short-lived and, other than establishing a diagnosis, achieves little in the way of long-term management. It is suggestive of punishment and rapidly leads to a loss of confidence in medical care, since withdrawal may be the patient's most feared event.

Impaired respiratory drive secondary to opiate excess is best managed by a naloxone infusion (2 mg in 500 ml, perhaps starting at around 10 ml/hour), with the aim of maintaining an acceptable level of oxygenation (as assessed by saturation or respiratory rate) but without necessarily fully restoring consciousness. Such an infusion may be required for up to 48 hours in those on methadone because of its relatively long half-life compared with other opiates.

Further investigations may in part depend on the latest immunological assessment and the local facilities. In Edinburgh, a CD4 count of perhaps <250 cells/mm³ would result in an attempt to obtain induced sputa, as would a failure to improve with the above regime. Elsewhere, a bronchoscopy might be considered as the initial investigation. In Edinburgh, a bronchoscopy is only considered if the patient is not improving and *P. carinii* is not obtained from an induced sputum. This regimen has reduced our bronchoscopy rate for around 400 HIV patients to only one to two per year, without any obvious detrimental effect on the patients [71].

If respiratory infection is ruled out, consideration should be given to echocardiography, in case the symptoms are due to pulmonary hypertension. Although in the UK to date tuberculosis has not been a major problem, our practice is to have all admissions with respiratory syndrome screened for tuberculosis.

References

1 White A.G. Medical disorders in drug addicts: 200 consecutive admissions. *Journal of the American Medical Association* 1973; **223**: 1469–1471.

2 Helpern M., Rho Y.M. Deaths from narcotism in New York City. *New York State Medical Journal* 1966; **66**: 2391–2408.

3 Louria D.B., Hensle T., Rose J. The major medical complications of heroin addiction. *Annals of Internal Medicine* 1967; **67**: 1–22.

4 Ritson A.B., Plant M.A. *Drugs and Young People in Scotland.* Edinburgh: Scottish Health Education Unit, 1977.

5 Robertson J.R., Bucknall A.B. *Heroin Users in a Scottish City—Edinburgh Drug Addiction Study.* Edinburgh: West Granton Medical Group, 1986.

6 Waldorf D., Biernachie P.J. Natural recovery from heroin addiction: a review of the incidence literature. *Journal of Drug Issues* 1979; **9**: 281–289.

7 Wille R. Processes of recovery from heroin dependence: relationship to treatment, social change and dry use. *Journal of Drug Issues* 1983; **13**: 333–342.

8 Cregler L.L., Mark H. Medical complications of cocaine abuse. *New England Journal of Medicine* 1986; **315**: 1495–1500.

9 Overland E.S., Nolan A., Hopewell P.C. Alteration of pulmonary function in intravenous drug abusers. *American Journal of Medicine* 1980; **68**: 231–237.

10 Tzu-Chin W., Tashkin D.P., Djahed B., Rose J.E. Pulmonary hazards of smoking marijuana as compared with tobacco. *New England Journal of Medicine* 1988; **318**: 347–351.

11 Silber R., Clerkin E.P. Pulmonary edema in acute heroin poisoning. *American Journal of Medicine* 1959; **27**: 187–192.

12 Troen P. Pulmonary edema in acute opium poisoning. *New England Journal of Medicine* 1953; **248**: 364–366.

13 Osler W. Oedema of the left lung in morphia poisoning. *Montreal General Hospital Reports* 1880; **1**: 291–292.

14 Siegel H., Helpern M., Ehrenreich T. The diagnosis of death from intravenous narcotism. *Journal of Forensic Sciences* 1966; **11**: 1–16.

15 Baden M.M. *Pathology of Addictive States in Medical Aspects of Drug Abuse.* Hagerstown: Harper and Row, 1975: 189–211.

16 Frand U.I., Shimm C.S., Williams M.H. Methadone-induced pulmonary edema. *Annals of Internal Medicine* 1972; **76**: 975–979.

17 Katz S., Aberman A., Frand U.I., Stein I.M., Fulop M. Heroin pulmonary edema. *American Review of Respiratory Disease* 1972; **106**: 472–474.

18 Citron B.P., Halpern M., McCarron M. *et al.* Necrotising angiitis associated with drug abuse. *New England Journal of Medicine* 1970; **283**: 1003–1011.

19 Gocke D.J., Hsu K., Morgan G. *et al.* Association between polyarteritis and Australia antigen. *Lancet* 1970; **ii**: 1149–1153.

20 Sergent J.S., Lockshin M.D., Christian C.L. Vasculitis with hepatitis B antigenaemia: long term observations in nine patients. *Medicine (Baltimore)* 1976; **55**: 1–18.

21 Travers R.L., Allison D.J., Brettle R.P., Hughes R.V. Polyarteritis nodosa: a clinical and angiographic analysis of 17 cases. *Seminars in Arthritis and Rheumatism* 1979; **8**: 184–199.

22 Krainer L., Breman E., Wishnick E. Parenteral talc granulomatosis: a complication of narcotic addiction. *Laboratory Investigation* 1962; **11**: 671.

23 Spain D.M. Patterns of pulmonary fibrosis. *Annals of Internal Medicine* 1950; **33**: 1150–1163.

24 Wendt V.E., Puro H.E., Shapiro J., Mathews W., Wolf P.L. Angiothrombotic pulmonary hypertension in addicts—'Blue Velvet' addiction. *Journal of the American Medical Association* 1964; **188**: 755–757.

25 Puro H.E., Wolf P.L., Skirgaudos J., Vazquez J. Experimental production of human 'Blue Velvet' and 'Red Devil' lesions. *Journal of the American Medical Association* 1966; **197**: 1100–1103.

26 Ben-Haim S.A., Ben-Ami H., Edoute Y., Goldstein N., Barzilai D. Talcosis presenting as pulmonary infiltrates in an HIV-positive heroin addict. *Chest* 1988; **94**: 656–658.

27 Taylor D.N., Wachsmuth I.K., Shangkuan Y.H. *et al.* Salmonellosis associated with marijuana. *New England Journal of Medicine* 1982; **306**: 1249–1253.

28 Scheidegger C., Zimmerli W. Infectious complications in drug addicts; seven-year review of 269 hospitalised narcotic abusers in Switzerland. *Reviews of Infectious Diseases* 1989; **2**: 486–493.

29 McGowan A., Steedman D., Schofield T.C., Robertson C.E. Parenteral drug misuse and the accident and emergency department. *Health Bulletin* 1984; **42** (5): 252–257.

30 Brettle R.P., Flegg P.J., MacCallum L. Injection drug use related HIV and AIDS. In: Harris W., Forster S. eds. *Recent Advances in STD and AIDS*, Vol. 4. London: Churchill Livingstone, 1991: 91–128.

31 Marantz P.R., Linzer M., Feiner C., Feinstein S.A., Kozin A.M., Friedland G.H. Inability to predict diagnosis in febrile intravenous drug abusers. *Annals of Internal Medicine* 1987; **106**: 823–828.

32 Calandra T., Francioli P., Glauser M.P., Baudraz-Rosselet F., Ruffieux C., Grigoriu D. Disseminated candidiasis with extensive folliculitis in abusers of brown Iranian heroin. *European Journal of Clinical Microbiology* 1985; **4**: 340–342.

33 Collignon P.J., Sorrell T. Disseminated candidiasis: evidence of a distinctive syndrome in heroin abusers. *British Medical Journal* 1983; **287**: 861–862.

34 Dupont B., Drouet E. Cutaneous, ocular, and osteoarticular candidiasis in heroin addicts: new clinical and therapeutic aspects in 38 patients. *Journal of Infectious Diseases* 1985; **152**: 577–591.

35 Mellinger M., De Beauchamp O., Gallien C., Ingold R., Taboada M.J. Epidemiological and clinical approach to the study of candidiasis caused by *Candida albicans* in heroin addicts in the Paris region: analysis of 35 observations. *Bulletin on Narcotics* 1982; **34**: 61–81.

36 Odds F.C. *Candida and Candidosis: A Review and Bibliography*, 2nd edn. London: Baillière Tindall, 1988.

37 Servant J.B., Dutton G.N., Ong-Tone L., Barrie T., Davey C. *Candida* endophthalmitis in Glaswegian heroin addicts: report of an epidemic. *Transactions of Ophthalmological Society UK* 1985; **104**: 297–308.

38 Himmelman R.B., Dohrmann M., Goodman P. *et al.* Severe pulmonary hypertension and cor pulmonale in the acquired immunodeficiency syndrome. *American Journal of Cardiology* 1989; **64**: 1396–1399.

39 Speich R., Jenni R., Opravil M., Pfab M., Russi E.W. Primary pulmonary hypertension in HIV infection. *Chest* 1991; **100**: 1268–1271.

40 Jacob A.J., Sutherland G.R., Bird A.G. *et al.* HIV heart muscle disease—prevalence and risk factors. *British Heart Journal* 1992; **68**: 549–553.

41 Diaz P.T., Clanton T.L., Pacht E.R. Emphysema-like pulmonary disease associated with human immunodeficiency virus infection. *Annals of Internal Medicine* 1992; **116**: 124–128.

42 Selik R.M., Starcher E.T., Curran J.W. Opportunistic diseases reported in AIDS patients: frequencies, associations, and trends. *AIDS* 1987; **1**: 175–182.

43 Stoneburner R.L., Des Jarlais D.C., Benezra D. *et al.* A larger spectrum of severe HIV-1 related disease in intravenous drug users in New York City. *Science* 1989; **242**: 916–918.

44 Haastrecht H.J.A., van dem Hoek A.J.A.R., Coutinho R.A. High mortality among HIV infected injecting drug users without an AIDS diagnosis: implications for HIV infection epidemic modellers? *AIDS* 1994; **8**: 363–366.

45 Galli M., Musicco M. for the COMCAT Study Group. Mortality of intravenous drug users living in Milan, Italy: role of HIV infection. *AIDS* 1994; **8**: 1457–1463.

46 Handwerger S., Mildvan D., Senie R., McKinley F.W. Tuberculosis and the acquired immunodeficiency syndrome at a New York City hospital. *Chest* 1987; **91**: 176–180.

47 Chaisson R.E., Schecter G.F., Theuer C.P., Rutherford G.W., Echenberg D.F., Hopewell P.C. Tuberculosis in patients with the acquired immunodeficiency syndrome: clinical features, response to therapy, and survival. *American Review of Respiratory Diseases* 1987; **136**: 570–574.

48 Centers for Disease Control Editorial. Tuberculosis and acquired immunodeficiency syndrome — New York. *Morbidity and Mortality Weekly Report* 1987; **36** (48): 785–790, 795.

49 Selwyn P.A., Hartel D., Lewis V.A. *et al.* A prospective study of the risk of tuberculosis among intravenous drug users with human immunodeficiency virus infection. *New England Journal of Medicine* 1989; **320**: 545–550.

50 Simberkoff M.S., El-Sadr W., Schiffman G., Rahal J.J., Jr. *Streptococcus pneumoniae* infections and bacteremia in patients with acquired immune deficiency syndrome, with report of a pneumococcal vaccine failure. *American Review of Respiratory Disease* 1984; **130**: 1174–1176.

51 Gilks G.F., Brindle R.J., Otieno L.S. *et al.* Life-threatening bacteraemia in HIV-1 seropositive adults admitted to hospital in Nairobi, Kenya. *Lancet* 1990; **336**: 545–549.

52 Selwyn P.A., Schoenbaum E.E., Hartel D. *et al.* AIDS and HIV-related mortality in intravenous drug users (IVDUs). In: *IV International Conference on AIDS*, Stockholm, Sweden, 1988: abstract 4526.

53 Selwyn P.A., Feingold A.R., Hartel D. *et al.* Increased risk of bacterial pneumonia in HIV-infected intravenous drug users without AIDS. *AIDS* 1988; **2**: 267–272.

54 Polsky B., Gold J.W., Whimbey E. *et al.* Bacterial pneumonia in patients with the acquired immunodeficiency syndrome. *Annals of Internal Medicine* 1986; **104**: 38–41.

55 Centers for Disease Control Editorial. Increase in pneumonia mortality among young adults and the HIV epidemic — New York City, United States. *Morbidity and Mortality Weekly Report* 1988; **37** (38): 593–596.

56 Redd S.C., Rutherford, III G.W., Sande M.A. *et al.* The role of HIV infection in pneumococcal bacteraemia in San Francisco residents. *Journal of Infectious Diseases* 1990; **162**: 1012–1017.

57 Slim J., Boghossian J., Perez G., Johnson E. Comparative analysis of bacterial endocarditis in HIV(+) and HIV(−) intravenous drug users. In: *IV International Conference on AIDS*, Stockholm, Sweden, 1988: abstract 8027.

58 Ruggeri P., Sathe S.S., Kapila R. Changing patterns of infectious endocarditis (IE) in parenteral drug abusers (PDA) with human immunodeficiency virus (HIV) infections. In: *IV International Conference on AIDS*, Stockholm, Sweden, 1988: abstract 8028.

59 Selwyn P.A., Hartel D.A., Wasserman W., Drucker E. Impact of the AIDS epidemic on the morbidity and mortality among intravenous drug users in a New York City methadone maintenance program. *American Journal of Public Health* 1989; **79**: 1358–1362.

60 Robertson J.R., Bucknall A.B.V., Welsby P.D.W. *et al.* An epidemic of AIDS-related virus (HTLV-III/LAV) infection amongst intravenous drug abusers in a Scottish general practice. *British Medical Journal* 1986; **292**: 527–530.

61 Brettle R.P., Nelles B. Special problems of injecting drug misusers. *British Medical Bulletin* 1988; **44**: 149–160.

62 Haw S., Liddell D. *Drug Problems in Edinburgh District: Report of the SCODA Fieldwork Survey*. London: SCODA.

63 Bisset C., Jones G., Davidson J. *et al.* Mobility of injection drug users and transmission of HIV. *Lancet* 1989; **ii**: 44.

64 Willocks L., Cowan F.M., Brettle R.P., Emmanuel F.X.S., Flegg P.J., Burns S. The spectrum of chest infections in HIV positive patients in Edinburgh. *Journal of Infection* 1992; **24**: 37–42.

65 Klein R.S., Selwyn P.A., Maude D., Pollard C., Freeman K., Schiffman G. Response to pneumococcal vaccine among symptomatic heterosexual partners of persons with AIDS and intravenous drug users infected with HIV. *Journal of Infectious Diseases* 1989; **160**: 826–832.

66 Parkin J.M., Helbert M., Hughes C.L., Pinching A.J. Immunoglobulin G subclass deficiency and susceptibility to pyogenic infections in patients with AIDS-related complex and AIDS. *AIDS* 1989; **3**: 37–39.

67 Klimas N.G., Blaney N.T., Morgan R.O. *et al.* Immune function and anti-HTLV-I/II status in anti HIV-1 negative intravenous drug users receiving methadone. *American Journal of Medicine* 1991; **90**: 163–170.

68 Tubaro E., Borelli G., Croce C., Cavallo G., Santiangeli C. Effect of morphine on resistance to infection. *Journal of Infectious Diseases* 1983; **148**: 656–666.

69 Anonymous. Editorial: opiates, opioid peptides, and immunity. *Lancet* 1984; **i**: 774–775.

70 Arora P.K., Fride E., Petitto J., Waggie K., Skolnick P. Morphine-induced modulation of the immune system: implications for AIDS. In: *IV International Conference on AIDS*, Stockholm, Sweden, 1988: abstract 8021.

71 Willocks L., Burns S., Cossar R., Brettle R.P. Diagnosis of *Pneumocystis carinii* pneumonia in a population of HIV positive drug users with particular reference to sputum induction and fluorescent antibody techniques. *Journal of Infection* 1993; **26**: 257–264.

8 Pulmonary tuberculosis in HIV infection

N.M. PRICE & M.A. JOHNSON

8.0 Epidemiology

Tuberculosis (TB) causes more deaths in the world each year than any other infectious agent [1]. It is also one of the most important diseases associated with HIV infection, and the various aspects of this relationship have been extensively reviewed [2–6]. On a global scale, HIV is the greatest risk factor for the development of active TB, and TB has emerged as a principal infection and cause of death in AIDS patients. The World Health Organization (WHO) has declared the alarming escalation in the incidence of TB around the world a 'global emergency'. The HIV epidemic is regarded as a central reason for this.

The interaction between HIV and TB is most devastating in areas where both diseases are common. As a result, the greatest strain of this enormous burden of disease falls on countries of the developing world [7–9]. The WHO has estimated that there are approximately 4 million people infected with both HIV and TB in the world, over three-quarters of these living in Africa [10]. In sub-Saharan Africa, where TB is one of the commonest infections and causes of mortality, 20–67% of patients with pulmonary TB are also HIV-positive [11]. Although there is currently less dual infection in Asia, many more people are infected with *Mycobacterium tuberculosis* than in Africa. As HIV is also increasing rapidly in Asia [12], ultimately HIV may have its greatest impact on the incidence of TB there.

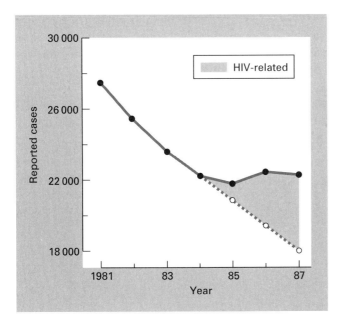

Fig. 8.1 Graph showing the number of reported cases of tuberculosis in the USA from 1981 to 1987. HIV-related cases (9226) are indicated by the tinted area. Reproduced with permission from [14].

While the overlap between HIV and TB also exists in the Western world, it is to a lesser extent. This is because TB generally has a lower prevalence and non-tuberculous opportunistic infections, such as *Pneumocystis carinii* pneumonia (PCP), are more frequently encountered. In the USA, the incidence of TB has been increasing since the mid-1980s. This has largely been attributed to the HIV epidemic [13,14] (Fig. 8.1), although poverty and the failure of TB control programmes are other important factors [1].

Across Europe, HIV infection has generally had much less impact upon the incidence of TB and the number of deaths from TB has fallen [15]. There has been a small rise in TB notifications in England and Wales recently, but this is thought to be mainly due to factors such as immigration and poverty. A survey of TB notifications from England and Wales in 1993 included anonymous HIV testing of patients aged 16–54; of these, only 2% were HIV-positive [16]. At present, 5–6% of AIDS patients in this country have TB, although TB may well be increasing in this group [17].

8.1 Pathogenesis

TB is usually transmitted via the respiratory route by inhalation of infected droplet nuclei. During the initial (primary) infection in immuno-competent individuals, alveolar macrophages engulf, process and present mycobacterial antigens to CD4 T cells. In turn, T cells release cytokines, which attract and stimulate further lymphocytes and macrophages to participate in the immune response. This response constitutes a cell-mediated immune reaction, which in approximately 90% of immunocompetent individuals is an effective defence, preventing clinically detectable infection from occurring. Of the remainder, active TB either develops soon after primary infection (5%) or years later, when cell-mediated immunity deteriorates because of old age or another immunosuppressive process (5%).

HIV infection is characterized by dysfunction and progressive depletion of CD4 cells, in addition to defective macrophage activity. As these cells play such a vital role in antimycobacterial defences, HIV infection facilitates the development of primary pulmonary TB, reactivation of latent TB and haematogenous spread to extrapulmonary sites. Tuberculosis complicating HIV disease is presumed to be mainly due to reactivation, although an increased susceptibility to primary infection is also likely [18]. There is, in addition, a suggestion that infection with TB may itself accelerate the course of HIV disease [19,20].

8.2 Clinical features

Unlike *P. carinii* and many other infections associated with AIDS, TB is infectious not only to the immunosuppressed but also to the immunocompetent. This presumably reflects its greater virulence as a pathogen. Because of this, TB is more likely to present in the early stages of HIV disease, typically with CD4 counts above 250 cells/mm^3. It is therefore recommended that HIV testing be performed in all patients with TB, regardless of known risk factors, since antiretroviral therapy and counselling to reduce HIV transmission can be initiated immediately in seropositive individuals [2]. Knowledge of a patient's HIV infection status can also allow TB treatment to be modified appropriately (see below).

In persons with dual infection, 74–100% will present as pulmonary TB [2], which since 1993 has been an AIDS-defining illness. (Extrapulmonary TB has always been AIDS-defining.) The clinical presentation is related to the stage of HIV-induced immunodeficiency (Fig. 8.2); the earlier TB develops, the more closely clinical features resemble 'normal' pulmonary TB [21]. Typical symptoms therefore include fever, sweats, cough, haemoptysis, chest pain, breathlessness and weight loss. In a large proportion of these cases there are no associated clinical features to suggest dual HIV infection at all [22].

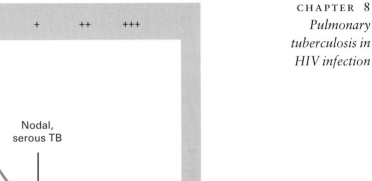

Fig. 8.2 Clinical and immunopathological course of HIV-associated TB. AFB indicates density of acid-fast bacilli, ranging from paucibacillary (0/+) to multibacillary (+++). PTB, pulmonary TB; TBM, TB meningitis; MTB, miliary TB. Reproduced with permission from [11].

Atypical presentations, with extrapulmonary spread, occur much more frequently in advanced HIV disease with low CD4 counts and clinically obvious immunosuppression [11,21]. Extrapulmonary TB usually occurs in addition to pulmonary disease, with lymphadenitis and bacteraemia being the most frequent manifestations. The gastrointestinal and central nervous systems are also often affected [21]. In Africa, disseminated TB is an important factor in the pathogenesis of 'slim' disease, which presents in advanced HIV disease with severe skeletal wasting, diarrhoea and fever [23]. Other specific examples of extrapulmonary TB in HIV-infected patients include brain abscesses, cerebral tuberculoma, meningitis, bone disease, pericarditis, peritonitis and gastric and scrotal TB [6].

8.3 Investigations

8.3.1 Tuberculin skin testing [24]

The inflammatory reaction to an intradermal injection of tuberculin (purified protein derivative), using either Heaf or Mantoux methods, is principally used to detect asymptomatic TB infection in HIV-positive individuals, with a view to offering preventive chemotherapy. The Heaf test is preferred to the Mantoux method, as it is technically more reproducible and easier to read reliably. However, skin reactions must be interpreted carefully, as results can be misleading.

The delayed hypersensitivity reaction seen in a positive tuberculin skin test is also an indicator of an individual's cell-mediated immune function. Tuberculin may therefore produce little or no response in advanced HIV disease and hence give rise to a false-negative result. However, in earlier stages reactivity may be preserved. Since there is an increased likelihood of a blunted skin test response, a lower 'cut-off' point of greater than 5 mm of induration is regarded as positive in patients with dual TB and HIV infection [24,25].

It is also important to be aware of the possibility of false-positive results in patients from populations which have undergone mass Bacillus Calmette–Guérin (BCG) vaccination, such as the UK. In this setting, positive reactions may indicate previous immunization rather than current infection. Tuberculin testing is not a routine practice in most HIV centres in the UK; however, if performed, it may suggest infection if there is a very strong positive reaction.

8.3.2 Chest radiographic appearances [2,26,27]

Coexistent HIV infection can alter the presentation of pulmonary TB, so that radiological features are varied and, again, dependent on the degree of immunodeficiency. Relatively non-immunosuppressed patients with positive tuberculin tests have features of 'reactivation' TB, including cavitation and upper-lobe shadowing, typically seen in immunocompetent individuals. In more advanced HIV disease, a miliary pattern, with hilar lymphadenopathy (similar to progressive 'primary' TB), is more commonly seen.

It can, on occasion, be difficult to distinguish between TB and other opportunistic infections. There may, for example, be interstitial infiltrates indistinguishable from PCP. Hilar lymphadenopathy, pleural fluid and cavitation are the most discriminating features suggesting TB, as they are rarely seen in PCP or cytomegalovirus pneumonitis. Pleural effusions and hilar lymphadenopathy are also seen in lymphoma and Kaposi's sarcoma, but there are usually extrapulmonary findings to support these diagnoses. Histoplasmosis and coccidioidomycoses also infrequently cause cavitation and pleural effusions, but a bilateral diffuse nodular infiltrate is a more common pattern. Rarely, the X-ray may appear normal in HIV-infected patients with pulmonary TB. Finally, combinations of opportunistic infections can also occur to complicate the radiological appearance.

8.3.3 Bacteriology and histology

Highly infectious patients can be rapidly identified by a positive acid-fast smear, using either auramine or Ziehl–Neelsen staining of clinical specimens. Approximately 60% of patients with HIV and pulmonary TB are reported to have positive acid-fast sputum smears and cavitary TB is associated with greater numbers of extracellular acid-fast bacilli and an increased likelihood of a positive smear. Despite the frequency of non-cavitating disease in HIV infection, similar positive sputum-smear rates are reported in both HIV- and non-HIV-infected individuals [28]. Sputum induction or bronchoscopy (which may reveal acid-fast organisms in lavage fluid or granulomas on biopsy) may improve the diagnostic yield. TB can also be isolated from blood cultures, more commonly in patients with advanced HIV disease and lower CD4 counts [21]. Specimens from other sites, such as lymph nodes, bone marrow and urine, may also be useful diagnostically.

If the bacillary load of a specimen is low, smears may be reported negative. In addition, in smear-positive cases it can be difficult to differentiate between species of mycobacteria on initial tissue staining. Since *M. tuberculosis* has a slow doubling time, the use of conventional culture techniques for detection of growth and speciation can take 6–10 weeks. Radiometric methods to detect early growth (such as the Bactec system) can shorten this to 2–3 weeks. The diagnostic process can be speeded up further with the additional use of deoxyribonucleic acid (DNA) probes, which can identify a culture growth as *M. tuberculosis* in a matter of hours [29].

8.3.4 Molecular biology techniques

The tools of molecular biology offer the possibility of yet more rapid diagnoses and speciation, in addition to providing greater information about the epidemiology of TB [29].

The polymerase chain reaction (PCR) can potentially give a direct diagnosis within several hours, without having to wait for a positive culture in a smear-negative case. The basis of this technique is the exponential amplification of a specific sequence of mycobacterial DNA, using appropriate oligonucleotide primers and a thermostable DNA polymerase. PCR is such a powerful technique that, in theory, genetic material from a single organism in a clinical sample could be amplified to a detectable level. (In practice, however, a minimum of 10–1000 organisms are usually required.) The insertion sequence IS6110, present 1–20 times in the genome of *M. tuberculosis*, is the most widely used target for amplification. The method also offers the potential to perform analysis on minute amounts of any tissue from which DNA can be extracted.

PCR-based assays perform well against culture methods, although PCR assays are reported as generally less sensitive. Problems with the technique include contamination of samples from previous amplifications, causing false-positives. Secondly, PCR assays give no indication of disease activity. The role of PCR is currently not established in everyday clinical practice. However, because of its rapidity and high specificity, PCR remains a valuable tool, in conjunction with the microbiology laboratory [29,30].

Restriction fragment length polymorphism (RFLP) is another powerful technique, which can be used to make a genetic distinction between different strains of *M. tuberculosis*. RFLP mapping makes use of naturally occurring copies of DNA sequences, which are randomly interspersed throughout the *M. tuberculosis* genome. Once again, IS6110 is a commonly used target. Digestion with a restriction enzyme, which cleaves these identical sequences wherever they arise, produces fragments of varying size, depending on the genetic composition of the particular strain being typed. These fragments are then separated by their different molecular weights, using gel electrophoresis, to produce a strain-specific pattern of bands. DNA fingerprints produced in this manner enable greater study of the transmission of TB. A cluster of new cases in a community caused by one strain will have the same fingerprint, for example, whereas cases caused by reactivation will have different fingerprints [29,31].

8.4 Treatment

8.4.1 Drug therapy

Pulmonary TB usually responds well to standard drug treatment [32]. However, HIV-positive patients have a greater risk of death during treatment compared with seronegative patients; this is attributable to other opportunistic diseases [7]. Standard regimens for at least 6 months are recommended [24] and should include isoniazid (300 mg/day), rifampicin (600 mg/day or 450 mg for persons weighing less than 50 kg), pyrazinamide (20–30 mg/day) and ethambutol (15 mg/kg/day) for the first 2

Table 8.1 Adverse reactions to antituberculous drugs.

Drug	Reaction
Isoniazid	Cutaneous hypersensitivity
	Peripheral neuropathy
	Hepatitis
	(May potentiate effects of anticonvulsants)
Rifampicin	Hepatitis
	Rash
	Gastrointestinal upset
	Flu-like syndrome
	Febrile reactions
	Thrombocytopenic purpura
	(Induction of hepatic enzymes)
Ethambutol	Optic atrophy
Pyrazinamide	Flushing
	Nausea, vomiting
	Anorexia
	Arthralgia, raised serum uric acid
Streptomycin	Rash (hypersensitivity)
	Giddiness, ataxia, vertigo
	Tinnitus, deafness
	(Avoid in babies, elderly, pregnant women and if renal impairment)
Thiocetazone	Gastrointestinal reactions
	Vertigo
	Conjunctivitis
	Hepatitis
	Severe skin reactions

months. Isoniazid and rifampicin should then be continued for at least another 4 months, depending on culture resistance patterns [33]. Empirical treatment may be indicated in smear-negative cases where the clinical suspicion of TB infection remains high.

The incidence of adverse reactions to antituberculous drugs is greater in patients with HIV infection (18% of cases) and may be very serious. Rifampicin is the most commonly implicated (12%); side-effects include a skin rash, hepatitis and gastrointestinal intolerance [32]. The important adverse reactions to the main antituberculous drugs are shown in Table 8.1. Thiocetazone is another antituberculous agent, which is an inexpensive and valuable companion drug, used particularly in developing-world treatment regimens. Very severe skin rashes occur more commonly in AIDS patients receiving thiocetazone and it is therefore avoided in HIV-positive individuals [34]. In general, antituberculous drugs should not be discontinued unless side-effects are serious.

Finally, it is important to be mindful of potential drug interactions, as HIV-positive patients are often taking many additional drugs on a daily basis [24]. For example, ketoconazole and fluconazole both interact with isoniazid and rifampicin, resulting in subtherapeutic serum concentrations and decreased antifungal activity. Ketoconazole can also interfere with the absorption of rifampicin and result in ineffective TB treatment. There does not appear to be a serious interaction between antituberculous and antiretroviral drugs [6].

8.4.2 Immunotherapy [35]

Immunotherapy is based upon the concept that the virulence of *M. tuberculosis* rests mainly in its ability to evoke an inappropriate immune response, rather than direct destructive action on host tissue by the organism itself. Evidence exists that interaction with some environmental mycobacteria may enhance or restore protective immunity against TB and suppress such deleterious tissue-necrotizing responses. The regulation of this balance is thought to be mediated by alterations in the cytokine profile. In turn, this influences the activity of functionally distinct T-helper-cell subsets to determine the immune response.

Mycobacterium vaccae, a harmless environmental saprophyte, is currently under investigation to see if it could have such a useful immunomodulatory role in a clinical setting. If successful, administration of *M. vaccae* could improve community TB control and offer an effective adjunct to chemotherapy, particularly in drug-resistant TB [36]. Moreover, such an approach is likely to be at a cost that developing countries could afford.

A small placebo-control trial in Nigeria showed that dually infected patients receiving adjunctive *M. vaccae* immunotherapy had increased survival and sputum clearance of TB, in addition to resolution of HIV-associated lymphadenopathy. A remarkable finding was that the two recipients of immunotherapy who were retested after 1 year had become seronegative for HIV infection, whereas patients in the placebo group remained seropositive [37]. The question of whether immunotherapy could help TB patients with coexistent HIV infection clearly needs further evaluation. Since dual infection appears to speed progression to full-blown AIDS, it is possible that promoting protective immunity to TB may also have a beneficial effect on the immunopathology of HIV infection.

8.5 Drug-resistant tuberculosis

Drug resistance is a serious problem and is well reviewed in the literature

[38–40]. Most drug resistance encountered involves loss of sensitivity to a single antimycobacterial agent. Multidrug-resistant TB (MDRTB) is defined as resistance to more than one drug (usually both isoniazid and rifampicin).

In New York City in 1991, 33% of TB cases were resistant to one drug and 19% were resistant to both isoniazid and rifampicin [41]. Drug resistance is much less of a problem in the UK in comparison, with 4% of cases reported resistant to one or more first-line drugs in a national survey. Outbreaks of MDRTB, which have occurred predominantly in HIV-positive patients, are a cause of great concern because the condition is virtually incurable. Even in immunocompetent individuals, only about a half of cases are successfully treated.

The molecular basis of drug resistance is spontaneous mutation of individual genes in the tubercle bacillus that confer insensitivity to specific antimicrobials. Drug resistance can occur through infection by organisms already resistant to antimicrobials (termed primary drug resistance); RFLP analysis shows that even advanced AIDS patients receiving treatment for drug-sensitive TB can be superinfected with MDRTB organisms [42]. Alternatively, resistance is acquired during treatment by selection of drug-resistant mutants, which arise because of inadequate therapy (secondary drug resistance).

Effective drug regimens depend on the pattern of resistance, but alternatives to standard treatment include ethionamide, cycloserine, aminosalicylic acid, streptomycin, capreomycin, amikacin, ofloxacin and ciprofloxacin. A physician experienced in managing such cases should supervise treatment. High-risk contacts and suspected new cases should be treated promptly with regimens based upon prevailing sensitivity patterns. In cases of MDRTB, duration of therapy is prolonged, often extending over 18 months or more. As in the treatment of TB in any context, single antituberculous agents should never be added to failing regimens. For prophylactic treatment, two or preferably three effective drugs should be used (see below).

Laboratory techniques which hasten the diagnostic process and provide drug sensitivity patterns rapidly are clearly desirable in the control of drug-resistant outbreaks. Molecular approaches, such as RFLP analysis and PCR-based assays, offer exciting possibilities and can be used to identify organisms containing DNA sequences indicating probable resistance to standard drugs at an early stage [29].

Clearly, in view of the difficulty in curing MDRTB, prevention and infection-control measures are of vital importance.

8.6 Prevention and control

8.6.1 Preventive chemotherapy

Chemoprophylaxis involves treatment of individuals identified as at risk, in order to prevent activation or reactivation of latent tuberculous infection. Preventive treatment can be divided into primary and secondary prophylaxis. The distinction between these, however, is not always clear and some overlap exists.

Primary chemoprophylaxis is mainly aimed at preventing active TB developing by reactivation of dormant disease in asymptomatic people. A positive tuberculin skin test may identify individuals with asymptomatic infection and there is evidence that isoniazid prophylaxis decreases the incidence of reactive TB in such patients. In addition, chemoprophylaxis may delay the progression of symptomless HIV-related disease [43]. It is therefore recommended that tuberculin skin testing is performed on all HIV-positive individuals and isoniazid given for at least 6 months to those considered at risk [24]. Preventive treatment should also be considered when the risk of exposure for HIV-positive individuals to TB is high. Primary prophylaxis may therefore be appropriate in close TB contacts or those from areas where TB is highly endemic. Blanket or mass chemoprophylaxis programmes for HIV-infected patients living in such areas in Africa, for example, may be an effective strategy, but requires further evaluation [44].

Secondary prophylaxis refers to treatment to prevent relapses of TB after successful therapy for active disease. Routine, lifelong, isoniazid prophylaxis is recommended on completing antituberculous therapy and is the usual practice, and it is effective in this respect [24].

8.6.2 Hospital-based control measures

RFLP analysis has shown that transmission readily occurs between patients in healthcare facilities [18]. It is therefore important that appropriate infection-control measures are taken to reduce transmission in hospitals and HIV units [45,46]. Efforts to identify patients with active TB as early as possible should be pursued vigorously. Sputum should be examined urgently by direct smear and, if negative but TB is still suspected, also by a PCR-based assay. Patients with suspected TB should be cared for in isolated rooms, ideally, kept at negative pressure, with removal of air to the building's exterior. Air filters and ultraviolet (UV) light may also be useful in reducing spread in the hospital environment. Cough-inducing procedures, such as bronchoscopy and nebulized pentamidine therapy, should take place in an adequately ventilated room or area occupied only by the patient. Face-masks may reduce microbial air contamination when a patient is being transported within or between hospitals and so protect staff from inhalation of bacilli. Such measures recognize that nosocomial infection of healthcare workers is a real cause for serious concern.

8.6.3 Community-based control measures

In the community, case finding and immediate effective treatment are the most important control measures of all. Notification of cases is a statutory legal requirement and contact screening should be initiated promptly. Well-organized control programmes are vital in the implementation of this, since delayed or inadequate treatment may facilitate spread of infection in the community and the emergence of drug resistance.

DNA fingerprinting can be used to show patterns of spread and has demonstrated that recent transmission rather than reactivation of TB is more common than had been suspected. In New York and San Francisco, for example, recent transmission gave rise to approximately 40% and 30% of new TB cases, respectively [47,48]. The San Francisco study showed that contact tracing missed 90% of cases related by RFLP analysis and one patient accounted for 6% of the cases evaluated. Hispanic ethnicity, black race, HIV infection and low-income neighbourhoods were identified as risk factors for infection. These studies therefore highlight environments and groups for the application of improved treatment and control measures, in addition to the importance of such strategies.

Finally, vaccination with BCG does not have a preventive role in HIV infection, because it is a live vaccine and the risk of developing disseminated BCG disease exists [45].

8.6.4 Compliance with drug treatment

Where the clinical response to chemotherapy is poor, a problem with treatment compliance should always be considered. Compliance can be assessed simply by testing urine (coloured orange by rifampicin), prescription checks or counting pills. Combination drug therapy with a single tablet makes taking medication easier and promotes compliance. The TB health adviser/nurse has a central role in ensuring completion of treatment.

If poor compliance is suspected, intermittent supervised or directly observed therapy (DOT) may be necessary [45]. DOT quite literally is where a healthcare worker watches while a patient swallows antituberculous drugs over the whole treatment course. Drug taking can be supervised daily or intermittently in a wide variety of settings, including homes, hospitals, clinics and schools.

In New York City from 1978 to 1992, the number of cases of TB had nearly tripled [41]. As a result of a concentrated effort, there was a 21% reduction in reported TB cases from 1992 to 1994 [49]. The widespread use of DOT and improved infection-control measures in institutions, such as hospitals, homeless shelters and correctional facilities, were the main reasons cited for this. Treatment completion rates rose from under 50% in 1989 to around 90% in 1994. Despite the apparent expense, programmes employing DOT are highly cost-effective [50].

8.7 Non-tuberculous opportunistic mycobacteria
[51–54]

Non-tuberculous mycobacteria (NTM) are common environmental organisms which are rarely pathological in immunocompetent persons, but cause serious opportunistic infection in HIV-positive patients and are classified as AIDS-defining diseases. The most important NTM is *Mycobacterium avium intracellulare* (MAI), which can be isolated from numerous sources, including soil and water. MAI complicates HIV infection at a more advanced stage of disease than TB (typically with CD4 counts of less than 50 cells/mm^3) and occurs in 30–50% of AIDS patients.

Although MAI can cause localized pulmonary disease, disseminated infection is a much more common presentation. Disseminated disease is preceded by colonization of the respiratory and gastrointestinal tracts (which are probably also the initial portals of entry) and is associated with a poor prognosis. Systemic features, such as fever, weight loss, fatigue and anaemia, are common clinically. Reports of specific pulmonary manifestations are few; a productive cough, pneumonia and X-ray abnormalities are occasional features. Chest-film findings are diverse and similarities between the radiographic appearances of TB and NTM in HIV infection exist. Chest X-ray patterns include focal consolidation, nodular infiltrates and cavitation [53,55]. Lymphadenopathy, hepatosplenomegaly and chronic diarrhoea are also recognized. Laboratory diagnosis is most commonly made from blood cultures and biopsy specimens from bone marrow, lymph nodes and liver.

MAI is resistant to all first-line antituberculous drugs, and treatment is aimed at restraining infection, rather than eradicating it. Effective oral regimens may involve combinations, including rifampicin, ethambutol, clarithromycin, clofazimine and ciprofloxacin among others. Sometimes it may be difficult to differentiate between TB and MAI, especially when acid-fast bacilli are identified in clinical specimens. Since TB is more often life-threatening and an infectious risk if untreated, drug therapy should initially be chosen to cover TB. Modification to treatment can be made later if necessary. Prophylaxis with rifabutin should be considered in patients with CD4 counts less than 100 cells/mm^3 to prevent colonization leading to disseminated disease [56].

Pulmonary infection caused by other NTM, including *M. kansasii, M. xenopi, M. gordonae, M. fortuitum, M. malmoense, M. chelonae* and *M. celatum*, have also been reported in AIDS patients. Clinical presentation is similar to MAI and treatment also usually involves combination chemotherapy.

References

1 Bloom B.R., Murray C.J. Tuberculosis: commentary on a reemergent killer. *Science* 1992; **257**: 1055–1064.

2 Barnes P.F., Bloch A.B., Davidson P.T., Snider D.E. Tuberculosis in patients with human immunodeficiency virus infection. *New England Journal of Medicine* 1991; **324**: 1644–1650.

3 Fitzgerald J.M., Allen E.A. The impact of human immunodeficiency virus infection on tuberculosis and its control. *Chest* 1991; **100**: 191–200.

4 Barnes P.F., Le H.Q., Davidson P.T. Tuberculosis in patients with HIV infection. *Medical Clinics of North America* 1993; **77**: 1369–1391.

5 Styblo K., Enarson D.A. The impact of infection with human immunodeficiency virus on tuberculosis. In: Mitchell D.M., ed. *Recent Advances in Respiratory Medicine*, Vol. 5. Edinburgh: Churchill Livingstone, 1991: 147–162.

6 Hopewell P.C. Tuberculosis in persons with HIV infection. In: Sande M.A., Volberding P.A. eds. *The Medical Management of AIDS*, 4th edn. Philadelphia: W.B. Saunders, 1995: 416–436.

7 Nunn P.P., Elliot A.M., McAdam K.P.W.J. Impact of human immunodeficiency virus on tuberculosis in developing countries. *Thorax* 1994; **49**: 511–518.

8 Grzybowski S. Tuberculosis in the Third World. *Thorax* 1991; **46**: 689–691.

9 Harries A.D. Tuberculosis and human immunodeficiency virus infection in developing countries. *Lancet* 1990; **335**: 387–390.

10 Raviglione M.C., Narain J.P., Kochi A. HIV-associated tuberculosis in developing countries: clinical features, diagnosis and treatment. *Bulletin of the World Health Organisation* 1992; **70**: 515–526.

11 De Cock K.N., Soro B., Coulibaly I.M., Lucas S.B. Tuberculosis and HIV infection in sub-Saharan Africa. *Journal of the American Medical Association* 1992; **268**: 1581–1587.

12 Lalvani A., Shastri J.S. HIV epidemic in India: opportunity to learn from the past. *Lancet* 1996; **347**: 1349–1350.

13 Centers for Disease Control. Update: tuberculosis elimination: United States. *Morbidity and Mortality Weekly Report* 1990; **39**: 153–156.

14 Murray J.F. The white plague: down and out, or up and coming? *American Review of Respiratory Diseases* 1989; **140**: 1788–1795.

15 Rieder H.L. Epidemiology of tuberculosis in Europe. *European Respiratory Journal* 1995; **8** (Suppl. 20): 620s–632s.

16 Watson J.M. on behalf of PHLS/BTS/DoH Collaborative Group. Results of a national survey of tuberculosis notifications in England and Wales in 1993. *Thorax* 1995; **50**: 442P.

17 Watson J.M., Meredith S.K., Whitmore-Overton E., Bannister B., Darbyshire J.H. Tuberculosis and HIV: estimates of the overlap in England and Wales. *Thorax* 1993; **48**: 199–203.

18 Daley C.L., Small P.M., Schecter G.F. *et al*. An outbreak of tuberculosis with accelerated progression among persons infected with human immunodeficiency virus: an analysis

using restriction fragment length polymorphisms. *New England Journal of Medicine* 1992; **326**: 231–235.

19 Toossi Z., Sierra-Madero J.D., Blinkhorn R.A., Mettler M.A., Rich E.A. Enhanced susceptibility of blood monocytes from patients with tuberculosis to productive infection with human immunodeficiency virus type 1. *Journal of Experimental Medicine* 1993; **177**: 1511–1516.

20 Wallis R.S., Vjecha M., Amir-Tahmasseb M. *et al*. Influence of tuberculosis on HIV: enhanced cytokine expression and elevated B2 microglobulin in HIV associated tuberculosis. *Journal of Infectious Diseases* 1992; **167**: 43–48.

21 Jones B.E., Summer M.M., Young D.A., Davidson P.T., Kramer F., Barnes P.F. Relationship of the manifestation of tuberculosis to CD4 cell counts in patients with human immunodeficiency virus infection. *American Review of Respiratory Diseases* 1993; **148**: 1292–1297.

22 Nunn P.P., Gicheha C., Hayes R. *et al*. Cross sectional survey of HIV infection among patients with tuberculosis in Nairobi, Kenya. *Tubercle and Lung Disease* 1992; **73**: 45–51.

23 Lucas S.B., De Cock K.M., Hounnou A. *et al*. Contribution of tuberculosis to slim disease in Africa. *British Medical Journal* 1994; **308**: 1531–1533.

24 Sub Committee of the Joint Tuberculosis Committee of the British Thoracic Society. Guidelines on the management of tuberculosis and HIV infection in the United Kingdom. *British Medical Journal* 1992; **304**: 1231–1233.

25 American Thoracic Society. Control of tuberculosis in the United States. *American Review of Respiratory Diseases* 1992; **146**: 1623–1633.

26 Goodman P.C. Tuberculosis and AIDS. *Imaging of Tuberculosis and Craniospinal Tuberculosis* 1995; **33**: 707–717.

27 Goodman P.C. The chest film in AIDS. In: Sande M.A., Volberding P.A., eds. *The Medical Management of AIDS*, 4th edn. Philadelphia: W.B. Saunders, 1995: 592–613.

28 Smith R.L., Bertowitz K.A., Aranda C.P. Factors affecting the yield of acid-fast sputum smears in patients with HIV and tuberculosis. *Chest* 1994; **106**: 684–686.

29 Marshall B.G., Shaw R.J. New technology in the diagnosis of tuberculosis. *British Journal of Hospital Medicine* 1996; **55**: 491–494.

30 Godfrey-Faussett P. Of molecules and men: the detection of tuberculosis, past, present and future. In: Porter J.D.H., McAdam K.P.W.J., eds. *Tuberculosis: Back to the Future*. Chichester: John Wiley and Sons, 1994: 79–98.

31 van-Soolingen D., Hermans P.W.M. Epidemiology of tuberculosis by DNA fingerprinting. *European Respiratory Journal* 1995; **8** (Suppl. 20): 649s–656s.

32 Small P.M., Schecter G.F., Goodman P.C., Sande M.A., Chaisson R.E., Hopewell P.C. Treatment of tuberculosis in patients with advanced human immunodeficiency virus infection. *New England Journal of Medicine* 1991; **324**: 289–294.

33 Joint Tuberculosis Committee of the British Thoracic Society. Chemotherapy and management of tuberculosis in the United Kingdom: recommendations of the Joint Tuberculosis Committee of the British Thoracic Society. *Thorax* 1990; **45**: 403–408.

34 Nunn P., Fibuga D., Gathua S. *et al*. Cutaneous hypersensitivity reactions due to thiacetazone in HIV-1 seropositive patients treated for tuberculosis. *Lancet* 1991; **337**: 627–630.

35 Stanford J.L., Grange J.M. The promise of immunotherapy for tuberculosis. *Respiratory Medicine* 1994; **88**: 3–7.

36 Etemadi A., Farid R., Standford J.L. Immunotherapy for drug-resistant tuberculosis. *Lancet* 1992; **340**: 1360–1361.

37 Stanford J.L., Onyebujoh P.C., Rook G.A.W., Grange J.M., Pozniak A. Old plague, new plague and a treatment for both? *AIDS* 1993; 7: 1275–1277.

38 Ellner J.J. Multidrug-resistant tuberculosis. *Advances in Internal Medicine* 1995; **40**: 155–196.

39 Hayward C.M.M, Herrman J.L., Griffin G.E. Drug-resistant tuberculosis: mechanisms and management. *British Journal of Hospital Medicine* 1995; **54**: 494–500.

40 Wood A.J.J. Treatment of multidrug resistant tuberculosis. *New England Journal of Medicine* 1993; **329**: 784–791.

41 Frieden T.R., Sterling T., Pablos-Mendez A., Kilburn J.O., Cauthen G.M., Dooley S.W. The emergence of drug-resistant tuberculosis in New York City. *New England Journal of Medicine* 1993; **328**: 521–526.

42 Small P.M., Shafer R.W., Hopewell P.C. *et al*. Exogenous reinfection with multidrug-resistant *Mycobacterium tuberculosis* in patients with advanced HIV infection. *New England Journal of Medicine* 1993; **328**: 1137–1144.

43 Pape J.W., Jean S.S., Ho J.L., Hafner A., Johnson W.D. Effect of isoniazid prophylaxis on incidence of active tuberculosis and progression of HIV infection. *Lancet* 1993; **342**: 268–272.

44 Walley J., Porter J. Chemoprophylaxis in tuberculosis and HIV infection. *British Medical Journal* 1995; **308**: 1621–1622.

45 Joint Tuberculosis Committee of the British Thoracic Society. Control and prevention of tuberculosis in the United Kingdom: code of practice 1994. *Thorax* 1994; **49**: 1193–1200.

46 Centers for Disease Control. Guidelines for preventing the transmission of tuberculosis in health-care settings, with special focus on HIV-related issues. *Morbidity and Mortality Weekly Report* 1990; **39**: 1–29.

47 Alland D., Kalkut G.E., Moss A.R. *et al*. Transmission of tuberculosis in New York City — an analysis of DNA fingerprinting and conventional epidemiologic methods. *New England Journal of Medicine* 1994; **330**: 1710–1716.

48 Small P.M., Hopewell P.C., Singh S.P. *et al*. The epidemiology of tuberculosis in San Francisco—a population based study using conventional and molecular based methods. *New England Journal of Medicine* 1994; **330**: 1703–1709.

49 Frieden T.R., Fujiwara P.I., Washko R.M., Hamburg M.A. Tuberculosis in New York City—turning the tide. *New England Journal of Medicine* 1995; **333**: 229–233.

50 Morse D.I. Directly observed therapy for tuberculosis. *British Medical Journal* 1996; **312**: 719–720.

51 Jacobsen M.A. Disseminated *Mycobacterium avium* complex and other bacterial infections. In: Sande M.A., Volberding P.A., eds. *The Medical Management of AIDS*, 4th edn. Philadelphia: W.B. Saunders, 1995: 402–415.

52 Rigsby M.O., Curtis A.M. Pulmonary disease from nontuberculous mycobacteria in patients with human immunodeficiency virus. *Chest* 1994; **106**: 913–919.

53 Kalayjian R.C., Toossi Z., Tomashefski J.F. *et al*. Pulmonary disease due to infection by *Mycobacterium avium* complex in patients with AIDS. *Clinical Infectious Diseases* 1995; **20**: 1186–1194.

54 Griffith D.E., Wallace R.J. Lung disease caused by non-tuberculous mycobacteria. In: Pennington J.E., ed. *Respiratory Infections: Diagnosis and Management*, 3rd edn. New York: Raven Press, 1994: 653–678.

55 Miller R.F., Birley H.D.L., Fogarty P., Semple S.J.G. Cavitary lung disease caused by *Mycobacterium avium-intracellulare* in AIDS patients. *Respiratory Medicine* 1990; **84**: 409–411.

56 Centers for Disease Control. Recommendation on prophylaxis and therapy for disseminated *Mycobacterium avium* complex for adults and adolescents infected with human immunodeficiency virus. *Morbidity and Mortality Weekly Report* 1993; **40**: 17–20.

9 Non-neoplastic lymphoproliferative disorders of the lung

S.J.G. SEMPLE

9.0 Spectrum of lymphoproliferative disorders of the lung in HIV infection: pulmonary lymphoid hyperplasia and lymphocytic interstitial pneumonitis

Hyperplasia of lymphoid tissue within the lung has been found following chemical or infective damage, in patients with rheumatoid arthritis and Sjögren's syndrome and in a variety of disorders of immunodeficiency. However, it may also be found without obvious cause and its precise role in the immune system in humans is unknown.

Hyperplasia of lymphoid tissue was described by Bienenstock *et al.* in two classic papers [1,2], largely based on animal studies, and this hyperplasia is now known as bronchus-associated lymphoid tissue (BALT). It has some, but not all, of the features of Peyer's patches, commonly referred to as gut-associated lymphoid tissue. In the majority of mammals, BALT develops postnatally and its development and expansion are a response to local stimulation from inflammation and inhaled environmental agents, which may or may not be antigenic. In humans, BALT is seldom seen in the normal lung, being encountered at autopsy in about 14% of examined lungs. In smokers, however, it was commonly identified in one series in 82% of lungs examined post-mortem [3].

In the lymphoproliferative disorders in HIV-infected people described in this chapter, the histological findings have many of the features of BALT [4]. It is possible, therefore, that HIV infection of the lung may be one of the several agents held responsible for the appearance and development of BALT and that BALT is involved in the lymphoproliferative disorders of the lung seen in HIV-infected people.

There are a series of conditions reported in patients who are HIV-infected where there is an infiltration and/or expansion of mononuclear cells within the lung, which are classified in this chapter under the general term pulmonary lymphoid hyperplasia (PLH). These conditions are follicular bronchitis/bronchiolitis, bronchiolitis obliterans organizing pneumonia (BOOP) and non-specific interstitial pneumonitis (NIP).

There are two other lymphoproliferative disorders considered in this chapter, namely lymphocytic interstitial pneumonitis (LIP) and the diffuse lymphocyte infiltrative syndrome. They are usually considered separately from PLH because of histological and clinical differences. First, there is extensive lymphocyte infiltration of alveolar septa and, second, the clinical presentation is of a more severe and widespread disorder.

9.1 Cell phenotypes and possible causation of lymphoproliferative disorders of the lung in HIV infection

It is possible that the lymphoproliferative disorders of the lung seen in some HIV-infected people are extensions of the lymphocytic alveolitis which was described and discussed in Chapter 2 (section 2.10.1). If this is so, it can be anticipated that the infiltrate of cells in the lung would contain T lymphocytes, some belonging to the CD8 subset. Analysis of the cell content of bronchoalveolar lavage (BAL) in two patients with LIP showed a high percentage and number of CD8 lymphocytes, with virtually no CD4 cells [5]. In biopsy specimens, both B and T cells have been identified [4,6], with, in one series, a predominance of T cells in both LIP and NIP [4]. In another report, in patients with NIP there was a similar mixture of cells but the B cells were in aggregates in bronchiolar walls and perivascular spaces. When the infiltrate of cells was more extensive and extended into the alveolar septa, there was a more diffuse infiltrate of T cells, which were CD4 and CD8 cells in approximately equal numbers [6]. In the diffuse infiltrative CD8 lymphocytosis syndrome, the dominant lymphocytes, as the name of the syndrome suggests, were of the CD8 subset [7]. This analysis of cell phenotype in NIP and LIP does suggest that they are extensions of the lymphocytic alveolitis reported in many HIV-infected people.

If these lymphoproliferative disorders in HIV-infected patients are an extension of the lymphocytic alveolitis described in Chapter 2, the question arises as to why some patients develop these disorders and others do not. The answer to this question is not known, but may be related to age, ethnic origin, different strains of HIV virus and the host response of the patient. For example, LIP is common in children seropositive for HIV but rare in adults. Likewise, LIP is rarely seen in white homosexual males but is more commonly seen in Afro-Caribbean patients, particularly from Haiti [8]. The evidence for a strain-dependent virus effect comes from a lentivirus other than HIV, namely the ovine lentivirus which infects sheep and produces pulmonary lesions similar to LIP and NIP. In this animal model of the effects of infection, the lymphocytes found in the lung were primarily T-cytotoxic/suppressor lymphocytes. In lambs artificially infected with the ovine lentivirus via the trachea, the lesions found in the lung were strain-dependent; those strains that caused cell lysis *in vitro* produced a LIP-like picture in the lambs, with extrapulmonary disease, while non-lytic strains produced a mild lymphocytosis within the lung similar to NIP [9].

The cause of the lymphoproliferative disorders is not known but the most plausible explanation is that they are due to infection of the lung with HIV and the immunological response to that infection. Evidence of lung infection by HIV has already been presented in Chapter 2 (section 2.8.2). In addition, there are two reports of the isolation of HIV from BAL in three patients with LIP [10,11]. In two of these patients with LIP, the ratio of HIV-specific immunoglobulin G (IgG) to total IgG was higher in BAL than in the peripheral blood, indicating a specific immune response locally in the lung [11]. HIV ribonucleic acid (RNA) has been detected in some, but not all, patients in lung biopsy specimens by *in situ* hybridization [4]. No evidence has been found to substantiate infection with Epstein–Barr virus, cytomegalovirus or herpes simplex virus 1 and 2 as a cause of LIP or NIP in adults [4,6].

9.2 Non-specific interstitial pneumonitis

9.2.1 Lung pathology in non-specific interstitial pneumonitis [4,6]

This consists of an interstitial infiltrate of mature lymphocytes, plasma cells and macrophages. Lymphocytes may be in aggregates (sometimes with germinal centres) in bronchiolar walls, perivascular spaces and interlobar and subpleural connective tissue. In the vicinity of the interstitial infiltrates, oedema fluid and macrophages may be seen in the alveoli.

Where the interstitium is expanded by infiltrates or oedema, type II pneumonocytic hyperplasia is often observed. Less common findings are an increase in eosinophils and patchy intra-alveolar changes of the type seen in BOOP [6] and, in one series of 46 patients with NIP, four had areas of diffuse alveolar damage [4]. However, these changes are uncommon and the overall picture is one of a mild chronic interstitial pneumonitis.

9.2.2 Clinical presentation of non-specific interstitial pneumonitis

Patients with NIP may be asymptomatic. This was most convincingly demonstrated in a study of 24 HIV-seropositive people with no pulmonary symptoms, a normal chest radiograph, no history of *Pneumocystis carinii* pneumonia (PCP) and no prophylaxis for PCP. The purpose of the investigation was to determine how often *P. carinii* organisms or other pathology could be detected in HIV-infected people with no respiratory symptoms and with normal chest radiographs. Transbronchial biopsy was carried out in the patients and chronic NIP was found in 11 out of 23 biopsies [12].

The presenting symptoms are cough or dyspnoea or both [6,13]. There are usually no constitutional symptoms or signs of HIV disease. The chest-radiograph changes are described as reticular, which may be nodular or diffuse. There may be a 'subtle' or fine perihilar loss of translucency and lung markings [6,14]. The terms reticular and reticulonodular, which are used here in this section and describe the changes seen in NIP, are probably equivalent to 'interstitial infiltrates' and 'diffuse loss of radiotranslucency with loss of lung markings', which are descriptive terms used in much of the radiology literature.

Rarely, there may be a pleural effusion. It is difficult to determine the frequency of this finding. In one report, a frequency of 11% [14] is quoted, but this must be accepted with some reservation. In this series, most biopsies were recorded as showing diffuse alveolar damage [13,14], which was not seen, or rarely seen, in two recent reports on 54 patients with NIP [4,6]. In addition, many of the patients in the earlier report had Kaposi's sarcoma or other possible causes of lung damage, in addition to NIP [13].

The arterial gas tensions may be normal or show mild hypoxaemia; the CD4 cell count is likely to be normal, as is the peripheral lymphocyte count [6].

The initial prognosis in these patients is good, in that the condition may remain stable or clear spontaneously [6]. A good response to steroids has been reported in two patients [6], but this has not established the benefit of this treatment because spontaneous resolution may occur. The results of follow-up of patients with NIP in two series showed that survival was poor, being less than 32 months in one study and 12 months in the other. The cause of death was due to one or more of the complications of AIDS and was unrelated to NIP [6,13].

9.3 Lymphocytic interstitial pneumonitis

LIP was originally named lymphoid interstitial pneumonia and was described as a diffuse lymphoreticular infiltration of the lung accompanied by abnormalities of the plasma immunoglobulins [15,16]. These changes were often associated with Sjögren's syndrome, and indeed it was considered possible that the cellular infiltration of the lung was an extension of that occurring in the salivary glands [16]. The disease was more common in women and was usually first diagnosed between the age of 40 and 60, but a few patients were in their teens or elderly. The onset was insidious, with cough, dyspnoea, weight loss and fever. When the illness was complicated by Sjögren's syndrome, there was keratitis sicca and xerostoma. The chest radiograph showed fine or coarse reticulonodular changes, usually most evident at the lung bases, which showed slow progression with time. No cause has been identified, but it is interesting, in view of the AIDS epidemic, that possible aetiological factors proposed were acquired immunodeficiency and/or a direct or indirect effect of viral agents [16]. Some caution is needed in extrapolating the original findings in LIP to the interstitial pneumonia or pneumonitis found in patients infected with the HIV. This is because the original description probably included some patients with lymphoma [16]. With advances in the ability to distinguish between monoclonal and polyclonal proliferation of cells, the separation of LIP from lymphoma can be made with greater certainty [17]. There are, however, rare reports of malignant lymphoma complicating LIP in patients not infected with HIV, which has been described as a 'monoclonal B-cell neoplasm arising in a polyclonal lymphoproliferative disorder' [18]. At the time of writing, we are not aware of LIP in an HIV-infected person progressing to lymphoma.

LIP prior to the AIDS epidemic was a rare disease. For example, during the period 1966–82, no cases of LIP were seen at one large hospital in North America, while, during 1982–86, 31 cases of LIP were documented [8]. Nevertheless, LIP is an uncommon manifestation of disease due to HIV in adults, which is not the case in children.

9.3.1 Lung pathology in lymphocytic interstitial pneumonitis [4,6]

The findings in biopsies of the lung in patients with LIP were the same as in NIP, but, in contrast to NIP, there were substantial alveolar septal lymphoid infiltrates in all specimens. Loose intraluminal fibrosis, protruding into bronchioles, alveolar ducts and alveoli, was seen in a few biopsies. Bronchiolar involvement, leading to bronchiolitis obliterans, has also been one of the less common histological findings.

Most of the reports in the literature state that the diagnosis of LIP was made on biopsy, without giving details of the histology, which presumably means the changes seen were consistent with previous findings in patients with LIP who were not infected with HIV. A more detailed description of pathology was given in a report on 16 patients with LIP and AIDS or AIDS-related complex (ARC) [8]. At open-lung biopsy, the abnormal areas of the lung were found to be nodular and adjacent to pulmonary vessels, lymphatics and interlobular septa. The lung interstitium was infiltrated with lymphocytes (polyclonal in origin), plasma cells and reticulum cells. Some of the biopsies had immunoblasts and histiocytes containing cellular debris in their cytoplasm. There were two features of the histology which deserve special mention. First, in some biopsies the process was more diffuse and less nodular and led to areas of consolidation of alveoli. Second, some aggregates of lymphocytes appeared to be leading to bronchiolar obstruction and were described as similar to bronchiolitis obliterans [8].

9.3.2 Clinical presentation of lymphocytic interstitial pneumonitis and outcome

The majority of the patients infected with HIV who develop LIP are black, often from Haiti. LIP occurs in homosexuals, bisexuals and intravenous drug users (IVDUs) and some of the patients in the latter group will be heterosexual. The illness has many of the features of LIP previously described in patients who had no evidence of infection with HIV. These include cough, dyspnoea, weight loss, night sweats and fatigue [5,7,8,19–21]. Some patients will have Sjögren's syndrome, with associated clinical manifestations. Polyclonal hypergammaglobulinaemia [20] is found in the serum, and reticulonodular shadows, predominantly in the basal region, which may be fine or coarse, are seen in the chest radiograph [8]. However, there are many differences in LIP in seronegative patients, presumably due to infection with HIV. Patients often present with generalized lymphadenopathy, hepatosplenomegaly and parotid-gland enlargement [5,7,8,20,21]. Additional features on the chest radiograph to the usual reticulonodular shadows have been noted. In one report of 16 patients with LIP, five had unexplained pleural effusions and four mediastinal lymphadenopathy [8]. Of the four patients with lymphadenopathy, one was due to Kaposi's sarcoma and one was probably due to *Mycobacterium avium intracellulare*, but the cause of the other two was not established [8]. Radiological findings point to evidence of areas of lung consolidation in a few patients, which are described as 'alveolar densities' and 'patchy alveolar infiltrates' [8,20,21].

There are no reliable means of distinguishing between LIP and opportunistic infection of the lung, so that diagnosis is made by transbronchial or open-lung biopsy. Lung-function tests may be normal or near normal and, when abnormal, show mild hypoxaemia, a reduced transfer factor and a restrictive defect of forced expiratory volumes [5,20,21]. Patchy uptake of gallium by the lung has been reported, so this test is of no value for distinguishing between LIP and other infections [7,20,21].

It is difficult to determine the prognosis and outcome of LIP in patients who are seropositive for HIV, because the illness may be profoundly affected by the latter infection. In one report of 16 patients with LIP, survival varied from 1 to 28 months, but in 12 patients the chest-radiograph abnormalities remained unchanged. All patients developed ARC or AIDS and, although the exact cause of death was not stated, it was (presumably) due to their HIV disease rather than LIP [8]. Several reports of patients with LIP record no change or improvement without specific therapy, sometimes with clearing of the chest-radiographic infiltrates [5,19,20]. There are individual reports of improvement on steroid therapy [5,19,20] and in one patient there was an exacerbation of symptoms when the dose of steroids was tapered [20]. In view of the favourable course of the illness in most patients without treatment, the efficacy of therapy with steroids must remain uncertain. However, the response to this treatment seems much more encouraging than that reported in patients with LIP before the advent of the AIDS. The role of zidovudine in the management of patients with LIP is similarly uncertain. Of two brief reports on its use, one records a favourable response in two patients [22] and the other records no change in the clinical condition of a single patient [23].

9.3.3 Diffuse infiltrative lymphocytosis syndrome

This syndrome, described in 17 patients who were seropositive for HIV [7], is characterized by persistent CD8 lymphocytosis and diffuse lymphocytic tissue infiltration. The tissues involved are predominantly the parotid glands and the lung, but the gastrointestinal tract and liver may also be infiltrated. The parotid glandular involvement leads to a Sjögren-like syndrome, while the histological changes in the lung are those of LIP.

Of the 17 patients described with this syndrome, 12 were black, two Hispanic and three Caucasian. Eight patients were IVDUs and six were homosexual; transmission of the virus was heterosexual in all the

Caucasian patients. All the patients had bilateral parotid-gland enlargement, 14 had xerostomia and six xerophthalmia or keratoconjunctivitis sicca. Nine of 11 patients imaged with gallium-67-citrate radiotracer had increased uptake in the parotid gland; uptake by the nasal mucosa was seen in all patients. Fourteen of the patients had generalized lymphadenopathy, most obvious in the cervical region. Ten patients had LIP proved on histology, four had neurological involvement and three had lymphocytic infiltration of the gastrointestinal tract.

None of the patients had AIDS but 14 could be classified as having ARC. All 17 patients had leucocyte counts greater than 4.0×10^9 cells/l and, although the CD4/CD8 cell ratio was less than 1, the patients had a higher mean number of CD4 cells than a comparable group of patients with AIDS or ARC. Fifteen patients had an absolute CD8 cell lymphocytosis, of which the majority of cells belonged to the CD8 CD29 subset. A polyclonal hypergammaglobulinaemia was present in all patients; five had positive rheumatoid or antinuclear factors. Of the 12 black patients, 10 expressed the major histocompatibility complex (MHC) group human leucocyte antigen (HLA)-DR5, a significantly higher proportion than that found in a matched control group of 45 black people. The authors speculated that the syndrome they described might reflect a distinctive host response to HIV which is dependent on a particular MHC class II allele.

Parotid-gland biopsies were carried out to exclude the diagnosis of lymphoma and the biopsies showed discrete foci of lymphocytes, which were predominantly made up of CD8-positive T cells. In some patients, there was complete preservation of the glandular architecture but, in others, there was atrophy of the duct epithelium, with fibrosis. The authors point out two factors which distinguish the diffuse infiltrative lymphocytosis syndrome from the classic Sjögren's syndrome in women. First, no autoantibodies to Ro/SS-A and La/SS-B were found in their patients and, second, the lymphocytes belonged to the CD8 subset rather than the CD4 group.

Of the 10 patients with LIP, four were treated for 'respiratory insufficiency'. Three patients received high-dose corticosteroids, with improvement in two but the third died of respiratory failure. A fourth patient was treated with chlorambucil, with complete resolution of the changes seen on the chest radiograph and the disappearance of parotid swelling. Follow-up of the remaining patients ranged from 6 to 72 months (median duration 26 months) and only two patients died, one from pneumococcal pneumonia and one from incidental head trauma. Three patients had complete resolution of their sicca symptoms, parotid enlargement and the pulmonary abnormalities seen on the chest radiographs. Only one patient developed an opportunistic infection and none developed Kaposi's sarcoma or lymphoma.

In our preceding description of LIP, we recorded that some patients had an associated Sjögren's syndrome and therefore these patients could be exhibiting the diffuse infiltrative lymphocytosis syndrome. Indeed, the syndrome may just be a description of a subset of patients with LIP who have a lymphocytic infiltration of the parotid gland and other organs, of which the lung is one. There is, for example, a report of five such patients with the persistent generalized lymphadenopathy syndrome who presented with the sicca complex (xeropthalmia and xerostomia) [24]. All patients had benign lymphocytic infiltrates in other organs, as well as the parotid glands, which included the lung (LIP), liver and kidney. The patients had IgG antibodies to Epstein–Barr virus antigens, but anti-nuclear antibodies, rheumatoid factor and antibodies against Ro/SS-A and La/SS-B antigens were not found. Although lymphopoenia occurred in three patients, there was a CD8 lymphocytosis in two patients. These five patients would appear to meet the criteria of the diffuse infiltrative lymphocytosis syndrome, but they were reported before the publication of the description of that syndrome.

9.4 Follicular bronchiolitis, lymphocytic bronchiolitis and bronchiolitis obliterans organizing pneumonia

9.4.1 Follicular bronchiolitis and lymphocytic bronchiolitis

Follicular bronchiolitis is rare and may occur without obvious cause. It has been reported following chemical or infective damage to the lung, in patients suffering from rheumatoid arthritis and Sjögren's syndrome and in a variety of disorders of immunodeficiency [25]. In follicular bronchiolitis, a concentric inflammatory infiltrate of lymphocytes and plasma cells surrounds the bronchioles, and lymphoid hyperplasia with abundant germinal centres are seen, which may extend along and into interlobular septa, subpleural regions and lymphatics. Hyperplastic follicles are frequently located between bronchioles and pulmonary artery and may compress the lumen into a slit. Immunodeficiency has been associated with follicular bronchiolitis and in one patient (quoted in [25]) the cause of the deficiency was AIDS. A lymphocytic bronchiolitis has been reported in a patient with AIDS which was shown to be lymphocytic on lung biopsy and on the cellular analysis of BAL [26]. The respiratory symptoms of the patient with lymphocytic bronchiolitis were dyspnoea and cough and the chest radiograph showed diffuse bilateral nodules 2–5 mm in diameter. The symptoms and chest radiographs were virtually unchanged over an 18-month period of observation [26].

9.4.2 Bronchiolitis obliterans organizing pneumonia

In idiopathic BOOP, there is a mononuclear cell infiltration of the walls of the terminal and respiratory bronchioles, with plugs of granulation tissue in the lumen and extending into the alveolar ducts. When the ducts are involved, the alveoli distal to them may be affected, with macrophages in the lumen and lymphocytes and plasma cells in the interstitium. This condition is different from bronchiolitis obliterans with irreversible obstruction and responds to corticosteroid treatment with complete clinical and physiological recovery [27].

There are now four HIV-infected people with BOOP reported in the medical literature [28,29]. The presenting symptoms were cough, dyspnoea and fever and one of the patients was hypoxaemic. A lymphocytosis was found in BAL, although in one patient there was a neutrophil predominance. The chest-radiograph findings were described as showing 'patchy alveolar and interstitial infiltrates'. The diagnosis was made on lung biopsy. Three of the four patients were treated with steroids, with resolution of the pneumonia, while in the fourth resolution was spontaneous.

Thus BOOP in HIV-infected people has a similar presentation and clinical course to those in patients not infected with HIV. This similarity extends to the response to steroid therapy. However, therapy is usually necessary for several months to ensure resolution of BOOP and this is a potential danger for those patients who are immunosuppressed. In these patients with BOOP, who received long-term treatment with steroids, in only one was it necessary to discontinue treatment because of the development of an opportunistic infection. In this patient, prednisone was stopped after 11 months because of retinitis due to cytomegalovirus.

The histological changes of BOOP have occasionally been noted in patients who have had open-lung biopsy for diagnostic purposes. However, these changes were in association with infection due to PCP and in one patient a pneumonia due to *Pseudomonas aeruginosa* [30,31]. The clinical presentation and response to treatment were consistent with the underlying infection, although treatment of the infection was supplemented with prednisolone.

9.5 Drug-induced lymphocytic interstitial pneumonitis

In patients with an unexplained interstitial pneumonitis, whether they be infected with HIV or not, it is always important to consider whether it is drug-induced. Phenytoin, for example, has been reported as a cause of LIP in a patient free of HIV [32], as well as in an HIV-infected patient (quoted in [4]).

9.6 Human T-cell leukaemia virus type I

Human T-cell leukaemia virus type 1 (HTLV-I), unlike HIV-1, is one of the tumour viruses and a member of the oncovirinae, which is one of the subfamilies of the retroviruses; it is associated with adult T-cell leukaemia/lymphoma. In this condition, the majority of patients suffer from pulmonary complications, which include leukaemic infiltration of the lung, interstitial fibrosis or infection with *P. carinii* [33]. However, most of those infected with HTLV-I are asymptomatic, in spite of it being a leukaemic virus. HTLV-I infection is also associated with two forms of chronic spastic paraparesis, namely tropical spastic paresis (H-TSP) and HTLV-I-associated myelopathy (H-AM). These disorders are found in equatorial regions and in Japan [33].

A bronchoalveolar lymphocytosis has been demonstrated by BAL in both H-TSP and H-AM [34,35]. The alveolitis in H-TSP is predominantly composed of CD8 and lymphocytes, while in H-AM both CD8 and CD4 cells are increased, leading to a normal CD4/CD8 ratio. The bronchoalveolar lymphocytosis reported in patients with H-TSP was not associated with any respiratory symptoms and the chest radiographs were normal [34]. This may also be the finding in H-AM, but in some patients the chest radiograph may show 'micronodular infiltrates' in the lower-lung fields, the transfer factor may be reduced and there may be mild hypoxaemia [35]. In H-AM patients, soluble interleukin-2 receptor (IL-2R) levels in BAL were significantly elevated and correlated with the number of CD4 cells in that fluid. The level was also nearly 13 times that found in serum. If production of IL-2R is accepted as an indicator of T-lymphocyte activation, these findings in BAL of H-AM patients suggest that lymphocytes are activated locally within the lung to produce IL-2R [35]. The bronchoalveolar lymphocytosis and elevated IL-2R levels are likely to be a reflection of the immunological response to a retrovirus infection of the lung.

References

1 Bienenstock J., Johnston N., Perey D.Y.E. Bronchial lymphoid tissue. I. Morphological characteristics. *Laboratory Investigation* 1973; **28**: 686–692.

2 Bienenstock J., Johnston N., Perey D.Y.E. Bronchial lymphoid tissue. II. Functional characteristics. *Laboratory Investigation* 1973; **28**: 693–698.

3 Richmond I., Pritchard G.E., Ashcroft T., Avery A., Corris P.A., Walters E.H. Bronchus associated lymphoid tissue (BALT) in human lung: its distribution in smokers and non-smokers. *Thorax* 1993; **48**: 1130–1134.

4 Travis W.D., Fox C.H., Devaney K.O. *et al.* Lymphoid pneumonitis in 50 adult patients infected with the human immunodeficiency virus: lymphocytic interstitial pneumonitis versus nonspecific interstitial pneumonitis. *Human Pathology* 1992; **23**: 529–541.

5 Solal-Celigny P., Couderc L.J., Herman D. *et al.* Lymphoid interstitial pneumonitis in acquired immunodeficiency syndrome-related complex. *American Review of Respiratory Disease* 1985; **131**: 956–960.

6 Griffiths M.H., Miller R.F., Semple S.J.G. Interstitial pneumonitis in patients infected with the human immunodeficiency virus. *Thorax* 1995; **50**: 1141–1146.

7 Itescu S., Brancato L.J., Buxbaum J. *et al*. A diffuse infiltrative CD8 lymphocytous syndrome in human immunodeficiency virus (HIV) infection: a host immune response associated with HLA-DR5. *Annals of Internal Medicine* 1990; **112**: 3–10.

8 Oldham S.A.A., Castillo M., Jacobson F.L., Mones J.M., Saldana M.J. HIV-associated lymphocytic interstitial pneumonia: radiologic manifestations and pathologic correlation. *Radiology* 1989; **170**: 83–87.

9 Lairmore M.D., Poulson J.M., Adducci T.A., DeMartini J.C. Lentivirus-induced lymphoproliferative disease: comparative pathogenicity of phenotypically distinct ovine lentivirus strains. *American Journal of Pathology* 1988; **130**: 80–90.

10 Ziza J.-M., Brun-Venet F., Venet A. *et al*. Lymphadenopathy-associated virus isolated from bronchoalveolar lavage fluid in AIDS-related complex with lymphoid interstitial pneumonitis. *New England Journal of Medicine* 1985; **313**: 183.

11 Resnick L., Pitchenik A.E., Fisher E., Croney R. Detection of HTLV-III/LAV-specific IgG and antigen in bronchoalveolar lavage fluid from two patients with lymphocytic interstitial pneumonitis associated with AIDS-related complex. *American Journal of Medicine* 1987; **82**: 553–556.

12 Ognibene F.P., Masur H., Rogers P. *et al*. Nonspecific interstitial pneumonitis without evidence of *Pneumocystis carinii* in asymptomatic patients infected with human immunodeficiency virus (HIV). *Annals of Internal Medicine* 1988; **109**: 874–879.

13 Suffredini A.F., Ognibene F.P., Lack E.E. *et al*. Nonspecific interstitial pneumonitis: a common cause of pulmonary disease in the acquired immunodeficiency syndrome. *Annals of Internal Medicine* 1987; **107**: 7–13.

14 Simmons J.T., Suffredini A.F., Lack E.E. *et al*. Nonspecific interstitial pneumonitis in patients with AIDS: radiologic features. *American Journal of Roentgenology* 1987; **149**: 265–268.

15 Carrington C.B., Liebow A.A. Lymphocytic interstitial pneumonia. *American Journal of Pathology* 1966; **48**: 36.

16 Liebow A.A., Carrington C.B. Diffuse pulmonary lymphoreticular infiltrations associated with dysproteinaemia. *Medical Clinics of North America* 1973; **57**: 809–843.

17 Julsrud P.R., Brown L.R., Li C.-Y., Rosenow E.C., Growe J.K. Pulmonary processes of mature appearing lymphocytes: pseudolymphoma, well-differentiated lymphocytic lymphoma, and lymphocytic interstitial pneumonitis. *Radiology* 1978; **127**: 289–316.

18 Banerjee D., Ahmad D. Malignant lymphoma lymphocytic interstitial pneumonia: a monoclonal B-cell neoplasm arising in a polyclonal lymphoproliferative disorder. *Human Pathology* 1982; **13**: 780–782.

19 Grieco M.H., Chinoy-Acharya P. Lymphocytic interstitial pneumonia associated with the acquired immune deficiency syndrome. *American Review of Respiratory Disease* 1985; **131**: 952–955.

20 Morris J.C., Rosen M.J., Marchevsky A., Teirstein A.S. Lymphocytic interstitial pneumonia in patients at risk for the acquired immune deficiency syndrome. *Chest* 1987; **91**: 63–67.

21 Lin R.Y., Gruber P.J., Saunders R., Perla E.N. Lymphocytic interstitial pneumonitis in adult HIV infection. *New York State Journal of Medicine* 1988; **88**: 273–276.

22 Bach M.C. Zidovudine for lymphocytic interstitial pneumonia associated with AIDS. *Lancet* 1987; **ii**: 796–797.

23 Helbert M., Stoneham C., Mitchell B., Pinching A.J. Zidovudine for lymphocytic interstitial pneumonitis in AIDS. *Lancet* 1987; **ii**: 1333.

24 Couderc L.-J., D'Agay M.-F., Danon F., Harzic M., Brocheriou C., Clauvel J.-P. Sicca complex and infection with human immunodeficiency virus. *Archives of Internal Medicine* 1987; **147**: 898–901.

25 Youssem S.A., Colby T.V., Carrington C.B. Follicular bronchitis/bronchiolitis. *Human Pathology* 1985; **16**: 700–706.

26 Ettensohn D.B., Mayer K.H., Kessimian N., Smith P.S. Lymphocytic bronchiolitis associated with HIV infection. *Chest* 1988; **93**: 201–202.

27 Epler G.R., Colby T.V., McLoud T.C., Carrington C.B., Gaensler E.A. Bronchiolitis obliterans organizing pneumonia. *New England Journal of Medicine* 1985; **312**: 152–158.

28 Allen J.N., Wewers M.D. HIV-associated bronchiolitis obliterans organizing pneumonia. *Chest* 1989; **96**: 197–198.

29 Sanito N.J., Morley T.F., Condoluci D.V. Bronchiolitis obliterans organising pneumonia in an AIDS patient. *European Respiratory Journal* 1995; **8**: 1021–1024.

30 Miller R.F., Pugsley W.B., Griffiths M.H. Open lung biopsy for investigation of acute respiratory episodes in patients with HIV infection and AIDS. *Genitourinary Medicine* 1995; **71**: 280–285.

31 Foley N.M., Griffiths M.H., Miller R.F. Histologically atypical *Pneumocystis carinii* pneumonia. *Thorax* 1993; **48**: 996–1001.

32 Chamberlain D.W., Hyland R.H., Ross D.J. Diphenylhydantoin-induced lymphocytic interstitial pneumonia. *Chest* 1986; **90**: 458–460.

33 Semenzato G., Agostini C. Human retroviruses and lung involvement. *American Review of Respiratory Disease* 1989; **139**: 1317–1322.

34 Conderc L.J., Caubarrere I., Venet A. *et al*. Bronchoalveolar lymphocytosis in patients with tropical spastic paraparesis associated with human T-cell lymphotropic virus type 1 (HTLV-1). *Annals of Internal Medicine* 1988; **109**: 625–628.

35 Sugimoto M., Nakashima H., Matsumoto M., Uyama E., Ando M., Araki S. Pulmonary involvement in patients with HTLV-1-associated myelopathy: increased soluble IL-2 receptors in bronchoalveolar lavage fluid. *American Review of Respiratory Disease* 1989; **139**: 1329–1335.

10 Pulmonary complications of HIV/AIDS in children

R. DINWIDDIE & V. NOVELLI

10.0 Introduction

Pulmonary complications are the most frequent manifestation of HIV/AIDS infection in children [1]. They frequently present as the first indication of HIV infection, which must now be suspected in all children who have pulmonary symptoms of an unusual aetiology or severity, especially in the first 6 months of life. A wide variety of infections occur, although *Pneumocystis carinii* pneumonia (PCP) is the major initial cause of morbidity and mortality in these children [2,3]. Virtually any other respiratory pathogen can also occur and lead to acute or chronic respiratory symptoms. Other non-infectious processes associated with HIV may also occur in older children and lead to chronic respiratory problems. In general, a small number of patients will die acutely from relentlessly progressive lung infection or its complications. Other children (the majority) will have chronic long-term disease, which leads to persistent parenchymal damage of the lung over a number of years; this is associated with increasing symptoms, such as exercise limitation, persistent cough, wheeze and sputum production, and ultimately leads to chronic respiratory failure. Despite the relatively poor prognosis, a wide variety of treatments are available to support these children throughout an illness which may last for many years [4].

Respiratory-tract infections are extremely common, even in normal children. Their response to these infections is dependent on a complex number of factors. These include the natural protection provided by maternal immunoglobulins and the normal maturation of the immune system, particularly during the first year of life. In the immunocompromised infant, these infections are much more likely to be severe and to cause long-term problems. Opportunistic lung infections are very common in this age group.

10.1 Epidemiology of HIV/AIDS in children worldwide and in the UK

10.1.1 Transmission to children—importance of vertical route

The epidemiology of HIV/AIDS in children varies considerably worldwide and also in the UK [5]. By the mid-1990s, the World Health Organization (WHO) has estimated that, worldwide, up to 3 million children may be infected with HIV, mostly in developing countries. In the UK, by late 1995, a cumulative total of 647 children had been reported with HIV infection; 232 had developed AIDS, of which 124 had died [6]. Vertical transmission (mother to child) of HIV, which may occur before, during or after delivery, is the major mode of acquisition in children. A proportion of patients acquire disease via contaminated blood or blood products; however, since screening of these products began in 1985, transmission via this route has virtually disappeared in most developed countries, including the UK. Direct transmission may also occur through sexual abuse, sexual activity and/or needle sharing in adolescents.

Among reported paediatric AIDS cases in the UK, some 80% of children have been infected through vertical transmission [6]. It may be difficult initially to prove infection in the child because of passively transferred maternal antibody, which can persist for many months after birth. The polymerase chain reaction (PCR) has now become the investigation of choice for confirmation of HIV status in infants [7]. It is estimated that about 14% of infants born to seropositive mothers are truly infected [8]. Vertical transmission is more likely if one infant in the family is already infected and also if the maternal CD4 count is particularly low. The most likely time of vertical transmission is during the intrapartum period [9]. Recent studies from the AIDS Clinical Trials Group 076 have shown that the use of zidovudine (azidothymidine — AZT) during pregnancy and birth and in the neonatal period can reduce vertical transmission by as much as two-thirds [10]. Caesarean section can also be a factor in reducing perinatal transmission of virus [11], although this is controversial. Breast-feeding may also be an important route of vertical transmission from mother to infant [12]. It is thought to increase the risk of perinatal transmission by as much as 14%, i.e. doubling the risk [13,14]. Despite vertically acquired HIV infection, more than 50% of children survive to 9 years of age [15].

10.2 Pulmonary complications of HIV/AIDS in children

The pulmonary complications of HIV/AIDS infection in children are extremely variable [2]. Some 60–80% will develop pulmonary disease, and in nearly half of them the pulmonary problem is the presenting feature. Infectious causes predominate, especially *P. carinii* and bacterial infections, although a wide variety of other pathogenic organisms, including viruses, such as cytomegalovirus (CMV), respiratory syncytial virus (RSV), herpes, influenza, parainfluenza and adenovirus, are not uncommon. Mycobacteria are also not infrequent. Fungal infection due to *Candida albicans* and *Aspergillus* is also well documented. Another frequent complication is the development of pulmonary lymphoid hyperplasia/lymphoid interstitial pneumonitis (PLH/LIP) [2]. Less frequently, malignant disease, with either Kaposi's sarcoma or pulmonary lymphoma, is also seen.

The immunological mechanisms for the susceptibility to lung disease are extremely complex and essentially multifactorial. Following initial HIV infection, considerable viral replication is thought to occur in the lymphoid tissue [1]. Eventually the major cell-mediated defect is shown in the reduction of CD4 lymphocytes, which, through lack of help provided to B cells, leads to an inability to deal with common pathogens. Despite the presence of a generalized hypergammaglobulinaemia, there is an inadequate specific antibody production in these patients [16]. Eventually, infected cells enter the lung, where alveolar macrophages become involved as well [17]. As HIV infection progresses, the function of the alveolar macrophages decreases. Tumour necrosis factor alpha (TNF-α) is also released by these cells, particularly during acute infections, and leads to facilitation of further HIV spread in the lungs. This in turn leads to alteration in function of other immunocompetent effector cells in the lung, as well as a progressive loss of pulmonary CD4 cells, resulting in infectious and non-infectious pulmonary complications.

Children in general and infants in particular are especially prone to upper and lower respiratory-tract infection, through which a great amount of natural immunity and immune memory of common organisms is acquired. In addition, at this age the immune system itself is immature, even in healthy individuals. The normal exposure to a wide variety of common organisms of all types is important for the development of natural immunity in this age group. The HIV-infected individual is much less able to cope with this major immune challenge in early life [18,19].

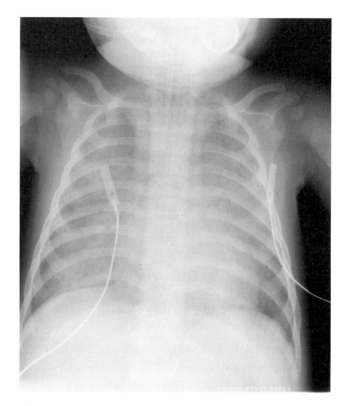

Fig. 10.1 Chest X-ray showing *Pneumocystis carinii* pneumonia (PCP) in an AIDS-affected infant.

Not only are these children prone to serious infection with common pathogens but they are highly susceptible to a variety of opportunistic organisms as well.

10.2.1 *Pneumocystis carinii* infection

PCP is the most common AIDS indicator disease in children with HIV, occurring in as many as 65% of patients during the first year of life. It is also responsible for as many as 82% of infant deaths [20]. By the age of 6, some 16% of children born to HIV-infected mothers will have developed significant *P. carinii* infection [21].

Affected patients present with tachypnoea, fever, dry cough, increasing exercise limitation and eventually cyanosis. The chest X-ray shows diffuse hazy shadowing bilaterally, which is commonly perihilar in the initial period (Fig. 10.1). The patient is hypoxaemic, with low levels of oxygen saturation and a normal or low carbon dioxide in the early phase. As respiratory failure progresses, respiratory difficulty increases. Auscultation of the chest reveals either no added sounds or fine bilateral crackles.

Diagnosis can now be made in as many as two-thirds of cases by immunofluorescence of nasopharyngeal secretions [20]. In those where this does not produce a definitive diagnosis, bronchoalveolar lavage (BAL) may be indicated if there is no response to empirical treatment with trimethoprim–sulphamethoxazole (TMP–SMX). In those patients who deteriorate rapidly and need ventilation from the outset, a BAL is performed immediately, along with the commencement of empiric therapy. Lung biopsy, either transbronchoscopic or open, is occasionally required if a definitive diagnosis cannot be made by the methods described and when other pulmonary pathology must be excluded.

The illness can be confused with bronchiolitis, especially during the epidemic season. PCP must now be considered in the differential diagnosis of all infants with persistent RSV-negative lower respiratory-tract infection [22,23]. Other differential diagnoses to be considered are pneumonitis due to viral agents (e.g. CMV, measles, Epstein–Barr virus (EBV)) or LIP.

Treatment consists of high-dose TMP-SMX (trimethoprim 20 mg/kg/day and sulphamethoxazole 100 mg/kg/day) for 21 days. If the patient fails to respond within 4–5 days, further confirmation of the diagnosis should be sought and therapy changed to pentamidine 4 mg/kg/day by slow intravenous infusion. This agent, however, is associated with a significant number of side-effects, including hypoglycaemia, hypotension and hepatic and renal toxicity, in as many as 50% of cases. Corticosteroids given as methylprednisolone 1 mg/kg 12-hourly contribute to a significant reduction in mortality in these children [24]. It is the author's practice to administer steroids to all patients with definite and documented PCP. The administration of pulmonary surfactant has also been used successfully in this condition [25]. The mortality rate for children with PCP is very high—between 50 and 80%—especially in infancy [26].

Prophylaxis against *Pneumocystis* is important for all potentially affected children. It should be given as co-trimoxazole 3 days per week to all infants of HIV-positive mothers from 4 weeks of age until the infection status is clearly known. It should also be given to all of those who have had an episode of proven infection in the past, and in those patients with an AIDS diagnosis or low age-related CD4 counts or CD4 percentages of total lymphocyte counts [27].

10.2.2 Viral infections

A number of viruses can cause significant lung disease in AIDS patients (Table 10.1). The common respiratory viruses will be seen at the same time as in non-affected children [28]. RSV, especially seen in the first year of life, does not usually cause more severe infection than in normal infants. Parainfluenza and influenza viruses are also seen in this age group

Table 10.1 Organisms causing respiratory infection in AIDS-affected children.

Pneumocystis carinii
Cytomegalovirus (CMV)
Respiratory syncytial virus (RSV)
Adenovirus
Measles
Epstein–Barr virus (EBV)
Varicella-zoster virus (VZV)
Mycobacterium tuberculosis
Mycobacterium avium intracellulare (MAI)
Streptococcus pneumoniae
Salmonella
Haemophilus influenzae
Enterococcus
Candida albicans
Aspergillus fumigatus

but do not often cause serious infection. Adenovirus has been associated with several fatal causes of disseminated disease and pneumonitis. CMV may be pathogenic in some patients and can cause a diffuse interstitial pneumonitis. In many children, concomitant infections due to *P. carinii* and other bacterial pathogens are present. However, patients often respond to treatment for PCP or bacterial pneumonia alone [29]. Diagnosis can be made either on pharyngeal aspirate or by BAL. The techniques of immunofluorescence, viral culture buffy-coat analysis, detection of early antigen by focus fluorescence (DEAFF) and urine culture for CMV may be helpful. The chest X-ray may show diffuse interstitial changes, but this is often on the background of chronic bilateral shadowing in the lungs due to LIP. This makes the interpretation of the X-ray difficult in determining acute change during intercurrent illness.

Specific antiviral agents should be used in those with severe disease. Ribavirin may be indicated for infants with RSV infection who develop significant respiratory failure. Ganciclovir is indicated for CMV disease, especially if there is multiorgan involvement. The use of steroids for the treatment of *Pneumocystis* infection can reactivate CMV in some susceptible individuals. Myelosuppression is the principal dose-limiting toxicity of ganciclovir.

Other viruses which can produce severe pneumonitis in these children include varicella zoster, which should be treated with intravenous aciclovir. Measles can also cause a severe and often fatal (giant-cell) pneumonia, which can be prevented by the use of measles vaccine. This should be given to all HIV-positive children.

10.2.3 Bacterial infections

Bacterial infection of the upper and lower respiratory tract is a very common problem in HIV- and AIDS-affected children, and is a consequence of B-cell dysfunction, mainly due to the immune dysregulation that occurs following CD4 and T-cell depletion [30]. Although activated, the B cells tend to respond poorly both to T-cell-dependent and T-cell-independent antigens. In some children, there is also evidence of immunoglobulin G_2 (IgG_2) subclass deficiency, further contributing to the likelihood of infection with encapsulated organisms [31].

Various studies have reported incidences of serious bacterial infection in HIV-infected children, ranging from 24 to 37% [32,33]. Acute pneumonia tends to be the most common clinically diagnosed entity [33]. Aetiological agents tend to be the encapsulated organisms, such as *Streptococcus pneumoniae* and *Haemophilus influenzae*. Less common organisms, such as *Salmonella*, Enterococcus and *Pseudomonas*, are also seen [1]. Although clinical signs of infection, including fever, tachypnoea, cough and sputum production, may be obvious, specific diagnosis can be difficult. Many patients have chronic long-standing changes, including those of LIP, on the chest X-ray, so that acute changes can be masked. A blood culture should be obtained and serum tested for the presence of antigens of *Pneumococcus* or *Haemophilus*. If these tests and a sputum culture fail to reveal a causative organism and if there is not a fairly rapid response to broad-spectrum antibiotic therapy, more invasive investigations, such as BAL, are indicated. A search should be made not only for common bacteria but also for mycobacteria, viruses, fungi and *Pneumocystis*.

Treatment is usually initiated with a third-generation cephalosporin, intravenously, in those patients requiring admission to hospital. This can be changed to an oral formulation, once there is a clinical response, to complete a 10-day course. Vaccination with *H. influenzae* type b (Hib) vaccine and also pneumococcal vaccine (Pneumovax) (>24 months) is an important prevention strategy. There is also evidence that daily co-trimoxazole (TMP–SMX) (for PCP prophylaxis) has a role in the prevention of recurrent bacterial infections in HIV-infected children. Regular infusions with intravenous immunoglobulins are usually only considered in those patients not able to take co-trimoxazole (TMP–SMX) [32].

Mycobacteria

Mycobacterial infection is a problem of increasing prevalence among HIV-positive children. *Mycobacterium tuberculosis* is also increasing generally in the child population worldwide and the HIV epidemic is thought to have contributed to some of this increase in recent years.

The infection is usually primary in type and is often acquired from parents who are themselves HIV-positive [34]. Diagnosis depends on culturing the organism from gastric washings or via BAL. A Mantoux test should be used, but may not always be positive, because of reduced cell-mediated immunity. A strong positive reaction >5 mm is probably indicative of active tuberculosis (TB) [35]. The typical chest-radiograph appearances may not be seen, due to overlying LIP.

Treatment consists of standard triple therapy — isoniazid, pyrazinamide and rifampicin — for 2 months, followed by rifampicin and isoniazid for up to 1 year. Success rates with this regime are high if compliance with treatment is maintained [36]. Quadruple therapy, with the addition of either streptomycin or ethambutol, is necessary in some cases where there is a high risk of drug resistance.

Bacillus Calmette–Guérin (BCG) vaccination should be given at birth to all infants, including those at risk of vertical HIV transmission, in areas of high prevalence. The risk of BCGosis in these infants appears to be extremely low. It must be remembered that HIV-infected adults with TB serve as potential reservoirs for TB infection for all children.

Atypical mycobacteria

Mycobacterium avium intracellulare (MAI) is another organism which not uncommonly infects HIV-positive children, being responsible for an AIDS diagnosis in about 4% of them. It is particularly seen in children with transfusion-acquired HIV infection and in those with low CD4 counts of less than 100 cells/mm3 [37]. Patients usually present with generalized systemic symptoms, increasing respiratory difficulty and diffuse bilateral shadowing on chest X-ray. The organism may be cultured directly from sputum and is also not infrequently grown from cultures of blood or bone marrow. BAL fluid should also be examined for this organism routinely. Treatment consists of the administration of a combination of three of more antibiotics with activity against the atypical mycobacteria group, i.e. clarithromycin, rifabutin, ciprofloxacin, ethambutol, clofazimine or amikacin.

10.2.4 Fungal infections

The most common infection in HIV/AIDS patients is oral/pharyngeal candidiasis. This is one of the classic presenting features of the illness and frequently causes persistent symptoms which can be difficult to eradicate. It is also a cause of pneumonia in these children [38]. Intrapulmonary candidiasis can be difficult to diagnose, especially in the presence of other chronic disease, such as LIP. Unless the patient is intubated, there may be contamination of specimens by upper-airway organisms. BAL is usually necessary to confirm the diagnosis. *Aspergillus* can also affect these patients, with localized or generalized intrapulmonary spread and a significant risk of disseminated systemic disease as well [39]. *Aspergillus* can cause widespread invasive damage to the lungs, including the formation of aspergillomatous fungal balls. Outside the UK, other fungi causing pulmonary problems include *Histoplasma capsulatum*, coccidioidomycosis and *Cryptococcus neoformans*.

Oral candidiasis is treated with nystatin or fluconazole. Treatment of pulmonary candidiasis is with one of the following antifungals: amphotericin, liposomal amphotericin or fluconazole. The treatment of choice for pulmonary aspergillosis is probably liposomal amphotericin; however, itraconazole is also often used.

10.2.5 Lymphoid interstitial pneumonitis

This condition, which is not usually seen until the second year of life, is a common complication of perinatally acquired HIV disease, occurring in 15% of children [40]. Although it is not now considered an AIDS-defining diagnosis, it used to rank as the second most common AIDS-indicator disease, affecting some 27% of paediatric cases reported to the Centers for Disease Control (CDC) [41]. It is rare in children with transfusion-associated HIV disease, in HIV-infected haemophiliacs and in adults with HIV infection. There is a spectrum of disease, ranging from classic LIP, which comprises a diffuse pulmonary interstitial infiltration with B lymphocytes (CD8 lymphocytes are also described), which do not cause major destruction of underlying lung structure, to PLH, which is a focal lymphocytic infiltration of the lung parenchyma and peribronchial areas. In many cases, there is overlap between LIP and PLH and hence the condition is often termed LIP/PLH. LIP/PLH is often seen in association with enlargement of lymphoid tissue elsewhere, especially the tonsils and adenoids, which can lead to significant upper-airway obstruction, sleep apnoea and even cor pulmonale. There may also be associated parotid-gland enlargement, hepatosplenomegaly and hypergammaglobulinaemia [42]. There is evidence that some patients may progress from LIP/PLH to a lymphoproliferative syndrome which is termed polyclonal, polymorphic B-cell lymphoproliferative disorder (PBLD) and considered intermediate between a benign and full-fledged malignant lymphoproliferation [42]. The pathogenesis of LIP/PLH may represent an atypical response to an inhaled or circulating antigen by a dysregulated immune system as a consequence of HIV infection. The role of Epstein–Barr virus (EBV) is not yet clear but it probably plays a significant part in the aetiology of this condition, since its presence can be documented in as many as 80% of cases [43,44].

The natural history of the disease is variable, ranging from spontan-

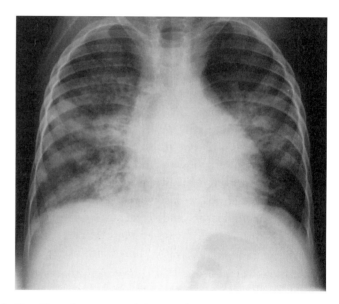

Fig. 10.2 Chest X-ray showing typical changes of lymphoid interstitial pneumonitis (LIP) in an HIV-infected child.

eous resolution to slowly progressive pulmonary disease that can result in respiratory failure. Typically, the condition presents with chronic cough and often with increasing breathlessness, especially on exercise. Eventually, there is evidence of more persistent chronic respiratory symptoms and finger clubbing. The chest X-ray shows diffuse bilateral reticulonodular infiltrates in the pulmonary interstitium, often much more severe in appearance than the degree of respiratory symptoms would suggest (Fig. 10.2). With disease progression, nodules increase in size and there is widening of the hilum and superior mediastinum. Ultimately, over a period of several years, bronchiectasis, pulmonary hypertension and cor pulmonale can develop. Throughout this period, there may be superadded bacterial or viral infections, causing exacerbation of pulmonary disease, with acute deterioration. It is our experience that this is one of the most common reasons for hospital admission in our paediatric HIV/AIDS population.

A presumptive diagnosis of LIP can usually be made clinically and by persistent chest X-ray findings lasting more than 2 months, not responding to antibiotics and without other documented cause. Miliary TB, with which LIP has often been confused, needs to be excluded, as does PCP. A lung biopsy is not usually performed, although, in some cases, where there is doubt about the diagnosis, BAL has been used to exclude an opportunistic infection.

A baseline chest X-ray is mandatory for each newly diagnosed HIV-infected child; subsequently, yearly chest X-rays are recommended to detect the early onset of LIP.

Treatment, if required, consists mainly of supportive therapy (oxygen, bronchodilators and physiotherapy). Broad-spectrum antibiotics, such as a third-generation cephalosporin, are given for any presumed associated bacterial superinfection. However, it is unusual to isolate a causative bacterial agent from the blood or respiratory secretions in these patients. Anecdotal reports also suggest that the use of oral steroids may be beneficial for severe cases [45]. Prednisolone, in a dose of 2 mg/kg/day for 4–6 weeks, is given, then reduced to an alternate-day regimen, if possible, and then stopped. Inhaled steroids are also widely used but have not been formally assessed. Bronchodilators and oxygen are given when necessary. The use of zidovudine is under investigation. The long-term prognosis is not yet known, but slowly deteriorating lung function, over several years in some patients, is the usual course. Diuretics may be required in the terminal phase of the illness. All patients with LIP/PLH should be immunized with the Hib and pneumococcal vaccines, as well as receiving, yearly, the current recommended influenza vaccine.

10.2.6 Kaposi's sarcoma and lymphoma

Kaposi's sarcoma is a complication of AIDS more commonly seen in adults but found in less than 1% of children with AIDS [46]. The putative agent is thought to be a new herpesvirus, named Kaposi's sarcoma herpesvirus (KSHV) or human herpesvirus 8 (HHV-8), which induces the proliferation of endothelial cells associated with Kaposi's sarcoma [47]. Presentation in children is often with marked lymphadenopathy and the appearance of purplish skin nodules and cutaneous plaques [48]. Respiratory symptoms and signs, such as a persistent cough, breathlessness, haemoptysis and blood-stained pleural effusions, may develop in these patients, consequent to visceral dissemination and lung involvement [49]. The chest X-ray shows interstitial shadowing and nodular infiltrates. Specific diagnosis is made by lung biopsy, although endobronchial lesions may be diagnosed at bronchoscopy. Treatment for lymphadenopathic, visceral and lung disease is with liposomal daunorubicin. Prognosis tends to be poor.

Lymphomas affecting the lungs are extremely rare. They can occur as part of a disseminated lymphoma, usually non-Hodgkin's lymphoma (NHL) (e.g. Burkitt's lymphoma) [50], or develop in the presence of other lung processes. As mentioned previously, a progressive B-cell lymphoproliferative disease (PBLD), induced by EBV, has been described in children with LIP/PLH. This may represent a progression of LIP/PLH or it may

Table 10.2 Investigations and management of acute respiratory exacerbations.

Investigation
Measure respiratory rate, temperature, oxygen saturation spirometry (if age >5 years)
Full blood count, CD4 count

Culture sputum for bacteria and microscopy/culture for mycobacteria
Evaluate respiratory secretions by immunofluorescence for PCP, RSV, influenza,
  parainfluenza, adenovirus (measles if clinically indicated)
Culture for CMV, buffy-coat analysis

Review chest X-ray
  Generalized reticular shadowing—may be LIP but secondary infection may be occult
  Focal shadowing—bacterial, fungal or mycobacterial infection
  Generalized granular shadowing in both lung fields—consider PCP or CMV

Bronchoalveolar lavage—bronchoscopic or non-bronchoscopic
  Directed to detection of PCP, CMV, mycobacteria, fungi or infection with more than one
  organism

Lung biopsy required if no response to standard treatment for infections mentioned above

Treatment
Broad-spectrum antibiotics, oral or intravenous, to cover common bacterial pathogens

Intravenous TMP/SMX if clinical suspicion of PCP
Use pentamidine after further confirmation, e.g. BAL, of PCP if no response within 4–5
  days

Ganciclovir for CMV if infection confirmed

Treat mycobacterial infection specifically if present

Underlying LIP may need treatment with oral steroids if CMV and TB are excluded

Continue long-term TMP/SMX prophylaxis for PCP 3 days per week after recovery from
  acute illness

PCP, *Pneumocystis carinii* pneumonia; RSV, respiratory syncytial virus; CMV,
cytomegalovirus; LIP, lymphoid interstitial pneumonitis; TMP, trimethoprim;
SMX, sulphamethoxazole; BAL, bronchoalveolar lavage; TB, tuberculosis.

arise *de novo* [42]. The possibility, then, is of further progression to the
development of a polyclonal or monoclonal malignant lymphoma.

10.3 Investigation and treatment of the HIV/AIDS child with acute pulmonary disease

A plan of investigation and treatment for the AIDS-positive child presenting with an acute exacerbation is set out in Table 10.2.

10.4 Conclusions

The emergence of HIV/AIDS as a serious infection in the paediatric age
group has presented a major challenge to those involved in the diagnosis

and care of affected children. A wide spectrum of disease is seen. Increasingly nowadays, initial presentation is in the young infant affected by vertical transmission from his or her HIV-infected mother. There has to be a high index of suspicion of the diagnosis in this age group, especially when the young child presents with persistent respiratory infection in the first few months of life. In this setting, PCP is most likely to be the underlying pathogen and specific measures should be taken for its diagnosis and treatment.

In the older child chronic lung disease is likely to supervene. This often consists of underlying LIP, with recurrent lower respiratory-tract infection causing exacerbations of underlying symptoms. Again, it is important to be constantly vigilant in the search for opportunistic pathogens, which may not be easy to identify unless a specific search is made for them.

Upper-airway obstruction due to hyperplasia of the adenotonsillar lymphoid tissue can lead to a major degree of sleep apnoea. This should be treated conventionally by adenotonsillectomy when clinically indicated.

Long-term treatment, including physiotherapy, to clear retained lung secretions and prevent or slow down the onset of chronic lung damage, including bronchiectasis, is important in those with persistent symptoms. Common respiratory conditions, including asthma, also occur in these children and should be treated in the normal way.

Effective therapy in this group of children can prolong life expectancy and greatly improve quality of life for increasing periods of time in this important group of patients.

References

1 Bye M.R. Human immunodeficiency virus infections and the respiratory system in children. *Pediatric Pulmonology* 1995; **19**: 231–242.

2 Marolda J., Pace B., Bonforte R.J., Kotin N.M., Rabinowitz J., Kattan M. Pulmonary manifestations of HIV infection in children. *Pediatric Pulmonology* 1991; **10**: 231–235.

3 Newell M.L., Peckham C., Dunn D., Ades T., Giaquinto C. ECS: natural history of vertically acquired HIV infection. *Pediatrics* 1994; **94**: 815–819.

4 Jones P. HIV in childhood. *British Medical Journal* 1994; **308**: 425–426.

5 Sotomayor J.L., Douglas S.D., Wilmott R.W. Pulmonary manifestations of immune deficiency disease. *Paediatric Pulmonology* 1989; **6**: 275–290.

6 CDSC. AIDS and HIV infection in the UK: monthly report. *Communicable Disease Report* 1996; **6**: 25–28.

7 Rogers M.F., Ou C.Y., Rayfield M. Use of the polymerase chain reaction for early detection of the proviral sequence of the human immunodeficiency virus in infants born to seropositive mothers. *New England Journal of Medicine* 1989; **320**: 1649–1654.

8 European Collaborative Study. Risk factors for mother to child transmission of HIV-1. *Lancet* 1992; **339**: 1007–1012.

9 Gabiano C., Tovo P.A., de Martino M. *et al.* Mother to children transmission of human immunodeficiency virus type 1: risk of infection and correlates of transmission. *Pediatrics* 1992; **90**: 369–374.

10 Connor E.M., Spercing R.S., Gelber R. *et al.* Pediatric AIDS Clinical Trials Group Proto-

col 076: study group reduction of maternal–infant transmission of human immunodeficiency virus type 1 with zidovudine treatment. *New England Journal of Medicine* 1994; 331: 1173–1180.

11 European Collaborative Study. Caesarean section and risk of vertical transmission of HIV1 infection. *Lancet* 1994; 343: 1464–1467.

12 Rubini N.H., Passman L.J. Transmission of human immunodeficiency virus infection from a newly infected mother to her two year old child by breast feeding. *Pediatric Infectious Disease Journal* 1992; 11: 682–683.

13 Dunn D.T., Newell M.L., Ades E.D., Peckham C.S. Risk of human immunodeficiency virus type 1 transmission through breast feeding. *Lancet* 1992; 340: 585–588.

14 Ziegler J.B. Breast feeding and HIV. *Lancet* 1993; 342: 1437–1438.

15 Turner B.J., Denison M., Eppes S.C., Houchens R., Fanning T., Markson L.E. Survival experience of 789 children with acquired immune deficiency syndrome. *Pediatric Infectious Disease Journal* 1993; 6: 310–320.

16 Bernstein L.J., Ochsh D., Wedgwood R.J., Rubenstein A. Defective humoral immunity in pediatric acquired immune deficiency syndrome. *Journal of Pediatrics* 1985; 107: 352–356.

17 Garner S., Markovits P., Markovits D.M., Kaplan M.H., Gallo R.C., Popovic M. The role of mononuclear phagocytes in HIV infection. *Science* 1988; 232: 215–219.

18 Wilfert C., Wilson C., Luzuriaga K., Epstein L. Pathogenesis of pediatric human immunodeficiency virus type 1 infection. *Journal of Infectious Disease* 1994; 170: 286–292.

19 Peters M.J., Klein N.J., Gibb D.M. HIV related lung disorders in infants and children, including lymphocytic interstitial pneumonitis. *European Respiratory Monograph* 1995; 2: 362–384.

20 Gibb D.M., Davison C.F., Holland F.J., Walters S., Novelli V., Mok J. *Pneumocystis carinii* pneumonia in vertically acquired HIV infection in the British Isles. *Archives of Disease in Childhood* 1994; 70: 241–244.

21 European Collaborative Study. CD4 cell count as predictor of *Pneumocystis carinii* pneumonia in children born to mothers infected with HIV. *British Medical Journal* 1994; 308: 437–440.

22 Tasker R.C., Wilkinson K., Slater T.J., Novelli V. Unsuspected *Pneumocystis carinii* pneumonia and vertically acquired HIV infection in infants requiring intensive care. *British Medical Journal* 1994; 308: 462–463.

23 Evans J.A., Marriage S.C., Walters M.D.S., Levin M. Unsuspected HIV infection presenting in the first year of life. *British Medical Journal* 1995; 310: 1235–1236.

24 Bye M.R., Cairns-Bazarian A.M., Ewig J.M. Markedly reduced mortality associated with corticosteroid therapy of PCP in children with AIDS. *Archives of Pediatric and Adolescent Medicine* 1994; 148: 638–641.

25 Slater A.J., Nichani S.H., Macrae D., Wilkinson K.A., Novelli V., Tasker R.C. Surfactant adjunctive therapy for *Pneumocystis carinii* pneumonitis in an infant with acute lymphoblastic leukaemia. *Intensive Care Medicine* 1995; 21: 261–263.

26 Bye M.R., Bernstein L.J., Glaser J., Klein D. *Pneumocystis carinii* pneumonia in young children with AIDS. *Pediatric Pulmonology* 1990; 9: 251–253.

27 Centers for Disease Control. Revised CDC guidelines for prophylaxis against *Pneumocystis carinii* pneumonia for children infected with HIV. *Mortality and Morbidity Weekly Report* 1995; 44: RR-4.

28 Hague R.A., Burns S.E., Hargreaves F.D., Mok J.Y.Q., Yap P.L. Virus infections of the respiratory tract in HIV-infected children. *Journal of Infection* 1992; 24: 31–36.

29 Jue S., Whitley R.J. Herpesvirus infections in children with HIV. In: Pizzo P.A., Wilfert C.M., eds. *Pediatric AIDS: The Challenge of HIV Infection in Infants, Children and Adolescents*, 2nd edn. Baltimore: Williams & Wilkins, 1994; 345–364.

30 Bernstein L.J., Kriegen B.Z., Novick B., Sicklick M.J., Rubinstein A. Bacterial infection in the acquired immunodeficiency syndrome of children. *Pediatric Infectious Disease Journal* 1985; 4: 472–475.

31 Church J.A., Lewis J., Spotkov J.M. IgG subclass deficiencies in children with suspected AIDS. *Lancet* 1984; i: 279.

32 Spector S.A., Gelber R.D., McGrath N., Pediatric AIDS Study Group. A controlled trial of IVIG for the prevention of serious bacterial infection in children receiving zidovudine for advanced human immunodeficiency virus infection. *New England Journal of Medicine* 1994; **331**: 1181–1187.

33 Krasinski K., Borkowsky W., Bonk S., Lawrence R., Chandwani S. Bacterial infections in human immunodeficiency virus-infected children. *Pediatric Infectious Disease Journal* 1988; **7**: 323–328.

34 Bakshi S.S., Alvarez D., Hilfer C.L. *et al*. Tuberculosis in HIV infected children: a family infection. *American Journal of Disease in Children* 1993; **147**: 320–324.

35 Committee on Infectious Diseases 1993–1994. Screening for tuberculosis in infants and children. *Pediatrics* 1994; **93**: 131–134.

36 Ackah A., Coulibaly D., Higben H. *et al*. Response to treatment, mortality and CD4 lymphocyte counts in HIV-infected persons with tuberculosis in Abidjan, Côte d'Ivoire. *Lancet* 1995; **345**: 607–610.

37 Rutstein R.M., Cobb P., McGowan K.L. *et al. Mycobacterium avium-intracellulare* complex in HIV-infected children. *AIDS* 1993; **7**: 507–512.

38 Vernon D.D., Holzman B.H., Lewis P., Scott G.B., Pirriel J.A., Scott M.B. Respiratory failure in children with acquired immune deficiency syndrome and acquired immune deficiency syndrome complex. *Pediatrics* 1988; **82**: 223–228.

39 Peravez N.K., Kleinerman J., Kattan M. *et al*. Pseudomembranous necrotising bronchiolitis in a patient with haemophilia and acquired immune deficiency syndrome. *American Review of Respiratory Diseases* 1985; **131**: 961–963.

40 Thomas P., Singh T., Williams R. *et al*. Trends in survival for children reported with maternally transmitted acquired immunodeficiency syndrome in New York City, 1982 to 1989. *Pediatric Infectious Disease Journal* 1992; **11**: 34–39.

41 Caldwell M.B., Rogers M.F. Epidemiology of HIV. *Pediatric Clinics of North America* 1991; **38**: 1–16.

42 Joshi V.V., Kauffman S., Oleske J.H. *et al*. Polyclonal polymorphic B-cell lymphoproliferative disorder with prominent pulmonary involvement in children with acquired immune deficiency syndrome. *Lancet* 1987; **59**: 1455–1462.

43 Andiman W.A., Eastman R., Martin K. *et al*. Opportunistic lymphoproliferations associated with Epstein–Barr viral DNA in infants and children with AIDS. *Lancet* 1985; ii: 1390–1393.

44 Katz B.Z., Berkman A.B., Shapiro E.D. Serological evidence of active Epstein–Barr virus infection in Epstein–Barr virus associated lymphoproliferative disorders of children with acquired immunodeficiency syndrome. *Journal of Pediatrics* 1991; **120**: 228–232.

45 Rubinstein A., Berstein L., Charytan M., Krieger B.Z., Ziprkowski M. Corticosteroid treatment for pulmonary lymphoid hyperplasia in children with the acquired immune deficiency syndrome. *Pediatric Pulmonology* 1993; **4**: 13–17.

46 Peterman T.A., Jaffe H.W., Beral V. Epidemiological clues to the etiology of Kaposi's sarcoma. *AIDS* 1993; **8**: 605–611.

47 Levy J. A new human herpesvirus: KSHV or HHV8? Lancet 1995; **34**: 786.

48 Connor E., Boccon-Gibod L., Joshi V. *et al*. Cutaneous acquired immunodeficiency syndrome associated Kaposi's sarcoma in pediatric patients. *Archives of Dermatology* 1990; **126**: 791–793.

49 McCarthy G.A., Kampmann B., Novelli V., Miller R.F., Mercey D.E., Gibb D. Vertical transmission of Kaposi's sarcoma. *Archives of Disease in Childhood* 1996; **74**: 455–457.

50 Young S.A., Crocker D.W. Burkitt's lymphoma in a child with AIDS. *Pediatric Pathology* 1991; **11**: 115–122.

11 Fungal infections of the lung in HIV-infected people

S.J.G. SEMPLE

11.0 Introduction

Many of the fungal infections of the lung are confined to certain geographical regions although with widespread facilities for travel they may present outside these areas. Three of the fungi are ubiquitous and occur worldwide. These are *Aspergillus* species, *Candida* and *Cryptococcus*.

11.1 Aspergillosis

Infection with *Aspergillus fumigatus* may present in the immunocompetent as allergic bronchopulmonary aspergillosis, aspergilloma and in the severely immunocompromised patient, such as in leukaemia, as invasive aspergillosis. *Aspergillus* species may colonize the respiratory tract as in patients with chronic obstructive airways diseases (COAD). However in this section attention is mainly directed at invasive disease in HIV-infected people.

Aspergillus species is a common pathogen in immunocompromised patients particularly in those patients who are neutropaenic following chemotherapy and systemic steroid therapy. Infection with *A. fumigatus* (or less commonly *A. flavus*) is a major and common problem in the treatment of patients with lymphoproliferative disorders and in transplant centres. In patients with AIDS it is uncommon, probably occurring in about 1% of patients. Aspergillosis was initially an AIDS-defining condition but this was subsequently withdrawn from the Centers for Disease Control (CDC) classification. The reason for the relatively low incidence of aspergillosis in AIDS compared with other groups of immunosuppressed patients is probably due to the protective mechanisms against this disease, which are dependent on granulocyte and macrophage function, rather than T-cell function and hence cell-mediated immunity. Of the reported patients with AIDS and aspergillosis, approximately half had neutropaenia or were receiving steroid therapy [1]. In some of these patients the neutropaenia was due to treatment with ganciclovir and zidovudine.

11.1.1 Clinical presentation and radiographic findings

The presentation of pulmonary aspergillosis in patients with AIDS has been described in a report of 36 patients, 30 of whom were identified in a review of the literature [1]. Fever, cough and dyspnoea were the most common presenting symptoms but pleuritic chest pain and haemoptysis were found in approximately one-third of the patients. The radiographic findings and clinical course of aspergillosis were divided into the following three groups.

1 *Cavitating upper lobe disease* was the most common radiographic finding seen in 13 of the 36 patients. Cavities could be unilateral or bilateral and single or multiple. An intracavity mass was seen in three patients which was mobile in two of them. These masses were not aspergillomas as they did not arise in a pre-existing cavity. They represent a mass of infected tissue separated from the surrounding lung. True aspergillomas did occur with *Aspergillus* species: *Aspergillus* infection involved pre-existing cavities in two patients; one was a pneumococcal pneumatocoele and the other a cavity due to previous *Mycobacterium kansasii* infection. Seven of the 13 patients died as a result of *Aspergillus* infection, five from fatal haemoptysis and five from disseminated aspergillosis. One patient

was cured of aspergillosis following surgical resection of a 'lingula cavitary infiltrate'. In view of the high mortality from haemoptysis, surgical resection should be considered as a therapeutic option in localized cavitating disease.

2 *Focal radiographic opacity*. Eight of the patients presented with a 'focal alveolar process' resembling bacterial pneumonia, several being noted as pleurally based. In three patients the disease progressed to involve both lungs and they died, one from disseminated aspergillosis and two from respiratory failure. Three patients responded favourably and radiographically to amphotericin B or itraconazole therapy.

3 *Bilateral opacities* were seen in 12 of the 36 patients reviewed and the radiographic findings were described as 'alveolar' which was diffuse or patchy and two patients had nodular or reticulonodular opacities. In three patients the opacities were secondary to bronchial obstruction and this condition will be referred to later. The clinical outcome, in those not due to bronchial obstruction, was poor; six of the patients died of aspergillosis.

4 *Airway disease due to aspergillosis*. Two of the 36 patients reviewed presented with normal chest radiographs but developed unexplained respiratory failure and died. In one of the patients, the presenting symptoms were cough and severe dyspnoea and widespread wheezes were heard on auscultation. Autopsy on both patients revealed pseudomembranes obstructing the central airways. Microscopically there was invasion of the bronchial walls and peribronchial tissue by *Aspergillus* organisms but no invasion of surrounding lung.

11.1.2 Tracheobronchitis due to infection with *Aspergillus*

Tracheobronchitis due to infection with *Aspergillus* in patients with AIDS has been reviewed in nine patients, of which four were seen by the authors [2]. (The review includes the two patients mentioned in the preceding section under group 4.) The presenting symptoms were usually cough, dyspnoea and fever and wheezes were heard in the chest in some but not all patients. Of the four patients directly studied, two had normal chest radiographs, one patient had a 'patchy perihilar infiltrate' and the other a 'patchy multinodular infiltrate'. Bronchoscopic examination revealed mild to moderate diffuse tracheobronchitis with erythematous, oedematous mucosa in three patients whilst in the fourth patient there was a single deep ulcer in the trachea close to the vocal cords. Several ulcers were seen in the first three patients some of which were grossly blackened and necrotic. Another bronchoscopic feature was raised, creamy-white plaques seen in the main stem bronchi. Culture of bronchoalveolar lavage (BAL) fluid was positive for *Aspergillus* species and *Aspergillus* was isolated from endobronchial or endotracheal biopsy specimens in all four patients. Histology of the endobronchial biopsies demonstrated acute and chronic inflammation with reactive mucosal metaplasia and ulceration of the surface mucosa. The remaining five patients, of the nine reviewed by the authors, demonstrated varying degrees of mucoid impaction, pseudomembrane formation, mucosal inflammation and ulceration and tissue invasion.

Three of the five patients reviewed in the preceding paragraph deserve special mention. They were originally reported in a study of 13 patients with pulmonary aspergillosis under the heading obstructing bronchial aspergillosis [3]. The three patients were acutely ill with cough, haemoptysis, chest pain, fever and hypoxaemia. Bronchial obstruction led to areas of atelectasis in the lung and in one patient there was mucus plugging of the airways. The onset of cough was progressive with the spontaneous production of fungal casts of the airways in two patients. Some of the features of the illness were consistent with a diagnosis of mucoid impaction of the bronchi, a syndrome which is considered a variant of allergic bronchopulmonary aspergillosis. However, in the three patients there was no asthma or other allergic symptoms characteristic of this syndrome. The authors of this paper [3] therefore suggested that the illness presented by these three patients was a new clinical entity related to large quantities of *Aspergillus* species in the airways and might be unique to people with AIDS.

11.1.3 Diagnostic procedures used where pulmonary aspergillosis is suspected

A definitive diagnosis of invasive aspergillosis has two components. The first is confirmation of the presence of the fungus which may be achieved by microscopical examination and culture of sputum and sputum casts or culture of BAL fluid or biopsy specimens for *Aspergillus* species. The second component is histological evidence of tissue invasion by fungus of lung or its airways.

A record of diagnostic procedures was made in a study of 13 patients with pulmonary aspergillosis and AIDS [3]. Ten patients were diagnosed as having invasive pulmonary aspergillosis and three as having obstructive bronchial aspergillosis. A definitive diagnosis of invasive aspergillosis was made on histology and a positive culture of *Aspergillus* species in seven patients, three by percutaneous aspiration of the lung in life and in three patients only at post mortem. In one patient diagnosis was established by aspiration from bone. A 'probable' diagnosis of invasive aspergillosis was made in three patients on radiographic findings and a positive culture for *Aspergillus* from BAL fluid. Bronchoscopy was otherwise normal in five patients who underwent this procedure. Transbronchial biopsy was carried out in three patients and was negative in all three at the time of diagnosis.

In the three patients with obstructing bronchial aspergillosis, microscopical examination and culture of sputum casts (expectorated in two patients) was diagnostic in each. All three patients underwent bronchoscopy; in one, fungal casts were seen; in another, the finding was that of a pseudomembrane; in the third, bronchoscopy was normal except for culture which grew copious amounts of *Aspergillus* species.

11.1.4 Outcome of treatment of aspergillosis in patients with AIDS

The report quoted in the section 11.1.3, on diagnostic procedures in patients with pulmonary aspergillosis and AIDS, provides the most reliable assessment of the results of treatment [3]. The number of patients treated in this report is small compared with the larger series of patients drawn from many centres [1], but it has the advantage of being carried out by one group of authors in a single institution with clearly defined criteria for diagnosis and a standard protocol for treatment. Ten patients were treated with amphotericin B or itraconazole or both; eight had invasive pulmonary aspergillosis and three had obstructing bronchial aspergillosis. Of the eight patients with invasive aspergillosis, one responded and survived the 10-month period of the study whilst another patient responded to treatment but was lost at follow-up. In the remaining six patients there was an initial clinical and/or radiological response, but five of these then relapsed and died of aspergillosis, the remaining patient dying of an unrelated cause.

In the three patients with obstructing bronchial aspergillosis there was a good response to treatment with sterilization of the sputum in two, but in the third there was no response and the patient died of aspergillosis.

11.2 Candidiasis

Infection of the oropharynx and oesophagus in HIV-infected people by *Candida* species is well known and is likely to affect all patients at some time in their HIV disease course. In contrast, candidiasis of the trachea, bronchi and lungs is rare in HIV infection as is candidaemia, disseminated candidiasis and deep focal candidiasis [4]. The likely explanation for this contrast is that while superficial candidiasis is prevented by T-lymphocyte function the defence against systemic candidiasis is humoral. An antibody response to the immunodominant 47 kDa antigen of

Candida albicans is found in patients with AIDS and occurs independently of mucocutaneous infection. It is postulated that this antibody production is part of the polyclonal B cell activation observed in HIV infection [5]. However, if the patient is neutropaenic for any reason and if there is a potential focus for infection, such as a central venous line, then infection with *Candida* species is possible. This may be a temporary candidaemia or a serious complication such as deep focal candidiasis or disseminated candidiasis.

Focal infection of the brain, meninges and gall bladder by *Candida* has been described in HIV-infected patients in single case reports [4]. In a review of the pulmonary complications of 70 patients with AIDS, *invasive* candidiasis was seen in just three patients, two of whom were only diagnosed at post mortem. The histological description of invasive candidiasis in this report was of spores and pseudohyphae invading bronchial walls and pulmonary parenchyma without a significant inflammatory reaction. Areas of haemorrhage and focal vascular invasion by the fungus was seen [6].

There are no specific features of the clinical presentation of pulmonary candidiasis. There are also no radiographic changes in the chest which are specific for pulmonary candidiasis and the chest radiograph may be normal or show 'bilateral patchy infiltrates'. Isolation of *Candida* from the sputum is not objective evidence of invasive disease because it may just represent colonization. However, there is some correlation between the recovery of a large quantity of fungus from BAL fluid of *Candida* species and the cause of an associated underlying pneumonia. In an HIV-infected patient with an unexplained abnormal chest radiograph, pulmonary candidiasis is one of the many differential diagnoses, especially if the patient is neutropaenic and has been receiving antibiotics. Indirect evidence for pulmonary involvement by *Candida* might come from a positive blood culture or a rising antibody titre to that fungus. In any event a positive blood culture would be an indication for antifungal treatment, as might be a rising antibody titre (especially if the initial titre was low in appropriate clinical circumstances). Unfortunately a high antibody titre alone is a less reliable diagnostic indicator of candidiasis and, in addition, antibodies may be absent or low in proven cases of invasive candidiasis in HIV-infected people. The only reliable means of diagnosing pulmonary candidiasis is a lung biopsy [7]. If the risk of this procedure, or the delay in carrying it out is not acceptable then the only alternative is a therapeutic trial.

The treatment of invasive candidiasis is with intravenous amphotericin B, until there is a clinical and mycological response, which may take 2–20 weeks [7]. There is preliminary evidence that fluconozole is equally effective as amphotericin B as therapy for candidaemia (primarily catheter-associated infection) in patients without neutropaenia [8]. However, in patients who are seriously ill, amphotericin B will remain the treatment of choice.

11.3 Pulmonary cryptococcosis

It is uncertain in what form the cryptococcus enters the lung because the spores isolated from the lungs of humans and mammals are too large and too wet to reach the alveoli. It could be that the cryptococcus enters those lung as a dessicated yeast or the spores are in a different form from those which have been isolated. Usually the 'spores' will be cleared by non-specific mechanisms although colonization of the respiratory tract may occur. If the infectious particles of the cryptococcus are not cleared and reach the alveoli, then elimination depends on cell-mediated immunity which in the immunocompetent will usually be successful. Failure of cell-mediated immunity leads to dissemination of the fungus throughout the body, most notably to the central nervous system (CNS).

Two strains of *Cryptococcus neoformans* of different pathogenicity have been isolated from humans [9]. These strains have been tested for pathogenicity in a murine model. Mice infected with one or other of the two strains respond quite differently. One strain, numbered 52, leads to an acute illness in the mice from which recovery is complete whilst the other strain, numbered 145, leads to disseminated cryptococcosis and is universally fatal. Recovery appears to be related, at least in part, to the cytokine and chemokine response to infection. Infection with strain 52 in mice leads to the early appearance of messenger ribonucleic acid (mRNA) for tumour necrosis factor alpha (TNF-α) and recovery of the chemokine-monocyte chemotactic protein-1 from BAL fluid. This response is delayed and reduced in animals infected with strain 145. Manipulation of the immunological response to infection with TNF-α antibodies delays and impairs the inflammatory response of mice to strain 52 so that the course of the disease is similar to that seen with strain 145, leading to disseminated cryptococcosis. Survival then appears to be dependent on a specific immunological response of the mice to the different strains. The reason for this difference is not apparent, although strain 145 produces melanin which strain 52 does not. Melanin *in vitro* inhibits production of TNF-α by macrophages and this is one possible mechanism whereby the immunological response to infection by the two strains is different [9]. The importance and interest of this experimental work is that it raises the possibility of using immunotherapy in the management of cryptococcosis in humans. At this stage it is too early and too speculative to judge whether this is likely to be a reality.

11.3.1 Frequency

Respiratory cryptococcal infection is an uncommon complication of HIV infection but is by no means rare [4,10–13]. In a major medical centre in North America between 1981 and 1989, 31 patients with combined infection with HIV and *C. neoformans* were identified. Twelve of these patients had primary pulmonary cryptococcosis [11]. A definitive diagnosis was made in 10 of these patients on the basis of an abnormal chest radiograph and culture of *C. neoformans* from either sputum, BAL fluid, pleural fluid and/or lung tissue. A presumptive diagnosis was made in two patients on the presence of symptomatic pulmonary disease with evidence of disseminated cryptococcosis and an abnormal chest radiograph [11]. In an urban reference hospital in Rwanda, Central Africa, pulmonary cryptococcosis was found not to be a rare complication of HIV-1 infection, being diagnosed in 37 patients over a 3-year period of which 29 patients (78%) had primary pulmonary cryptoccosis [12]. From a study in the same institution of HIV-infected patients with pulmonary disease, 13% were found to have pulmonary cryptococcosis. In studies of HIV-positive patients from North America, cryptococcal pneumonia has accounted for between 2 and 15% of all AIDS-related pneumonia. In contrast, this infection has only rarely been reported in the UK [13].

The most common and well known complication of cryptococcal infection in HIV-infected people is meningitis. However, in a review of fungal infections in HIV-infected people on behalf of the American Thoracic Society, '. . . extraneural cryptococcal disease, including cryptococcaemia, pneumonia and ulcerative skin lesions or umbilicated papules mimicking molluscum contagiosum is present in 25–50% of cases . . .' [4]. The cryptococcus may involve bone and bone marrow, and the prostate may be a 'silent' reservoir of this fungus.

Defining the incidence and presentation of primary uncomplicated pulmonary cryptococcosis is difficult because it may be associated with Kaposi's sarcoma, bacterial infection or other copathogens such as *Mycobacterium tuberculosis* and *Pneumocystis carinii* [13,14].

11.3.2 Clinical presentation

The clinical presentation and radiological findings in pulmonary cryptococcosis described here are derived from data on patients where the primary illness was pulmonary and was not complicated by a copathogen(s) and/or Kaposi's sarcoma.

The most common presenting symptoms are cough, fever, dyspnoea and weight loss. Other less common symptoms are headache, haemoptysis and chest pain [10–13]. The duration of symptoms is highly variable, ranging from a few days to several weeks [10]. The findings on clinical examination include fever, tachypnoea and lymphadenopathy and crackles may be heard on auscultation of the chest. Two patients have been reported to have developed the adult respiratory distress syndrome one of whom recovered on treatment [15].

Patients may be normoxic or hypoxaemic; in a report of 12 patients with pulmonary cryptococcosis the arterial Po_2 ranged from 28 mmHg (3.73 kPa) to 103 mmHg (13.73 kPa) with a mean of 72 mmHg (9.60 kPa) [11].

The most common finding on the chest radiograph is interstitial infiltrates which may be focal or diffuse, unilateral or bilateral. Less common findings are masses, mediastinal and/or hilar lymphadenopathy, nodules and pleural effusion(s) [5,11–13]. Hilar and mediastinal lymphadenopathy have been recorded in one patient without evidence of parenchymal involvement [9].

The pleural effusions, when present, are described as small, obliterating the costophrenic angles and are usually bilateral [13].

Alveolar involvement occurs with a more diffuse loss of radiotranslucency which may be extensive, leading to the characteristic description of a 'white out'. In one study of 14 patients with pulmonary cryptococcosis, a 'ground-glass' appearance was noted in six patients. Also in this study, two of the patients had normal chest radiographs [13].

It will be apparent from this description of the clinical presentation of pulmonary cryptococcosis that it is highly variable, non-specific and indistinguishable from other pulmonary infections, both opportunistic and non-opportunistic.

11.3.3 Diagnosis

Diagnosis rests in the microscopic identification of *C. neoformans* after staining with Indian ink and/or mucicarmine, as well as culture of the fungus from either sputum, BAL fluid, pleural fluid or biopsy specimen. Serum cryptococcal antigen is usually raised to high titres but may, on occasion, fail to act as an indicator of primary pulmonary cryptococcosis [12].

In pulmonary cryptococcosis in HIV-infected people it is likely that the fungus will be disseminated and can be cultured from blood and CSF. In a study of 11 patients with pulmonary cryptococcosis, *C. neoformans* was cultured from the CSF of all 11 patients [11]. Plainly a lumbar puncture is required for all patients with cryptococcosis whether or not they have neurological symptoms or signs [4].

11.3.4 Treatment

Drugs used in the treatment of cryptococcosis are amphotericin B (with or without flucytosine), itraconazole and fluconazole. Whilst the use of itraconazole may have a successful outcome in primary pulmonary cryptococcosis [12] fluconazole is the better and more reliable of the two azoles both for treatment and secondary prophylaxis [16]. An operational policy for the treatment of cryptococcosis in HIV-infected persons is to use amphotericin B initially in the most seriously ill and fluconazole for the remaining patients. After induction therapy all patients should have permanent suppressive therapy with fluconazole at a dose of 400 mg daily. In a trial of chronic suppressive therapy in 12 patients who presented without meningitis, five out of six patients receiving either itraconazole or fluconazole at 200 mg daily developed meningitis whilst none of the six patients on fluconazole 400 mg daily did so [16].

Where there is evidence of pulmonary and meningococcal cryptococcosis then the treatment regimen will be that for meningitis. An operational policy for the treatment of cryptococcal meningitis is to use amphotericin B initially in the most seriously ill and fluconazole for the remaining patients [16]. The combined use of flucytosine is controversial. Although this combination may be the preferred regimen for cryptococcal meningitis in non HIV-infected patients there is a high incidence of drug-induced cytopaenia in patients with AIDS especially if there is already bone-marrow suppression [4]. Nevertheless there is evidence that the relapse rate of meningitis may be reduced by adding flucytosine to the initial treatment. On this basis it is desirable to use flucytosine where it can be administered with safety. After induction, permanent suppressive therapy will be required.

11.4 The endemic mycoses

The main burden of disease from the endemic mycoses occurs in North America. The common fungi are *Histoplasma capsulatum*, *Coccidioides immitis* and *Blastomyces dermatitidis* which are particularly prevalent in the Ohio and Mississippi River valleys. Histoplasmosis also occurs in central and South America, the Caribbean islands and South-East Asia. Coccidioidomycosis is endemic to south-western USA, including southern California, northern Mexico and parts of Central and South America (Brazil, Argentina) whilst Blastomycosis has a northern extension into central Canada. Although the endemic mycoses are encountered outside north America, as would be expected in similar environments, the 'burden of disease' appears to be considerably less than in North America. Sarosi has suggested that the reason for this is that although infection of humans by the fungi undoubtedly occurs, the disease is overshadowed by other more prevalent infections such as tuberculosis (TB) [17].

Even within the regions of the endemic mycoses there are areas where fungal infection is common, yet only a few miles away it is absent and fungus can only be cultured with difficulty or not at all. This difficulty occurs even when the temperature and moisture are appropriate for fungal growth so that there remain as yet unknown factors necessary for fungal survival.

The spores of the endemic mycoses live in dirt or soil (especially when contaminated by bird or bat excrement) in the hyphal form at a temperature of around 23°C. The route of infection for humans is the lung, as the spores are readily inhaled. Fungal spores are of the right size (2–5 μm) to reach the alveoli and there they are usually eliminated by polymorphonuclear cells and alveolar macrophages. If they are not eliminated, which is especially likely to occur with a heavy burden of inhaled spores, then the fungus, which is dimorphic, converts from its hyphal or mould form to its parasitic (yeast) form which is too large to be coughed up and the infected person is not infectious. At this stage elimination can only be achieved by T-cell mediated immunity. When cell-mediated immunity is intact, the usual outcome is recovery from infection and progression to disease is only likely when this immunity is impaired or lost.

The defences against the endemic mycoses depend on a combination of mechanisms acting in concert. There is the physical/mechanical protection provided by the filtering of air in the nasopharynx, the pH of airway secretions and mucociliary clearance. Humoral mechanisms include naturally occurring antimicrobial compounds in airway secretions as well as antibody formation and complement. The epithelial lining of the airways provides a physical barrier to fungal penetration whilst the lymphocytes, dendritic cells and alveolar macrophages within the lung parenchyma are involved in cell-mediated immunity providing the final defensive mechanism against fungal disease.

Dissemination in HIV-infected persons of *H. capsulatum* and *C. immitis* are AIDS-defining conditions (CDC, category C; see Chapter 1, section 1.1.).

11.5 Histoplasmosis

In endemic areas for histoplasmosis the majority of persons living there will have been infected as shown by skin testing with histoplasmin.

11.5.1 Histoplasmosis in the immunocompetent

In the immunocompetent primary pulmonary infection may pass unnoticed or consist of a mild febrile illness which might be attributed to a 'cold' or 'influenza'. It is only a very small minority that progress to pulmonary histoplasmosis and this progression may be related to a heavy burden of inhaled spores as may occur during wood cutting, excavations, cave explorations and demolition work. The respiratory presentation (14–21 days after infection) may be that of an atypical pneumonia or focal pneumonia and the chest radiograph may show hilar lymphadenopathy, diffuse interstitial infiltration or multiple nodules. This may be accompanied by erythema nodosum or erythema multiforme. Recovery is usual without treatment.

Dissemination, if it occurs, is to the reticuloendothelial system, namely the liver, spleen, bone marrow and adrenals. Calcification in the lung, mediastinal lymph node, liver and spleen may be the residuum of previous infection.

Chronic histoplasmosis is mainly seen in the USA, it is more common in males and smokers and there is often underlying pulmonary emphysema [7]. It has many of the characteristics of pulmonary TB (except it is non-infectious) leading to lung cavities and fibrosis. The exuberant immunological response in the immunocompetent may be responsible for the chronic damage to the lung, leading to widespread fibrosis, bronchiectasis and atelectasis. Fibrosis may also lead to tracheal, mediastinal or oesophageal obstruction as well as vascular occlusion which may ultimately result in pulmonary hypertension.

11.5.2 Progressive disseminated histoplasmosis and AIDS

Progressive disseminated histoplasmosis (PDH) is an uncommon manifestation of infection with *H. capsulatum* in the immunocompetent. The risk factors are age, namely being over 54 years, and immunosuppression, whether this is due to malignancy, cytotoxic drugs, glucocorticoids [18] or, more recently, AIDS. Histoplasmosis in AIDS is both disseminated, which in the immunocompetent is usually contained, and progressive and therefore not contained and requires treatment. Histoplasmosis occurs in at least 5% of patients with AIDS residing in endemic areas in the USA and tends to occur early in HIV infection and is the AIDS-defining illness in at least half of the cases [19,20]. However, PDH has also been reported from New York City [21] and other non-endemic areas, including Europe [19,22,23], although most of the patients had lived near or in endemic areas such as the Caribbean or Puerto Rico for part of their lives. It is uncertain whether histoplasmosis in non-endemic areas is due to reactivation of dormant histoplasmosis or due to recently acquired infection. In favour of reactivation are reports of histoplasmosis outside endemic areas which have usually been in people who have at one time lived in or visited those areas. However there are reports of histoplasmosis in people who have never lived in or visited these areas [19]. *H. capsulatum* may be found in the environment of river valleys in temperate climates. Patients with AIDS who work in the construction or demolition industries, or whose leisure activities bring them into contact with areas contaminated with *H. capsulatum* such as caves, farms and bird roost sites are particularly at risk for developing histoplasmosis [19]. In Indianopolis there is a particularly high rate of histoplasmosis in patients with AIDS, which is due to recurrent outbreaks of histoplasmosis in that city. Epidemiological studies of these outbreaks have not established with statistical certainty whether reactivation or exogenous exposure to *H. capsulatum* was the primary cause of histoplasmosis in patients with AIDS. However there was a substantial rise in histoplasmosis in AIDS patients during the autumn of 1988, the time of the last outbreak of histoplasmosis in Indianapolis, favouring exogenous infection rather than reactivation [19].

11.5.3 Presentation of progressive disseminated histoplasmosis in AIDS

In a review of 230 patients with PDH, drawn from patients presenting in Houston and Indiana, combined with a review of the literature, the most common presenting symptoms were fever and weight loss with respiratory symptoms occurring in about half of the patients [20]. The respiratory symptoms were usually mild and consisted of cough (usually non-productive) and dysponea [21]. On examination, hepatosplenomegaly was the most common finding and mucosal and skin ulcers and rashes were seen in a minority [20]. Gas exchange was usually well maintained with a normal Po_2 [21] but hypoxaemia occurred in the more seriously ill [24].

The usual presentation of PDH is with a subacute illness but presentation in about 10% of cases may be fulminant with all the clinical features of sepsis [19]. Involvement of the reticuloendothelial system by *H. capsulatum* may lead to anaemia which is thought to be due to impaired release of iron derived from the catabolism of haemoglobin [24]. Other haematological abnormalities seen include the presence of lupus anticoagulant factor, disseminated intravascular coagulopathy and thrombocytopaenia. Ulceration of the gastrointestinal tract may lead to abdominal pain or bloody diarrhoea [19,24,25].

The chest radiograph is normal in about a third of the patients. A characteristic finding is of nodules, 2–4 mm in diameter, throughout both lung fields. Otherwise the radiographic changes are non-specific and include interstitial infiltrates, reticulonodular changes and diffuse loss of radiotranslucency suggesting alveolar consolidation. Occasional findings are of single or multiple calcified granulomata and occasional small pleural effusions.

Patients presenting with histoplasmosis may have other concurrent opportunistic infections; in a report of 72 patients, 38% had other infections which included *P. carinii* pneumonia, *Mycobacterium avium intracellulare*, *Candida* oesophagitis, *Cryptococcal* meningitis, *Cryptosporidum* gastroenteritis and disseminated cytomegalovirus (CMV) infection [19].

H. capsulatum may disseminate to the CNS leading to meningo-encephalitis or focal lesions of the brain. Unusual manifestations of histoplasmosis include pericarditis, rhabdomyolysis, pancreatitis, chorioretinitis, colonic masses and mesenteric nodules [19].

11.5.4 Diagnosis

Several approaches are usually necessary to establish a diagnosis of PDH. These include Wright-stained smear of peripheral blood or Giemsa staining of bone marrow, lymph nodes, sputum, BAL fluid, lung biopsy specimen or skin lesions. Culture and identification of the fungus in its yeast form is the most reliable diagnostic method but takes time. The success rate of culture is enhanced by lysing the blood, centrifuging the specimen and plating the sediment on agar plates (the lysis-centrifugation blood culture technique) [26]. The time taken for identification of the fungus has been considerably reduced by the use of specific deoxyribonucleic acid (DNA) probes [27] but the complete process of culture and identification may take about 1 week [25].

A radioimmunoassay to detect *H. capsulatum* variety *capsulatum* polysaccharide antigen has a high sensitivity for diagnosis of PDH as well as for the early detection of relapses occurring on prophylaxis [28,29]. This test may not be widely available. False-positive results have been noted in patients with blastomycosis and coccidioidomycosis due to a cross-reacting antigen. These false-positive results are still diagnostic of one of these three fungal diseases for which the treatment is broadly the same. Finally, there are serological tests for histoplasma antibodies by complement fixation or immunodiffusion, but these may be negative in the immunosuppressed.

The sites of positive identification of disseminated *H. capsulatum* infection are the blood and bone marrow. Histoplasmosis is a disease of the reticuloendothelial system and the bone marrow is the most accessible tissue of this system. Other sites of identification include sputum, BAL fluid, transbronchial biopsy and biopsy of skin and lymph glands. In a review of the source of diagnosis in 48 patients with AIDS, culture of the bone marrow provided a positive result in 69% and blood culture gave

Table 11.1 Culture of *Histoplasma capsulatum* from different sources in 48 patients with progressive disseminated histoplasmosis and AIDS. *H. capsulatum* was cultured in some patients from more than one site but each number is expressed as a percentage of the 48 patients. Reproduced from [30].

	Number	Percentage
Bone-marrow biopsy	33	69
Blood	13	27
Lung biopsy	12	25
Bronchoscopy	8	17
Sputum	4	8
Liver biopsy	5	10
Lymph node biopsy	5	10
Skin biopsy	5	10
Cerebrospinal fluid	2	4
Intestinal biopsy	2	4

the diagnosis in 27% of patients. *H. capsulatum* was cultured from more than one site and these are shown in Table 11.1 [30].

In a university hospital setting in Indiana with a high intake of patients with histoplasmosis, positive fungal cultures provided the diagnosis in 65 of 72 cases (90.3%) and in the remaining seven patients the diagnosis was established by the detection of high levels of *Histoplasma* polysaccharide antigen. Blood culture using the lysis-centrifugation method was positive in 32 of 35 cultures (91%) and *H. capsulatum* was isolated from the bone marrow in 19 of 21 patients (91%) and from the respiratory tract in 18 of 21 patients (86%). Serological tests demonstrated increased levels of antibodies against *H. capsulatum* by immunodiffusion or complement fixation in 25 of 36 cases (69%) [19]. The problem with all these diagnostic methods is the time delay between the diagnostic procedure and the completion of culture and identification of *H. capsulatum*. Antibodies against *H. capsulatum* can be absent at the start of the illness and may remain so in patients with AIDS. This stresses the importance of careful microscopic examination of blood and marrow for fungi following appropriate staining.

11.5.5 Treatment

Amphotericin B is highly effective as an initial treatment but ketoconazole is not [20]. Out of 65 patients receiving amphotericin B, 57 responded and these responders had received at least a total of 500 mg. The remaining eight patients died before they received 500 mg [19].

Suppressive therapy is needed to prevent relapse. A very high relapse rate was found using ketoconazole which has necessitated the use of amphotericin for suppression; 50–80 mg being given intravenously each week or each other week [20]. The most promising suppressive therapy is itraconazole [31] which may well replace the use of amphotericin for this purpose. After initial treatment with amphotericin B (15 mg/kg) over 4–12 weeks, 42 patients with AIDS were given itraconazole 200 mg daily by mouth. The median follow-up was 109 weeks and the minimum 52 weeks. Two relapses occurred (5%, 95% confidence interval (CI) 0.5–16%), one in a patient withdrawn from the study and another through poor compliance. One patient had persistent hypokalaemia and discontinued itraconazole but otherwise no side-effects were recorded [31]. Patients with high levels of *H. capsulatum* antigen at the start of the study showed a reduction or clearing of antigen from blood and urine [31].

11.5.6 Is infection with *Histoplasma capsulatum* always disseminated and progressive in HIV-infected people?

There is surprisingly little information available to answer this question. In a report of 72 cases of histoplasmosis in patients with AIDS only three presented with isolated pulmonary infection and one subsequently experienced disseminated disease. Two remained well after 16 months while receiving ketoconazole, a rather poor suppressive agent. The degree of immunosuppression in these patients is not recorded [19].

We are not aware of any reports of *H. capsulatum* in otherwise asymptomatic HIV-infected people with well maintained cell-mediated immunity and with CD4 cell counts unequivocally in the normal range. It may be that the course of infection would be the same as in the immunocompetent and pass unnoticed or present with a self-limiting illness. Should such patients, if infection with *H. capsulatum* is detected, receive suppressive therapy to guard against reactivation of histoplasmosis when their cell-mediated immunity becomes impaired or lost? Probably not, because in those HIV-infected persons with prolonged survival suppressive therapy would be needed for many years. Careful follow-up of such patients would be a rational alternative.

11.6 Coccidioidomycosis during HIV infection

C. immitis is a fungus which lives in the soil, often in semi-desert conditions, but which is more widely disseminated by dust storms. Agricultural and oil-rig workers are particularly susceptible to infection. As with histoplasmosis, between 80 and 90% of people living in endemic areas develop positive skin tests without overt disease. Acute pulmonary, chronic pulmonary and disseminated coccidioidomycosis are possible clinical outcomes of pulmonary infection with *C. immitis*. Disseminated coccidioidomycosis occurs in persons who are immunosuppressed from whatever cause including persons with AIDS.

11.6.1 Frequency

A prospective study was carried out to determine the incidence of active coccidioidomycosis in HIV-infected people living in an endemic area, namely in Tucson and Phoenix, Arizona, USA [32]. One hundred and seventy HIV-infected people were followed up for a median of 11.3 months (range 0–44 months). Thirteen subjects had a history of coccidioidomycosis and 35 (22.3%) had a positive skin test to spherulin at the start of the investigation. Of the 102 subjects with a negative skin test, 18 (17.6%) developed a positive test in follow-up. Thirteen people developed active coccidioidomycosis during the period of follow-up. From a Kaplan–Meier plot of the percentage of people free of coccidioidomycosis over time, the product-limit estimate for the development of active coccidioidomycosis after 41 months was 24.6% (95% confidence limits were 8.2 and 41.4%). The risk factors for development of infection were a CD4 count less than $0.25 \times 10^9/l$ and a diagnosis of AIDS. In Tucson, approximately 30% of individuals living in the area are infected with *C. immitis*, based on skin-testing, but only a small number develop clinically apparent infection (probably under 1% per annum). Therefore, the finding of an estimated rate of symptomatic coccidioidomycosis of 24.6% over 41 months shows that this fungal infection is a significant opportunistic infection for HIV-infected people living within the endemic area.

Factors associated with prior infection, such as a positive skin test, prolonged residence in the endemic area and a previous history of coccidioidomycosis were not associated with the development of active coccidioidomycosis in this cohort. In two cases active disease did appear to be due to reactivation of a previously acquired infection. This study, however, did not distinguish the proportion of cases due to acute infection from that due to reactivation of previously acquired coccidioidomycosis [32].

A retrospective review of cases of coccidioidomycosis and AIDS arising in the years 1981–1989 in the state of Arizona has been made. In this state 804 cases of AIDS were identified, of whom 49 had disseminated coccidioidomycosis (6%), thus it was the most frequently reported opportunistic infection following *P. carinii* pneumonia (PCP) and oesophageal candidiasis [33].

11.6.2 Clinical presentation and diagnosis of coccidioidomycosis in HIV-infected people

The clinical presentation of this fungal infection is very variable. In a review of 77 HIV-infected patients with coccidioidomycosis 51 patients presented with a respiratory illness. The precise nature of the respiratory infection was not defined but on the basis of the chest radiograph they were divided up into those with focal and those with diffuse pulmonary disease [33].

Focal pulmonary disease

This group comprised 20 patients who presented with the following radiographic abnormalities (numbers of patients in parentheses): focal alveolar infiltrates (13), hilar adenopathy (4), pulmonary cavity (3) and bilateral pleural effusions (1). In this group of patients the fungus was isolated from respiratory secretions in nine patients, mediastinal or cervical lymph nodes in four and the urine in one patient. Histological examination of respiratory secretions revealed *C. immitis* in two patients. A focal pulmonary infiltrate on the chest radiograph and positive coccidioidal serology provided the diagnosis in 4 patients.

Diffuse pulmonary disease

The remaining 31 patients with a respiratory illness presented with a chest radiograph showing diffuse reticular pulmonary infiltrates in both lungs. In 21 patients *C. immitis* was identified in respiratory secretions with no evidence of extrapulmonary coccidioidomycosis. Of these 21 patients, the diagnosis was established by culture of the sputum but in 16 patients bronchoscopy was necessary to make a diagnosis, presumably by culture of aspirated secretions or BAL fluid. Evidence of dissemination of the fungus was found in 9 of the 31 patients as *C. immitis* was grown from blood, urine or other extrapulmonary sites. In one patient, the diagnosis was based on a raised coccidioidal complement-fixing antibody titre and a chest radiograph showing diffuse pulmonary infiltrates.

Twelve of the 77 patients had PCP at the time of diagnosis of coccidioidomycosis; 10 patients had diffuse pulmonary disease, one patient had focal infiltrates and, in one patient, the diagnosis was based on biopsy of a lymph node.

Twenty-six of the 77 patients reviewed presented with a variety of manifestations of coccidioidomycosis which was cutaneous in four, localized extrathoracic lymph node or liver involvement in seven and meningitis in six. In six patients no identifiable focus of infection was found and the diagnosis was based on positive coccidioidal serology determined by complement-fixing antibody or the immunodiffusion technique for tube precipitin antibody. Twelve of these 26 patients also had abnormal chest radiographs showing focal or diffuse pulmonary infiltrates.

The CD4 cell count was obtained in 55 of the 77 patients, the median count was 0.101×10^9 cells/l with a range of 0.005 to 0.670×10^9 cells. The median cell count for those patients with focal pulmonary disease was 0.143×10^9/l and with diffuse pulmonary infection it was 0.044×10^9/l.

Diagnosis of coccidioidomycosis requires the recovery of fungus on culture or visualization of the organism in biological material or in histopathological sections [4]. Cytological identification of spherules in BAL fluid using Papanicolaou or Grocott's methenamine silver stain may be achieved in about 40% of proven cases of coccidioidomycosis whilst culture of the fluid is usually positive after 3–5 days. In patients with diffuse pulmonary disease where an early diagnosis is required it may be necessary to carry out a transbronchial biopsy for histological examination of the tissue. Standard serological tests are frequently positive in patients with active infection and they are also useful to monitor progress on treatment [4].

11.6.3 Outcome and treatment

The median follow-up for the 77 patients was 6 months with a range of 0 (diagnosis made at postmortem) to 32 months. Thirty-two of the 77 patients died (42%) and the mortality was highest in patients with diffuse pulmonary involvement (70%). Amphotericin B and ketoconazole were the main therapeutic agents used with fluconazole being used in patients with meningitis. Three patients developed active coccidioidomycosis on ketoconazole started previously for other conditions which, together with the data on its use in patients with histoplasmosis, suggests it is not a satisfactory antifungal agent for suppressive therapy. Only two patients in this series received itraconazole [33]. The current recommendations for treatment are that amphotericin B should be used for patients with diffuse pulmonary infiltrates and also in those patients where focal lesions outside the chest are progressing rapidly. Fluconazole is the treatment of choice for patients with meningitis both acutely and for suppressive therapy for life. Where the illness is more indolent, fluconazole or itraconazole are effective [4,8,34].

11.7 Blastomycosis

Blastomycosis is caused by the dimorphic fungus *B. dermatitides* which may infect humans and also dogs. It is the least common of the endemic mycoses, the incidence being about one-tenth that of histoplasmosis. The tissue response of the host to infection is granulomatous as occurs with histoplasmosis, but unlike histoplasmosis there is a significant pyogenic component. The result is that pulmonary blastomycosis usually leads to cough with mucopurulent sputum in which fungi can be frequently seen and cultured.

Blastomycosis is not a common infection in HIV-infected people even in endemic areas and disseminated blastomycosis is not an AIDS-defining condition.

11.7.1 Presentation of blastomycosis in HIV-infected people

In a report of 15 patients who were seropositive for HIV, blastomycosis occurred late in their disease in that 14 patients had an AIDS-defining condition (according to the 1993 CDC Revised Classification System) and all 14 had CD4 cell counts under 0.20×10^9/l [35].

Blastomycosis presented in two forms, pulmonary and disseminated. Cough, fever, dyspnoea and weight loss were the symptoms of pulmonary blastomycosis which occurred in seven patients. One of these patients had severe respiratory failure leading to the adult respiratory distress syndrome. All seven patients had abnormal chest radiographs including focal pneumonia in three, miliary or diffuse interstitial changes in three and bilateral nodules in one. In addition to these chest radiographic changes, one patient had cavitatary disease and one a pleural effusion.

Eight patients with disseminated disease also had diffuse pulmonary blastomycosis with widespread interstitial infiltrates. In six of these eight patients more than one organ was involved, including the spleen, liver, kidneys, skin, bone marrow, lymph nodes and thyroid. Five of the six patients had cerebral or meningeal blastomycosis including one patient with large cerebral abscesses.

Two of the eight patients with disseminated blastomycosis had disease limited to one site. One patient had multiple small facial papular lesions and a large paranasal crusting lesion. The other of these two patients presented with meningitis.

11.7.2 Diagnosis

The diagnosis of blastomycosis was confirmed by culture of *B. dermatitides* in 14 of the 15 patients including all eight patients with disseminated disease. *B. dermatitides* was cultured from bronchoscopic specimens in nine patients, skin in three patients and blood in two patients. Organisms consistent with *B. dermatitides* were identified on histology of at least one clinical specimen before the results of culture were available. Cytology and histology are important diagnostic methods for early diagnosis as cultures may take 2–4 weeks to develop. In only one of the 15 patients was fungus not cultured. This patient presented with lower lobe pneumonia and right pleural effusion and *B. dermatitides* was identified on histology of the pleura, but culture of the pleural fluid and tissue were negative.

11.7.3 Outcome and treatment

Six patients died within a short period varying from a few hours to 21 days after admission; all died of disseminated blastomycosis. Only three of the patients received antifungal treatment. Two patients received amphotericin B but the total dosage achieved was only 300 mg and 800 mg respectively. The third patient, who refused amphotericin B, was given ketoconazole 400 mg daily but died after 9 months of treatment.

Of the nine patients who survived for longer than a month, two patients were alive at the end of the study. The remaining seven patients died after a mean time interval of 11 months (range 4–24 months), two patients from blastomycosis and five patients from other AIDS-related causes [35].

Amphotericin B is the recommended treatment for blastomycosis in patients who are HIV-infected, with a total dose of 1–2 g usually being adequate to control the infection. Itraconazole is recommended for chronic maintenance therapy [4].

11.8 Oral azole drugs as systemic antifungal therapy

Amphotericin B is a naturally occurring compound produced by *Streptomyces nodosus* whilst the azoles are synthetic compounds. The azoles are classed as imidazoles (ketoconazole) or triazoles (fluconazole and itraconazole) according to whether they contain 2 or 3 nitrogen atoms in the 5-membered azole ring. The azoles inhibit ergosterol synthesis which impairs cell membrane structure and function leading to increased permeability and inhibition of cell growth and replication.

11.8.1 Pharmacology

The bioavailability of itraconazole is 2–3 times higher when taken with food than when taken on an empty stomach. The peak plasma concentrations of this drug are 3–5 times higher after 7–14 days of treatment than after a single dose. In serious infections a loading dose of 200 mg of itraconazole three times daily for 3 days is recommended. A loading dose of fluconazole is also recommended as it takes 6–10 days to reach a steady state peak concentration of the drug.

Ketoconazole and itraconazole are extensively bound to plasma proteins but the unbound drug distributes well throughout most tissues. Fluconazole is highly water soluble, is minimally bound to protein and its volume of distribution is close to total body water. The peak cerebrospinal fluid (CSF) concentrations of fluconazole in fungal meningitis range from 70 to 90% of peak plasma concentrations.

Ketoconazole and itraconazole are extensively metabolized in the liver and excreted in the faeces and urine. Because these drugs are metabolized, little ketoconazole or itraconazole are excreted in the urine so the dosage does not need to be adjusted for patients with renal impairment. This is not true for fluconazole which is minimally metabolized and 80% is excreted unchanged in the urine. Dosage should be reduced in patients with glomerular filtration rates below 50 ml/min.

11.8.2 Activity of azoles and resistance

The three azoles are active against *C. neoformans, C. albicans, C. immitis, H. capsulatum, B. dermatitides, Paracoccidioides brasiliensis* and *Sporothrix schenckii*. Itraconazole is more active against *Aspergillus* species than any other azole drugs.

Resistance to treatment with azoles after long courses are rare although there is increasing evidence of resistance of oropharyngeal and oesophageal candidiasis to fluconazole in HIV-infected patients who are receiving intermittent or continuous fluconazole therapy. In general, the *in vitro* testing of sensitivity of fungal organisms to antifungal drugs is of doubtful value because of the poor correlation of the results with clinical response.

11.8.3 Adverse effects

Gastrointestinal complications are the most common side-effects of the three azoles and consist of nausea and vomiting (occurring in 5% to 10% of patients). At dosages up to 400 mg a day it is rarely necessary to discontinue therapy. Patients may experience rashes and pruritis and fluconazole may rarely cause an exfoliative dermatitis. In about 10% of patients there may be an asymptomatic rise in plasma aminotransferases and liver function studies should be measured before treatment and periodically thereafter especially at the start of treatment. Azole therapy should be discontinued in patients who develop symptomatic hepatitis or laboratory evidence of progressive or persistent hepatic dysfunction. Ketoconazole in doses over 400 mg a day may reversibly inhibit the synthesis of

Table 11.2 Drug interactions involving oral azole antifungal drugs. Reproduced after modification from [8].

Decreased plasma concentrations of azole	
Cause	*Drugs*
Decreased absorption of ketoconazole and itraconazole	Antacids. H$_2$-receptor-antagonists. Sucralfate
Increased metabolism of ketoconazole	Isoniazid
Increased metabolism of ketoconazole and itraconazole	Phenytoin
Increased metabolism of ketoconazole, itraconazole and fluconazole	Rifampicin

Increased plasma concentration of coadministered drug	
Azole	*Coadministered drug*
Ketoconazole, itraconazole, fluconazole	Cyclosporine
Ketoconazole, fluconazole, itraconazole	Phenytoin
Ketoconazole, fluconazole, itraconazole	Sulphonylurea drugs especially tolbutamide
Ketoconazole, itraconazole	Terfenadine
Ketoconazole, fluconazole, itraconazole	Warfarin

testosterone, oestradiol and cortisol. Endocrine disturbances include impotence, loss of libido, menstrual irregularities and occasionally adrenal insufficiency. A few patients taking itraconazole may develop hypokalaemia, hypertension and oedema.

11.8.4 Drug interactions

Drug interactions with the azoles are shown in Table 11.2 but these interactions are very variable, some are clinically important whereas others are less likely to interact, as judged by controlled studies and limited observations on patients [8,36]. Because the effect on the patient is unpredictable, the ideal procedure would be to monitor the plasma concentration of the azole and interacting drug but this is usually impractical in practice.

References

1 Miller W.T., Sais G.I., Frank I., Gefter W.B., Aronchick J.M., Miller W.T. Pulmonary aspergillosis in patients with AIDS. *Chest* 1994; **105**: 37–44.
2 Kemper C.A., Hostetler J.S., Follansbee S.E. *et al*. Ulcerative and plaque-like tracheobronchitis due to infection with *Aspergillus* in patients with AIDS. *Clinical Infectious Diseases* 1993; **17**: 344–352.

3 Denning D.W., Follansbee S.E., Scolaro M., Norris S., Edelstein H., Stevens D.A. Pulmonary aspergillosis in the acquired immunodeficiency syndrome. *New England Journal of Medicine* 1991; **324**: 654–662.

4 American Thoracic Society. Fungal infection in HIV-infected persons. *American Journal of Respiratory and Critical Care Medicine* 1995; **152**: 816–822.

5 Mathews R., Smith D., Midgley J. *et al.* Candida and AIDS: Evidence for protective antibody. *Lancet* 1988; ii: 263–266.

6 Marchevsky A., Rosen M.J., Chrytal G., Kleinerman J. Pulmonary complications of the acquired immunodeficiency syndrome: a clinicopathologic study of 70 cases. *Human Pathology* 1985; **16**: 659–670.

7 Hay R.J., Mackenzie W.R. Fungal infections (mycoses). In: Weatherall D.J., Ledingham J.G.G., Warrell D.A. (eds). *Oxford Textbook of Medicine Volume 1*, 3rd edn. 1996; 807–808. Oxford University Press, Oxford.

8 Jackson A.C., Dismukes W.E. Oral azole drugs as systemic antifungal therapy. *New England Journal of Medicine* 1994; **330**: 263–272.

9 Huffnagle G.B. Mechanisms of pulmonary host defense against fungi. Oral, unpublished communication. In: *Symposium, Update on fungal pneumonias*. American Thoracic Society Meeting, May 15th 1996.

10 Wasser L., Talavera W. Pulmonary cryptococcosis in AIDS. *Chest* 1987; **4**: 692–695.

11 Cameron M.L., Bartlett J.A., Gallis H.A., Waskin H.A. Manifestations of pulmonary cryptococcosis in patients with acquired immunodeficiency syndrome. *Reviews of Infectious Diseases* 1991; **13**: 64–67.

12 Batungwanayo J., Taelman H., Bogaerts J. *et al.* Pulmonary cryptococcosis associated with HIV-1 infection in Rwanda: a retrospective study of 37 cases. *AIDS* 1994; **8**: 1271–1276.

13 Friedman E.P., Miller R.F., Severn A., Williams I.G., Shaw P.J. Cryptococcal pneumonia in patients with the acquired immunodeficiency syndrome. *Clinical Radiology* 1995; **50**: 756–766.

14 Clark R.A., Greer D., Atkinson W., Valainis G.T., Hyslop M. Spectrum of *Cryptococcus neoformans* infection in 68 patients infected with human immunodeficiency virus. *Reviews of Infectious Diseases* 1990; **12**: 768–777.

15 Murray R.J., Beker P., Furth P., Criner G.J. Recovery from cryptococcaemia and the adult respiratory distress syndrome in the acquired immunodeficiency syndrome. *Chest* 1988; **93**: 1304–1306.

16 Nelson M.R., Fisher M., Cartledge J., Rogers T., Gazzard B.G. The role of azoles in the treatment and prophylaxis of cryptococcal disease in HIV infection. *AIDS* 1994; **8**: 651–654.

17 Sarosi G.A. (1996) Oral unpublished presentation to American Thoracic Society at a symposium, *Update on fungal pneumonias*, May 15th.

18 Wheat L.J., Slama T.G., Norton J.A. *et al.* Risk factors for disseminated or fatal histoplasmosis. *Annals of Internal Medicine* 1982; **96**: 159–163.

19 Wheat L.J., Connolly-Stringfield P.A., Baker R.L. *et al.* Disseminated histoplasmosis in the acquired immune deficiency syndrome: Clinical findings, diagnosis and treatment and review of the literature. *Medicine (Baltimore)* 1990; **69**: 361–374.

20 Sarosi G.A., Johnson P.C. Disseminated histoplasmosis in patients infected with human immunodeficiency virus. *Clinical Infectious Diseases* 1992; **14**: S60–S67.

21 Saltzman S.H., Smith R.L., Aranda C.P. Histoplasmosis in patients at risk for the acquired immunodeficiency syndrome in a nonendemic setting. *Chest* 1988; **5**: 916–921.

22 Brivet F., Roulot D., Naveau S. *et al.* The acquired immunodeficiency syndrome: B cell lymphoma, histoplasmosis, ethics and economics. *Annals of Internal Medicine* 1986; **104**: 447.

23 Dietrich P.-Y., Pugin P., Regamey C., Bille J. Disseminated histoplasmosis and AIDS in Switzerland. *Lancet* 1986; **2**: 752.

24 Hassoun P.M. Case 43-1991. *New England Journal of Medicine* 1991; **325**: 1228–1238.

25 Basgoz N. Case 4-1994. *New England Journal of Medicine* 1994; **330**: 273–286.

26 Paya C.V., Roberts C.D., Cockerill F.R. Laboratory methods for the diagnosis of disseminated histoplasmosis. Clinical importance of the lysis-centrifugation blood culture technique. *Mayo Clinic Proceedings* 1987; **62**: 480–485.

27 Padhye A.A., Smith G., McLaughlin D., Standard P.G., Kaufman L. Comparative evaluation of a chemiluminescent DNA probe and an exoantigen test for rapid identification of *Histoplasma capsulatum*. *Journal of Clinical Microbiology* 1992; **30**: 3108–3111.

28 Wheat L.J., Kohler R.B., Tewari R.P. Diagnosis of disseminated histoplasmosis by detection of *Histoplasma capsulatum* antigen in serum and urine specimens. *New England Journal of Medicine* 1992; **314**: 83–88.

29 Wheat L.J., Connolly-Stringfield P., Blair R., Connolly K., Garringer T., Katz B. Histoplasmosis relapse in patients with AIDS: Detection using *Histoplasma capsulatum* variety *capsulatum* antigen levels. *Annals of Internal Medicine* 1991; **115**: 936–941.

30 Johnson P.C., Khardori N., Najjar A.F., Butt F., Mansell P.W.A., Sarosi G.A. Progressive disseminated histoplasmosis in patients with acquired immunodeficiency syndrome. *American Journal of Medicine* 1988; **85**: 152–158.

31 Wheat J., Hafner R., Wulfsohn M. *et al*. Prevention of relapse of histoplasmosis with itraconazole in patients with the acquired immunodeficiency syndrome. *Annals of Internal Medicine* 1993; **118**: 610–616.

32 Ampel N.M., Dols C.L., Gagliani J.N. Coccidioidomycosis during human immunodeficiency virus infection: Results of a prospective study in a coccidioidal endemic area. *American Journal of Medicine* 1993; **94**: 235–240.

33 Fish D.G., Ampel N.M., Gagliani J.N. *et al*. Coccidioidomycosis during human immunodeficiency virus infection. *Medicine (Baltimore)* 1990; **69**: 384–391.

34 Gagliani J.N., Catanzaro A., Cloud G.A. *et al*. and the NIAID-Mycoses study group. *Annals of Internal Medicine* 1993; **119**: 28–35.

35 Pappas P.G., Pottage J.C., Powderly W.G. *et al*. Blastomycosis in patients with the acquired immunodeficiency syndrome. *Annals of Internal Medicine* 1992; **116**: 847–853.

36 Heylen R., Miller R.F. Adverse effects and drug interactions of medications commonly used in the treatment of adult HIV positive patients. *Genitourinary Medicine* 1996; **72**: 237–246.

Index